The Only Vet-Approved Homemade Dog Food Cookbook You'll Ever Need [2 Books In 1]:

150+ Simple, Allergy-Friendly Recipes for All Sizes and Ages That Improve Health and Save You Thousands on Vet Bills

By: Charles Shepherd

TABLE OF CONTENTS

INTRODUCTION

"Dogs do speak, but only to those who know how to listen."
Orhan Pamuk

If you're here, you must love your dog like family. You want the absolute best for them — and you've probably done everything you can to make sure they're healthy, happy, and full of life. You've read the labels. You've bought the "premium" food brands. You've followed your vet's advice and trusted that what you were feeding your dog was good enough.

And yet... something feels off. Your dog has itchy skin that never seems to clear up. They are a little less playful than they used to be. Or they have recurring digestive issues that no "sensitive stomach" kibble seems to fix. If this sounds familiar, you're not alone, and you are definitely not failing your dog.

The truth is, most commercial dog food — even the expensive stuff — isn't as healthy as it's marketed. It's processed, stripped of natural nutrients, and loaded with fillers your dog's body was never meant to digest. Feeding your dog highly processed food every day is like eating fast food for every meal — eventually, it takes a toll.

But here's the good news: There's a better way — and it's much simpler (and more rewarding) than you think.

Why I Wrote This Book

Hi, I'm Charles Shepherd. I've spent years working with dogs — training them, helping them through anxiety, and building trust and confidence between pets and their owners. But no matter how good the training was, I kept seeing a frustrating pattern. Dogs who should've been bouncing with energy were sluggish. Dogs who should've been calm and focused were anxious and restless. Owners who did everything "right" still saw health problems creep in.

At first, I thought it was just bad luck or breed genetics. But the more dogs I worked with, the more obvious it became — nutrition was at the heart of everything. No matter how much you train a dog, you can't out-train a poor diet. Just like you can't expect a child to focus at school if they're living on candy and soda.

I started researching canine nutrition. I read everything I could, worked with holistic vets, and experimented with home-cooked meals for the dogs under my care. The results were unbelievable. Dogs who were once lethargic started running circles around the yard. Skin issues cleared up. Digestive problems disappeared. And, most amazing of all, their behavior improved. The dogs were calmer, happier, and more focused.

Food wasn't just fuel. It was the foundation. That's why I wrote this book. Because once you understand what real nutrition is and how easy it is to provide it — you'll never look at a bag of kibble the same way again.

The Problem We're Solving

Dogs were never meant to eat highly processed, dry pellets day after day. Their bodies crave fresh, real food packed with nutrients. Commercial kibble is filled with cheap fillers like corn, soy, wheat (which can cause allergies), meat by-products, mystery meats, artificial preservatives, colors, and flavors.

It's no wonder so many dogs today suffer from chronic allergies, digestive issues, obesity, and even behavioral problems. Feeding your dog the wrong food isn't just about poor ingredients — it's about everything they're missing out on: more energy, better moods, fewer trips to the vet, and extra years by your side.

The Solution

The solution is simple. It starts with homemade meals that are balanced, safe, and tailored to your dog's needs. And the best part? You don't need to be a professional chef to do it. You don't need to spend hours slaving over a stove. And you certainly don't need to spend a fortune on trendy boutique dog food brands. What you need is the right knowledge, the right recipes, and a practical, easy-to-follow system.

That's exactly what this book gives you.

What You'll Learn in This Book

This isn't just another cookbook. It's a complete, practical guide to nourishing your dog the way nature intended. Here's what you'll find inside:

- The foundations of canine nutrition — what your dog's body truly needs, from proteins and fats to vitamins and minerals.
- A safe transition plan — step-by-step guide on how to shift your dog to homemade meals without upsetting their stomach.
- Over 150 vet-approved recipes — delicious, balanced meals for puppies, adult dogs, and seniors, plus allergy-friendly and special health condition meals.
- Special diets — including low-fat, diabetic-friendly, and anti-inflammatory meals.
- Time-saving meal prep methods — batch-cooking, freezer-friendly storage, and fast cooking techniques to make life easier. Additionally, there're budget-friendly tips to secure quality ingredients without breaking the bank.
- Structured meal plans ¬¬— to help you feed your dog based on their age, size, and activity level. Whether your dog is a picky eater, a sensitive soul, or a happy-go-lucky pup, there's something for every four-legged friend.

Why This Book?

This book is for dog owners who want to take control of their dog's health, understand what goes into their bowl, and see real improvements in their well-being. It's for people who are ready to invest a little time and love into their dog's nutrition — and enjoy the amazing results.

This book is not for people looking for a quick fix. It's not for those who believe dogs can eat anything and be fine, and it's not for anyone unwilling to learn the basics of balanced feeding.

If you read this book, follow the simple steps inside, and make small changes to your dog's diet, you will see a difference. Not overnight. Not with magic powders or miracle claims. The changes may come quietly, but they'll be undeniable — in the way your dog moves, plays, and greets each new day. And you'll carry the deep comfort of knowing you chose the best for them.

Let's Get Started

The time has come to change your dog's energy and behavior. To let go of the frustrations you have endured over the years. Do not wait for small problems to become bigger and cause serious health issues. Your dog depends on you — and you have what it takes to make a difference.

So, if you're ready to ditch the guesswork, leave the guilt behind, and give your dog the life they deserve — turn the page.

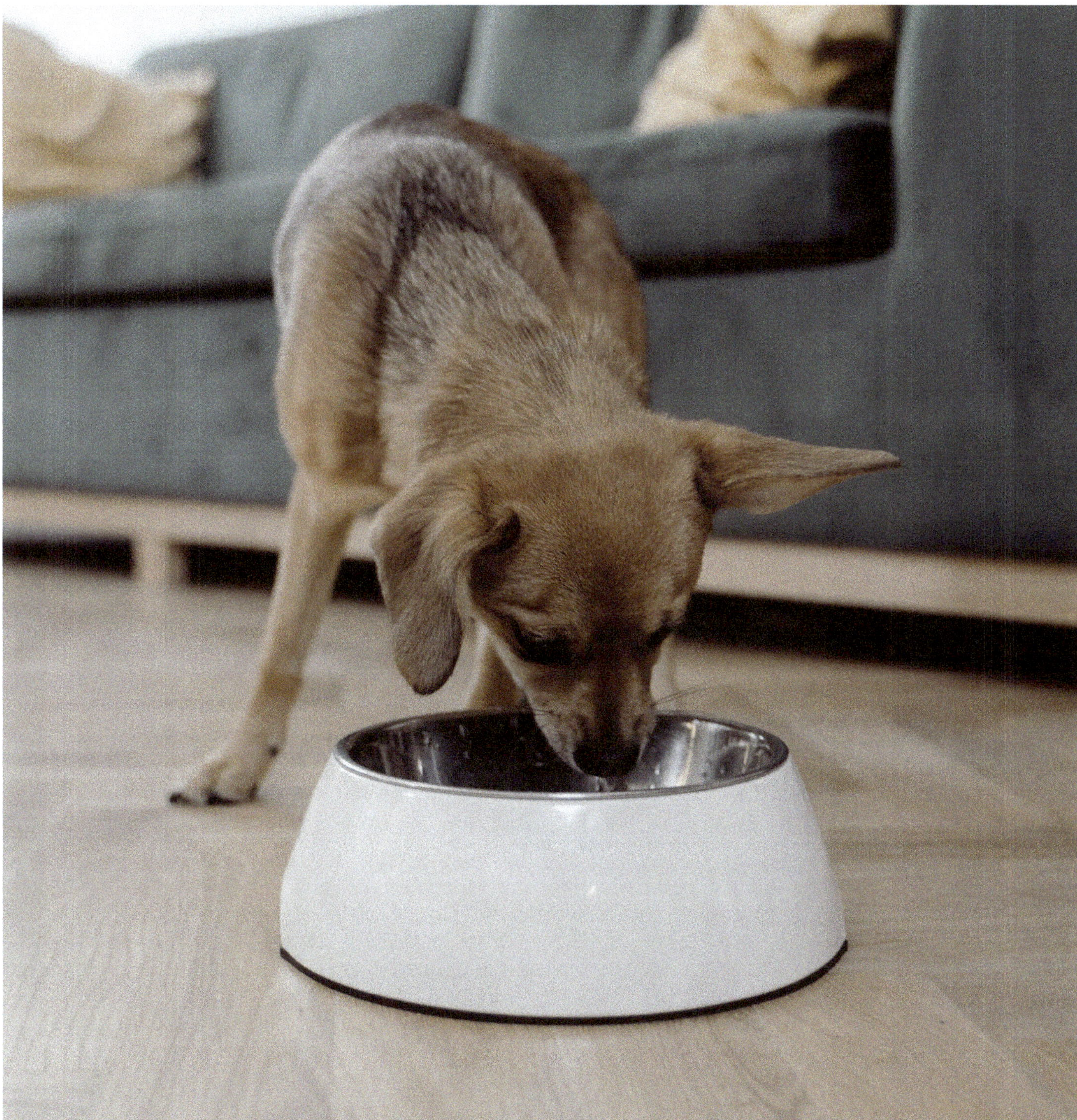

CHAPTER 1:

The Science of Canine Nutrition What Your Dog Really Needs

"Dogs are not tiny humans. Their dietary needs are entirely different from ours yet many pet owners make the mistake of feeding them like they would a person."

A well-balanced diet is the key to a healthy life, and dogs need a balance of proteins, fats, carbs, and micronutrients to live a long and active life. However, many dog owners assume that what is healthy for them is also good for their dogs — a misconception that can be harmful to a dog's health.

Here's a breakdown of the essential nutrients (proteins, fats, carbohydrates, vitamins, and hydration) to ensure you make the best dietary choices for your pup.

1. Essential Nutrients Every Dog Needs

Proteins:

Proteins play a key role in maintaining your dog's muscle health. Proteins facilitate the formation of cartilage, tendons, ligaments, skin, hair, nails, and blood. Proteins also provide the necessary amino acids, which promote cell growth, enzyme production, and boost the immune system. Without adequate protein in their diet, dogs suffer from muscle loss, poor immunity, and slower recovery from injuries. Their fur becomes brittle and skin flaky, leading to a poor coat that lacks shine and protection against parasites.

Protein meals include muscle meat, organs, poultry, grains, and oilseeds. However, puppies need more protein-rich food for proper nourishment. According to Dr. Tiffany Tupler, a veterinarian with expertise in shelter medicine and animal behavior, growing dogs need at least 18% protein (dry matter), while adult dogs need at least 8%, preferably from a high-quality source (Tupler, 2024). Likewise, older dogs, gestating or lactating dogs, and dogs with various conditions need protein-rich meals to meet their nutritional requirements. However, all protein sources are not equal, as animal-based proteins offer more nutritional value and better digestion than plant-based ones.

Fats:

Crucial in a dog's diet, fats provide a concentrated source of energy that improves the dog's fur and supports their overall health. Fats promote good vision, bone health, immune function, and cell protection. They also supply sustained fuel that keeps your dog active all day. Dogs may suffer from a weakened immune system and low energy levels without proper fat intake.

According to the National Research Council of the National Academies (2006), fat requirements vary based on a dog's life stage and condition. Puppies weighing 12 to 33 pounds at maturity need 21 grams of total fat per day, while an average 33-pound adult dog requires 14 grams. Pregnant or nursing dogs have higher energy demands, needing between 29 to 67 grams of fat daily to support their own health and their puppies' growth (National Research Council, 2006).

However, many dog owners confuse a fat-rich diet with obesity, but in reality, fats are just as important as protein. A diet with insufficient fats results in dry, coarse hair and skin, increasing the risk of your furry friend contracting infections. In a research involving 27 Beagle puppies during their rapid growth phase (two to seven months of age), researchers found that puppies on a low-fat diet showed faster fat deficiency symptoms like poor skin and coat health, lower essential fatty acids, and metabolic imbalances. However, puppies who were fed adequate fat had normal growth and healthy skin (Wiese et al., 1962). Such drastic differences show the importance of fats in a dog's diet, as fats support healthy growth, energy production, and healthy skin and coat.

Carbohydrates:

Carbohydrates are a quick source of energy that support your dog's overall metabolism. While they are not as important as proteins and fats, they are beneficial in limited quantities. For active dogs or working breeds, carbs are a good source of energy to meet nutritional requirements. Moreover, carbs are needed to maintain stable blood sugar levels (glucose). As Dr. Tiffany Tupler states, the body needs glucose from carbs, and without enough carbs, it will divert amino acids from other essential processes in the body (Tupler, 2024). When amino acids are diverted due to insufficient carbs in the diet, your dog can suffer from muscle breakdown, weakened immune function, and slower recovery from injuries; as amino acids are essential for building and repairing tissues.

The recommended daily carb intake depends on your dog's age, activity level, and health condition. Studies show that an adult dog's diet can have up to 50% carbohydrates, with 2.5–4.5% from fiber, 5.5% from fats, and 10% from protein (National Research Council, 2006). However, not all dogs require a high-carbohydrate diet. They can get their energy from proteins and fats, which is why they can sustain low-carb diets. For dogs with obesity or diabetes, carbohydrate intake through proteins and fats avoids unnecessary weight gain and blood sugar fluctuations. Puppies and highly active dogs, on the other hand, should be fed moderate carbs for sustained energy.

Dog owners should choose high-quality sources of carbohydrates over refined carbs. Natural sources like sweet potatoes, brown rice, and vegetables provide essential nutrients and fiber, while refined carbs offer little nutritional value and can cause blood sugar spikes.

2. The Importance of Vitamins and Minerals

In addition to proteins, fats, and carbs, a dog needs vitamins and minerals to stay healthy. Micronutrients like calcium, phosphorus, and zinc support bone strength, immune function, and overall well-being. However, many commercial and even homemade meals can lack these essential micronutrients due to poor cooking, processing, or storage methods. This is why many dog owners give supplements to their furry friends to ensure optimal health. According to a Packaged Facts report, pet owners most commonly purchased supplements for joint health, heart function, skin and coat condition, digestion, and omega fatty acids (American Veterinary Medical Association, 2015).

However, do not feed your dog a ton of supplements as overfeeding has its side effects. Instead, certain factors like a dog's age, breed, activity level, and specific health conditions determine if supplements are necessary. Dogs going through aging, breed genetics, or higher activity levels (large breeds) experience common joint issues like arthritis, hip dysplasia, and muscle stiffness. In such cases, supplements provide essential vitamins and minerals to support long-term mobility, comfort, and overall well-being. A study in The Veterinary Journal found that after 70 days of treatment, dogs given glucosamine and chondroitin sulfate (common ingredients in dog supplements for joint pain) experienced less pain and improved mobility (McCarthy et al., 2007). Dogs with dietary restrictions or medical issues that limit their nutrient absorption also need supplements to fill nutritional gaps. Without enough micronutrients, they can suffer from nutritional deficiencies that lead to long-term health problems.

Dr. Russell, a board-certified veterinarian in Canine and Feline Practice with expertise in canine rehabilitation, says that common dog supplements include (Russel, 2023):

- **Glucosamine and chondroitin supplements** — to support joint cartilage, heal and support the fluid that lubricates the joints, and treat conditions like hip dysplasia, osteoarthritis, loose joints, or cartilage damage.
- **Antioxidant supplements** — protect cells from free radicals in the body, which reduces inflammation, supports the immune system, and keeps the aging body healthy.
- **Fish oil (omega-3) supplements** — to make the coat shinier, keep the skin healthier, strengthen heart muscles, and promote healthy brain development.
- **Probiotic supplements** — to rebalance and maintain good flora levels in the gastrointestinal tract to treat chronic diarrhea, help absorb nutrients, and reduce collateral damage during or after antibiotic therapy.

When choosing supplements for your dog, prioritize supplements rich in essential vitamins and minerals. According to researchers Kazimierska and Biel from the West Pomeranian University of Technology, your dog needs key minerals like calcium, phosphorus, potassium, sodium, and magnesium; and essential micronutrients such as copper, iron, manganese, selenium, and zinc. They also stress the importance of antioxidant-rich vitamins E and C, and vitamin D and B-group vitamins to keep your dog healthy and active, especially if they are highly energetic or involved in sports (Kazimierska and Biel, 2020). Here is a quick breakdown of these vitamins and minerals:

- **Calcium & Phosphorus** — for strong bones and teeth for growing puppies and active dogs.
- **Potassium** — boosts muscle function, nerve signals, and maintains hydration.
- **Sodium** — for regulating fluid balance and blood pressure; recommended in limited quantities.
- **Magnesium** — promotes muscle and nerve function, and increases enzyme activity and energy production.
- **Copper** — fosters red blood cell formation, supports immune health, and enhances coat pigmentation.
- **Iron** — transports oxygen to the blood and protects against anemia.
- **Manganese** — helps with bone development, joint health, and metabolism.
- **Selenium** — acts as an antioxidant and protects cells from damage.
- **Zinc** — enhances skin and coat health, promotes faster wound healing, and boosts immune function.
- **Vitamin E & Vitamin C** —act as antioxidants, support the immune system, and improve skin health.
- **Vitamin D** - improves bone health by regulating calcium and phosphorus absorption in the body.
- **B-group Vitamins like B2, vitamin B9, and vitamin B12**- boost energy metabolism, nervous system function, and red blood cell production.

Without these micronutrients, dogs can develop deficiencies like weaker bones, poor cell function, and bad immunity. Homemade meals sometimes lack key vitamins and minerals like vitamins B, E, and D.

Poor nutrition can cause lethargy, poor digestion, weak bones, joint pain, bad vision, and neurological issues. To avoid these deficiencies, plan your dog's meals to ensure a balanced nutrition, and include supplements when necessary.

3. Hydration: The Overlooked Nutrient

Hydration is a necessity, but sometimes dog owners overlook its importance. Water performs many functions, including regulating your dog's body temperature, lubricating joints, and breaking down carbs, protein, and fats for easy absorption. Without adequate hydration, dogs cannot get the full benefit of their diet. This is why The Association of American Feed Control Officials (AAFCO) has listed water as one of the six essential nutrients for dogs (Rotat 2016).

A dog's recommended water intake depends on the dog's size, activity levels, diet, and environment. However, a general rule of thumb is to provide water 2.5 times the amount of dry matter they eat. PetMD suggests giving your dog approximately 1 ounce of water (⅛ cup) per pound of their body weight every day. However, there is no need to calculate the amount of water your dog drinks unless directed by a pet physician. Just remember to provide fresh, clean water and let your dog drink to its fill (Pignatro 2024).

Remember that hydration needs increase during summer, exercise, or after eating low-moisture (dry) food. Puppies, lactating, and senior dogs drink more water than adult dogs. So, ensure that your dog has access to plenty of clean and fresh water all the time.

You can also keep track of your dog's hydration by watching for any signs of dehydration, including:

- Dry gums
- Excessive panting without increased activity
- Loss of skin elasticity
- A dry nose
- Sunken eyes
- Unusual lethargy
- Dark yellow urine

These signs signal dehydration. However, you can perform a simple test to confirm; gently lift the skin at the back of their neck — if the skin does not snap back into its prior position instantly, your dog needs more water. Immediately provide clean, fresh water to save your dog from kidney failure and other life-threatening illnesses. For picky drinkers, try flavored water, ice cubes, or a pet fountain to encourage water intake. Lastly, dogs who are sick, recovering from illness, or experiencing vomiting and diarrhea are at a higher risk, so owners should be extra cautious in such cases and provide adequate hydration.

Chart: Balanced Nutrition

Dogs need a mix of everything — proteins, fats, carbs, minerals, and vitamins — to support their well-being. Dog owners who prefer feeding their pets homemade meals often struggle to find reliable resources and guidance on proper nutrition. To make things easier, here is a chart outlining key nutrients and their best food sources, along with a list of foods that should always be avoided.

Nutrient	Food Sources	Purpose
Lean Proteins	Chicken, Turkey, Beef, Fish, Lamb	Building muscle, boosting the immune system, and providing energy.
Whole Grains	Brown Rice, Quinoa, Oats, Barley	Fiber for digestion and sustaining energy production.
Vegetables	Carrots, Spinach, Sweet Potatoes, Peas, Broccoli	Rich in vitamins, minerals, and antioxidants for enhancing immune and digestive health.
Fruits	Blueberries, Apples, Bananas, Pumpkin, Watermelon	Vitamins and hydration benefits; act as natural antioxidants to prevent inflammation.
Healthy Fats	Fish Oil, Flaxseed Oil, Olive Oil	Support skin and coat health; improve brain function and joint mobility.
Dairy	Yogurt, Cottage Cheese (in moderation)	Calcium and probiotics for good gut health - should be fed in small amounts.
Herbs & Spices	Parsley, Turmeric, Ginger, Basil, Cilantro	Anti-inflammatory properties prevent inflammation and help in better digestion.
Foods to Avoid	Chocolate, Grapes, Onions, Garlic, Avocado	**Toxic and cause serious health issues.**

Key Takeaways:

- Dogs need proteins, fats, and carbohydrates to stay healthy. Each nutrient plays a different role in muscle health, energy production, and metabolism.
- Proteins support muscle development, immunity, and cell growth, while fats provide sustained energy and maintain skin and coat health.
- Carbohydrates are a quick energy source but should be given in moderation, especially for dogs with obesity or diabetes.
- Dogs require micronutrients like calcium, phosphorus, zinc, and B-group vitamins for bone strength, immunity, and well-being.
- Supplements can be given to dogs to fill nutritional gaps, especially for aging dogs, large breeds, or those with dietary restrictions.
- Key supplements for dogs include glucosamine for joint health, antioxidants for immune support, fish oil for coat health, and probiotics for digestion.
- Look for vitamins and minerals like calcium, phosphorus, magnesium, potassium, copper, iron, selenium, zinc, and vitamins C, E, D, and B (B2, B9, and B12) in dog supplements.
- Water is essential for regulating body temperature, lubricating joints, and nutrient absorption.
- Dehydration can lead to lethargy, poor digestion, and severe health issues, so watch out for lethargic movements, excessive panting, extra yellowish urine, dry gums and nose, and sunken eyes.
- Let your dog drink as much as it needs unless directed by a vet; keep plenty of fresh and clean water available.

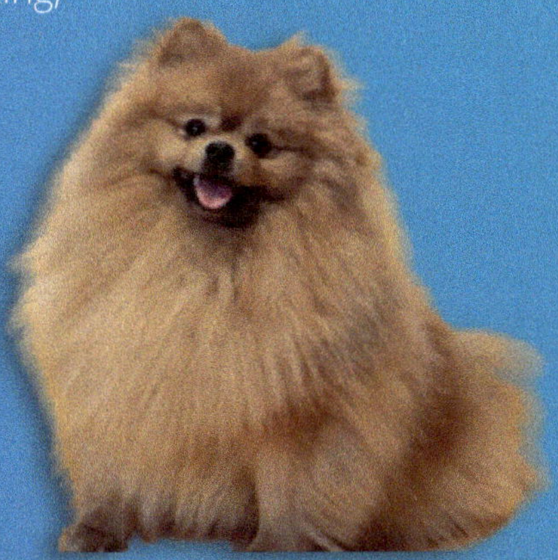

Now that you know what goes into a balanced diet, it's time to put that knowledge into action. From selecting high-quality ingredients to adjusting portions, the most important thing is to transition your dog to homemade food. The next chapter is a guide to a smoother transition, featuring tips and tricks to make the switch easier. With the right approach, your dog is going to love a yummy, nutritional, homemade meal!

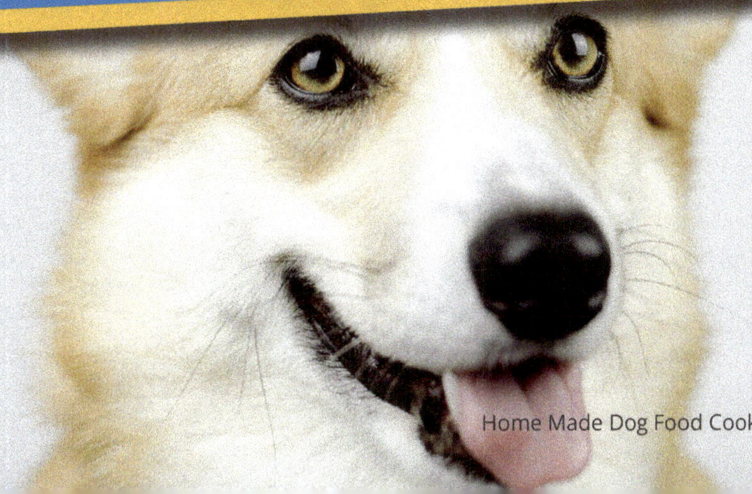

Get Your 5 Exclusive Bonuses—FREE!

Congratulations on taking the first step toward giving your dog a longer, healthier life with real, nourishing food made right in your kitchen. But before you dive into Chapter 2, I want to give you a special set of tools to help you on your journey.

What's in it for me?

☑ ***Homemade Dog Treats Cookbook*** - Keep your pup happy between meals with nutritious, easy-to-make treats that pair perfectly with their new homemade diet.

☑ ***Weekly Dog Meal Planner*** - Plan ahead with confidence! Map out balanced, vet-approved meals for your dog, save time in the kitchen, and eliminate guesswork.

☑ ***Dog Health Tracker*** - Track your dog's weight, energy, and digestion so you can quickly identify what's working—and spot any red flags early.

☑ ***Dog Potty Training eBook*** - Whether you're starting fresh or retraining, this guide provides fast, effective techniques to end indoor accidents for good.

☑ ***How to Prepare for a New Puppy In Your Home*** - Bringing a new dog into the family? This expert guide helps you puppy-proof your home, set a routine, and build a healthy foundation from day one.

Simply follow the instructions below, and your bonuses will be on their way!

SCAN THE QR CODE

Once you're set up, head into Chapter 2 to learn exactly how to transition your dog to a homemade diet without digestive issues or stress. Let's get cooking—the right way!

CHAPTER 2:

Transition to a Homemade Diet THE RIGHT WAY!

"Switching to homemade food is one of the best decisions for your dog but do it wrong, and you could cause more harm than good."

Switching to homemade food is a big step, and it's not as simple as swapping out kibble for home-cooked meals overnight. Changing your pup's diet suddenly can cause digestive issues, nutrient imbalances, or even food intolerance. This is why a careful, gradual transition is important to keep your dog healthy and avoid any digestive issues.

According to the American Kennel Club, you have to consider factors like your dog's eating history, weight, and overall health before switching to homemade food (2024). These considerations foster a smoother transition without digestive issues or nutrient imbalances. For example, by tracking portion sizes, nutrient intake, and preferred textures, you can create meals that meet your dog's needs while maintaining familiarity. Additionally, incorporating familiar elements makes the shift easier.

The first step, therefore, is to understand your dog's unique dietary needs. So, note down the following:

- **The type of food they eat -** kibble, wet/dry food, raw, or mixed diet.
- **Daily nutritional content —** protein, carbs, fats, minerals, vitamins, etc.
- **Eating habits and preferences —** meal timings, portion size, food preferences, picky eating.
- **Sensitivities —** food allergies, intolerances, medical conditions.
- **Stool quality** — firm, well-formed, loose, etc.

It may seem like a lot, but you've got this! Just grab a paper and pen and follow our complete guide to easily break down your dog's current dietary needs. Here we go!

1. Identifying the Type of Food Your Dog Currently Eats

Is it commercial kibble, canned food, or a mixed diet? Generally, dogs follow different diets, and each one affects the transition to homemade food differently:

- **Commercial Kibble** — dry dog food with low moisture content; sometimes contains fillers and artificial preservatives. Your dog will require a gradual transition to adjust to homemade meals' softer consistency and increased hydration.
- **Wet/Canned Food** — higher moisture content, often more palatable, but can differ in quality based on ingredients. Transition is easier due to similar texture and moisture but can also result in ingredient sensitivities.
- **Raw Diet** — fresh, unprocessed meats and bones. This type of diet requires a more gradual transition due to different digestion rates.
- **Mixed Diet** — Dogs that eat a combination of kibble and wet food adjust well to a home-cooked diet but need careful portioning to avoid digestive upset.

The transition period differs for each dog depending on their dietary needs. Dogs already familiar with wet food switch faster than dogs on a dry/raw diet. Don't worry, we have a plan for each case to make the switch easier.

2. Analyzing the Nutritional Content

The amount of protein, carbs, and fats your dog consumes in a day is directly related to the transition's success. Any imbalance between your dog's previous diet and homemade meals can cause digestive upset, weight fluctuations, or nutrient deficiencies.

For example, dogs that mostly consume high-carb kibble struggle more with a protein-rich homemade diet. Dogs on high-fat raw diets need a gradual reduction to prevent pancreatic stress. Therefore, matching the new diet's macronutrient profile to your dog's previous intake and adjusting slowly is important to maintain gut health, energy levels, and overall well-being during the transition.

What to do:

- **Protein:** note down which protein source your dog consumes daily, meat- (chicken, fish, beef) or plant-based. Make sure to note any allergies or sensitivities.
- **Fat:** Identify fat sources and how much your dog consumes in a day (meat, eggs, oils, or seeds).
- **Carbs:** Note if your dog eats a high or low-carb diet, like kibble (high), wet food (moderate), or a raw diet (low), as this affects how their body adapts to homemade meals.
- **Vitamins and minerals:** Look at the supplements (if any). Commercial diets have added vitamins and minerals to meet a dog's nutritional needs, which are not naturally present in the ingredients. Tracking how much micronutrients your dog needs daily helps balance the overall nutritional intake in homemade meals.
- **Moisture content:** Note if your dog eats more dry or wet food, as transitioning from dry to homemade food (which has higher moisture) requires gradual adjustments to water intake.
- **Water:** Not really necessary, but still important if your dog is dehydrated, eats dry food, or has an active lifestyle.

3. Evaluating Your Dog's Eating Habits and Preferences

Once you've tracked your dog's food intake and nutrient levels, evaluate their eating habits and dietary preferences, such as:

- **Meal Timings:** How often does your dog eat? Free feeding or scheduled meals?
- **Portion Size:** How much food is served in a single meal?

- **Food Preferences:** Does your dog have a food preference like crunchy kibble or soft wet food? This helps to ensure that your dog will like homemade meals with similar textures.
- **Picky Eating:** Transition takes more time and effort for picky eaters. Note the food types and textures your dog likes so you can incorporate them in homemade meals.

4. Checking for Digestive Sensitivities and Health Issues

You don't want to switch your dog's food only to end up dealing with an upset stomach, allergies, or worse. Some dogs have sensitive stomachs, and certain ingredients just don't sit well with them. If your dog has a history of digestive issues or health conditions like kidney disease or pancreatitis, the wrong food can make things worse. Therefore, note any past reactions—like itching, loose stools, or vomiting—to help you avoid ingredients that might trigger an adverse reaction.

In short, remember the following to make the transition smoother and save a lot of stress later:

- **Previous Digestive Problems:** If your dog often has diarrhea, vomiting, or bloating; what causes that?
- **Food Allergies or Intolerances:** Common allergens like chicken, beef, grains, and dairy, so you can avoid any adverse reactions later.
- **Weight and Body Condition:** Helps track if homemade meals are keeping your pup healthy and not causing weight gain or nutrient imbalances. Also, overweight dogs need a lower-calorie homemade diet while underweight dogs require calorie-dense meals.
- **Medical Conditions:** Dogs with kidney disease, diabetes, pancreatitis, or other health issues need specialized nutritional adjustments.

5. Monitoring Stool Quality and Digestion

Your dog's poop is a good indicator of how well they're handling the new diet. Note down the condition of their poop so you can tweak meals before small issues turn into bigger problems.

Here is how you can determine your pup's digestion by observing the stool:

- **Firm and well-formed stool** means the pup has a balanced diet.
- **Loose stools or diarrhea** suggest food sensitivities or improper digestion.
- **Excessive gas** indicates difficulty digesting certain ingredients.
- **Constipation** indicates lack of fiber or moisture.

By observing the stool condition, you can easily adjust their diet for a smoother transition.

Bonus: Diet Info Template

Keeping track of everything your dog eats, their habits, and any health concerns can be overwhelming. A seemingly small mistake can create tummy troubles or even serious health issues. To help ease your troubles, here is an easy-to-use tracker.

Simply **screenshot/copy-paste and print it, fill it out, and keep it in your kitchen.** With your dog's important dietary info available at a glance, meal prep and transitions will be a lot smoother.

Diet Info Chart

Category	Options	Your Dog's Info
Current Diet Type	☐ Kibble ☐ Wet/Canned ☐ Raw ☐ Mixed Diet	
Protein Source(s)	☐ Chicken ☐ Fish ☐ Beef ☐ Plant-Based	
Fat Source(s)	☐ Meat ☐ Eggs ☐ Oils ☐ Seeds	
Carb Intake	☐ High (Kibble) ☐ Moderate (Wet) ☐ Low (Raw)	
Vitamins & Minerals	☐ Commercial Supplements ☐ Natural (Food-Based)	
Moisture Content	☐ Mostly Dry ☐ Mostly Wet	
Water Intake	☐ Low ☐ Normal ☐ High	
Meal Timings	☐ Free Feeding ☐ 2 Meals ☐ 3+ Meals	
Portion Size (Per Meal)	☐ Small ☐ Medium ☐ Large	
Food Preferences	☐ Crunchy ☐ Soft/Wet ☐ Warm ☐ Cold	
Picky Eater?	☐ Yes ☐ No	
Digestive Issues?	☐ diarrhea ☐ Vomiting ☐ Gas ☐ Bloating ☐ None	
Food Allergies	☐ Chicken ☐ Beef ☐ Dairy ☐ Grains ☐ None	
Weight Condition	☐ Underweight ☐ Normal ☐ Overweight	
Medical Conditions	☐ Kidney Issues ☐ Diabetes ☐ Pancreatitis ☐ None	
Current Stool Condition	☐ Firm ☐ Loose ☐ Constipated ☐ Gassy ☐ Normal	

Step-by-Step Transition Guide

Dr. Jennifer Coates, a seasoned veterinarian and animal welfare expert, recommends two methods to successfully switch your dog's diet. These methods — gradual and quick — greatly minimize the chances of complications like food refusal, diarrhea, vomiting, and gassiness (Coates, 2022).

In a gradual transition, you take things slowly and switch to a homemade diet in a period of 7 to 21 days. On the other hand, a quick transition process skips the gradual adjustment phase and shifts your dog to homemade food within a few days. However, the quick method is only recommended for adult and healthy dogs who can safely skip a few meals before switching to a homemade diet.

Let's explore both transition methods in detail—benefits, risks, and step-by-step guidelines—so you can choose the best approach for your dog.

1. Gradual Transition Method

A gradual transition involves slowly introducing homemade food into your dog's diet over a set period. Start by giving your dog a smaller portion of homemade food mixed with a larger portion of their previous diet. This method helps your pup's body learn to digest new food before completely switching to a different diet. The transition period gives the dog's digestive system enough time to adjust to new ingredients, textures, and nutrients without causing stomach upset, diarrhea, or refusal to eat.

Moreover, a gradual transition is necessary for dogs on commercial/raw diets as their bodies take longer to adapt to homemade meals. Kibble has dry texture and less moisture content while home-cooked meals are often high in moisture content. Raw diets are high in protein, taking dogs longer to transition to nutritionally balanced meals. By taking it slow, you ensure that your furry friend remains comfortable and enjoys their new diet without distress.

1.1. Time Frame of Gradual Transition

The ideal time frame in a gradual transition varies from 7 to 21 days, although it may take less or more time depending on your dog's sensitivity. As a rule of thumb:

- 7-day transition — better for dogs with really strong digestion.
- 14-day transition — good for most dogs as a steady transition fosters better gut adaptation.
- 21-day transition — great for dogs with food sensitivities, past digestive problems, or senior dogs.

However, even if your dog has really great digestion, we recommend you go for a 21-day transition period to minimize complications as much as possible. By slowly introducing homemade meals into your pup's diet, you ensure their digestive health remains stable and comfortable.

1.2. Step-by-Step Guide Transition Guide

Switching your dog to a homemade diet shouldn't be rushed. A slow and steady approach prevents digestive upset, making the transition smoother for your pup. As mentioned previously, the timeline depends on your dog's digestive sensitivity—some adjust quickly, while others need more time to adapt.

Here are the 7, 14, and 21-day transition timelines, with step-by-step instructions to implement them:

7-Day Transition (For Dogs with Strong Digestion)	
Day 1	10% homemade food / 90% current food
Day 2	20% homemade food / 80% current food
Day 3	30% homemade food / 70% current food
Day 4	40% homemade food / 60% current food
Day 5	60% homemade food / 40% current food
Day 6	80% homemade food / 20% current food
Day 7	100% homemade food

14-Day Transition (For Most Dogs)	
Day 1-2	10% homemade food / 90% current food
Day 3-4	20% homemade food / 80% current food
Day 5-6	30% homemade food / 70% current food
Day 7-8	40% homemade food / 60% current food
Day 9-10	60% homemade food / 40% current food
Day 11-12	80% homemade food / 20% current food
Day 13-14	100% homemade food

21-Day Transition (Best approach for preventing digestion problems)	
Days 1-3	10% homemade food / 90% current food
Days 4-6	20% homemade food / 80% current food
Days 7-9	30% homemade food / 70% current food
Days 10-12	40% homemade food / 60% current food
Days 13-15	60% homemade food / 40% current food
Days 16-18	80% homemade food / 20% current food
Days 19-21	100% homemade food

Usually, it takes no more than three weeks to fully transition your pup to homemade meals. However, this timeline can vary depending on how well your dog adapts to the new diet. To stay on the safer side, adopt a feeding strategy that gradually introduces new ingredients to your pup — explained below!

1.3. Practical Transition Strategies

When transitioning your pup to homemade meals, follow these practical strategies to increase their interest in the new diet:

- Layer the food strategically: Place the new food at the bottom of the bowl and the old food on top. This way, your dog starts with what's familiar, making them more likely to accept the new food as they reach it.
- Use a favorite treat as encouragement: Sprinkle a bit of your dog's favorite treat over the new food before adding the old food on top. This reinforces a positive association with the new meal and they are less likely to reject their new diet.
- Introduce new aromas gradually: If your dog is really picky, try placing the new food slightly away from the old food in the bowl. At first, give only a tablespoon of the new food, so your dog can get used to the smell without feeling pressured to eat it. If they show interest, increase the new food slightly and start moving the portions closer together.
- Warm up the food: Though it's best to serve food at room temperature, you can try warming homemade food slightly (not too much). This enhances the aroma of food, making it more appealing to picky eaters.
- Hand-feed small amounts: If it's really hard for your dog to accept new food, first build a safe connection with their new diet. Feed your pup small bites of the new food from your hand so they know it's safe and feel more encouraged to try it willingly.
- Stick to a consistent feeding schedule: Dogs thrive on routine, so keeping mealtimes the same can make them more inclined to eat new foods.

You can follow one or more of these strategies to practically introduce new food to your pup. Remember to be patient as it takes time for your furry friend to adjust to new textures and aromas.

2. Quick Transition Method

Sometimes, you have to switch your dog's diet immediately for various reasons. Maybe it's an unexpected dietary restriction, or the vet recommended their old food to be discontinued. In such situations, a gradual transition method is not viable as you cannot mix old food with new food. So, what to do? According to Dr. Jennifer Coates, dog owners can try the quick transition method (Coates, 2022).

The quick transition method is for healthy adult dogs that can handle a direct switch. In this approach, feed your dog small portions of the new food directly while monitoring their response. Usually, the dog refuses to eat the new food at first, but eventually, they accept their new diet. It takes no less than 48 hours to switch to a completely new diet with this method. However, if your dog refuses to eat for more than 48 hours or experiences vomiting or diarrhea, reconsider the food choice or consult a veterinarian.

Important: The quick transition method is **not safe for puppies or dogs with health conditions.** As this method involves offering new food directly, it is common for dogs to skip a few meals before accepting their new diet. While healthy adult dogs can safely avoid a few meals, this can be dangerous for puppies or sick dogs.

1.1. Time Frame of Quick Transition

A quick transition takes no more than one to two days. Your dog may refuse to eat at first, but soon, they will start eating when no other food is available. It is also common for dogs to eat a smaller portion than their regular diet. The quick transition method works on direct acceptance or refusal of the new food. If your dog eats the food, well done; but if they refuse, don't offer anything until the next meal.

The ideal time frame for a quick transition looks like this:

- **Day 1:**
    - First meal: Introduce a small portion of the new food.
    - If eaten, increase the portion in the next meal.
    - If refused, remove the food after 30 minutes and wait for the next meal.

- **Day 2:**
    - If your dog ate well the previous day, increase the portion further.
    - By the end of Day 2, most dogs will be eating full meals of the new food.

By day 3, your dog should be fully transitioned. If they still refuse the new food or show signs of illness, seek professional advice.

If you are worried about your dog skipping meals, know that it's completely fine. Dr. Rhiannon Koehler, a veterinarian and medical writer, says that most adult dogs can go three to five days without eating as long as they're still drinking water (Koehler, 2024). So, don't worry if your dog does not eat on the first day of the quick transition. Switching takes time and the wait is worth it.

1.2. Step-by-Step Transition Guide

Before you start the quick transition, answer the following:

- Is your dog healthy, with no underlying medical conditions that require a specialized diet?
- Is your dog an adult?
- Has your dog had any digestive issues (vomiting, diarrhea, gas) in the past? If yes, gradual transition is best.
- Are you in contact with your vet in case your dog refuses the new food?

If you answered yes to all the questions, you can start with the quick transition:

- **Day 1 – Meal 1**
    - Offer only a small portion of the new food (around ¼ of a regular meal).
    - If your dog doesn't eat within 30 minutes, remove the bowl and do not offer anything else until the next meal.

- **Day 1 — Meal 2**
    - If your dog ate Meal 1, increase the portion slightly.
    - If they refused Meal 1, offer another small portion of the new food. Again, if not eaten in 30 minutes, remove it.

- **Day 1 — Meal 3**
    - If your dog is eating well, increase the portion again.
    - If they refused previous meals, continue offering small amounts at each mealtime.

- **Day 2 - Meal 1**
    - If your dog ate the last meal well, offer a bigger portion.
    - If they refuse, offer a small portion of the new food. If not eaten, pick up the bowl in 30 minutes. Note if there are any signs of distress.

- **Day 2 — Meal 2**
    - If your dog ate the last meal well, offer a bigger portion.
    - If they refuse, this is the last chance before intervening. Monitor for symptoms of distress.

- **Day 2 — Meal 3 (Final Step)**
    - If your dog has been eating, offer a full portion of the new food.
    - If they are still refusing or showing signs of digestive issues, consult a vet.

A successful quick transition ends on day 2, so if your dog still refuses to eat by that time, it could be due to several reasons, such as:

- Discomfort with sudden change.
- Digestive upset, as a sudden switch can cause mild nausea or an upset stomach.
- Your dog might simply dislike the new taste or texture.

What You Can Do:

✔ Offer their previous food (if it's not toxic or unsafe for them) to check if they are willing to eat.

✔ Monitor for symptoms like vomiting, diarrhea, or lethargy. If you notice these symptoms, consult a vet immediately.

✔ Try gradual transitioning by mixing small amounts of the new food with their old food to encourage them to eat and adapt to their new diet.

1.3. Practical Transition Strategies

Since the quick transition method relies on immediate change, you can use a few tricks to encourage your dog to accept the new food faster:

- **Warm up the food slightly:** Dogs are more likely to accept food that smells familiar or appetizing. Lightly warm the homemade meal (but not too much) to enhance its aroma.
- **Use a "hunger boost" approach:** Since dogs can safely skip one or two meals, let their appetite build up naturally. This increases the likelihood that they will eat the new food at the next mealtime. However, constantly monitor for signs of distress.
- **Mix in a treat:** This is a personal favorite that usually works! If your dog is hesitant to eat new food, top it with a small amount of their favorite treat. It could be anything from boiled chicken, a small piece of cheese, to an irresistible dog-friendly topping. This can encourage them to take the first bite.

- **Hand-feed the first few bites:** Some dogs respond better if you hand-feed them the new food at first. Offer small amounts by hand to get them started before putting the rest in their bowl.
- **Use a new feeding bowl:** Dogs associate their usual bowl with their old food. If your dog refuses the new meal, try using a different bowl to prevent them from expecting their old food.
- **Reduce distractions during mealtime:** Provide a quiet, stress-free environment so your dog can focus on the new food instead of getting distracted.

Just like a gradual transition, a quick transition to homemade food requires patience and careful monitoring. You need to be more cautious with this method because your dog may refuse and skip meals. Make sure to keep an eye on their reactions, and if they refuse the food for too long or show signs of digestive distress, consult a vet.

Bonus: Find the Right Transition Method for Your Dog!

Each dog has unique dietary needs, so you have to carefully choose the right transition method. It can be a bit tricky, but we've made it easy for you! Our practical comparison chart is created to help you choose the best transition method based on your dog's health, eating habits, and sensitivity levels.

Simply screenshot/copy-paste, and print this chart, and fill it out with your dog's details. It'll give you a clear idea of which method suits your pup best, so you can transition them smoothly with confidence!

Transition Method Chart

Transition Method Chart	Options	Your Dog's Info
Is your dog generally picky with food?	☑ Yes → Use this method	☒ No → Use this method
Does your dog have a sensitive stomach? (e.g., frequent vomiting, diarrhea, gas)	☑ Yes → Use this method	☒ No → Use this method
Is your dog currently eating a completely different type of food? (e.g., kibble to homemade, raw to cooked, etc.)	☑ Yes → Use this method	☒ No → Use this method
Does your dog have health issues (e.g., diabetes, kidney disease, pancreatitis, or other chronic conditions)?	☑ Yes → Use this method (consult vet first)	☒ No → Use this method
Can your dog safely skip 1-2 meals without getting weak or sick?	☒ No → Use this method	☑ Yes → Use this method
Do you need to switch your dog's food immediately? (e.g., food recall, allergies, urgent diet change)	☒ No → Use this method	☑ Yes → Use this method
How patient is your dog with new foods?	● Will take time to accept → Use this method	● Will eat anything → Use this method
Are you okay with monitoring stool consistency for a longer period?	☑ Yes → Use this method	☒ No → Use this method

Can you mix old and new food in each meal?	☑ Yes → Use this method	☒ No → Use this method
Will your dog stop eating completely if they dislike the new food?	☑ Yes → Use this method	☒ No → Use this method

Essential Guidelines for Switching to Homemade Dog Food

Switching your dog to homemade food is an exciting step, but it's important to get it right. Regardless of the transition method you choose, there are important factors to consider to ensure your dog stays healthy and adapts smoothly. For instance, you have to carefully select the ingredients for the first few recipes. The ingredients should be familiar to your dog's previous diet to increase the chances of a successful transition. Likewise, watching for digestive or behavioral symptoms can save trouble in the long run.

It's just a few things you must take care of. Let's make this switch smooth, healthy, and stress-free for both you and your furry friend!

1. Choosing the Right FIRST Homemade Meals

The FIRST homemade meals you feed your dog matter the most. They should be easily digestible, or else things might go south. You want to make sure the ingredients in the first few recipes resemble your pup's current food. For example, if your dog's current diet is:

- **Kibble –** Start with lightly cooked meals that include lean meats (like chicken or turkey) and small amounts of easily digestible carbs (like rice or sweet potatoes). Keep the texture firm by reducing moisture initially.
- **Raw meat –** Introduce gently cooked meats instead of jumping straight to fully cooked meals. Stick to familiar protein sources and slowly add in cooked veggies.
- **Wet/canned food –** Use soft, moisture-rich meals with similar textures, like stews or slow-cooked meats with broth. Start with ingredients found in their usual wet food to avoid refusal.
- Matching familiar textures and ingredients makes the transition process easier, as:
- Your dog will like the homemade food more if it tastes and feels as familiar as their previous diet.
- Starting homemade meals will be successful with minimal food rejection.
- There will be lower chances of digestive upset, diarrhea, or vomiting due to gradual changes. The gut easily adapts to new nutrients without shock.
- There will be no sudden drops in energy from drastic dietary changes.
- A familiar diet keeps mealtime stress-free for both you and your pup.

Therefore, start with what your dog already likes and avoid using ingredients or textures they are not familiar with.

2. Watching for Digestive or Behavioral Reactions

Transition is not easy; one missed step can result in adverse reactions. If you don't want your dog to fall sick, you have to be very observant when feeding a new diet. Whether you choose the gradual or quick transition, monitor these symptoms:

- **Mild digestive reactions:** A little bit of loose stool or extra gas isn't usually a big deal. It just means your pup's gut bacteria are adjusting to the new food. However, if it lasts more than a few days or gets worse, change the ingredients.
- **Severe intolerance signs:** Vomiting, persistent diarrhea, excessive itching, or lethargy signal the need to slow the transition or reconsider ingredients. Consult a vet immediately if things go south.
- **Appetite changes:** If the dog refuses homemade food, ensure it's palatable and not too different from previous meals. It's okay if your dog skips the first few meals but don't let it go on for more than two days (and only if your dog is an adult and healthy).

3. Adapting to Nutritional Gaps

Yes, we've mentioned this plenty of times, and guess what? We're saying it again—you need nutritionally balanced homemade meals to save your pup from deficiencies! Your key considerations should be:

- **Calcium & Phosphorus Ratio:** Dogs need calcium for bone health. Use ground eggshells, bone meal, or vet-approved supplements.
- **Essential Fatty Acids:** Omega-3s (fish oil) and Omega-6s (flaxseed or sunflower oil) support skin and coat health.
- **Fiber for Digestion:** Vegetables like carrots and zucchini provide prebiotic fiber.

Also, take note of hydration. If your dog previously ate dry food/kibble, they are likely to drink less water due to the increased moisture content in homemade food. However, you should still monitor hydration through:

- Normal urine color (should be light yellow, not dark).
- Skin elasticity (pinch the skin at the back of their neck; if the skin does not snap back immediately, your dog needs more water).
- Daily water intake based on weight (approximately 1 oz per pound of body weight, though no limitations if your pup drinks more).

4. Monitoring Long-Term Health

Once the dog is fully on homemade food, you can gradually expand protein sources and carbohydrates for variety. Every few days, you can introduce new ingredients one at a time to watch for reactions. If your pup remains healthy and stable, you can continue adding the tested ingredients to their daily diet. Also, keep monitoring the following factors to ensure their long-term health:

- Coat quality (should be shiny, no excessive shedding).
- Digestive health (should be firm stools, no bloating).
- Energy levels (consistent, no lethargy).
- Weight maintenance (not gaining/losing rapidly).

Over time, your dog will get used to home-cooked meals—it just takes a little patience and careful observation. Sure, there might be a few bumps along the way, but in the end, you're giving them fresh, nutritionally balanced meals made with love. And really, what more could a pet parent ask for?

Key Takeaways:

- Switching to homemade food can be great for your dog, but doing it wrong can cause health issues.
- Your dog's eating history, weight, and health should be considered before making changes.
- Tracking portion sizes, nutrients, and food textures makes the switch easier.
- Dogs on different diets (kibble, wet food, raw, mixed) need different transition plans.
- Matching homemade meals to your dog's previous nutrient intake is great for preventing digestive upset.
- Some dogs are picky eaters, so keeping familiar textures can make the change easier.
- Watching for allergies, sensitivities, and past digestive issues avoids reactions from escalating. Checking stool quality is good for tracking how well your dog is adjusting to the new diet.
- Gradual and quick are two transition methods to switch dogs to homemade food while avoiding digestive issues.
- The Gradual Transition Method takes 7 to 21 days, slowly introducing homemade food to prevent stomach upset and food refusal. Techniques like layering food, using treats, warming meals, and hand-feeding encourage dogs to accept new food.
- The Quick Transition Method is only for healthy adult dogs, requiring a direct switch to homemade food over 1–2 days.
- Quick transitions can be risky for dogs with health issues or puppies, as missing meals can be dangerous.
- Healthy adult dogs can safely go 3–5 days without eating, as long as they stay hydrated.
- Choose initial homemade meals that match your dog's previous diet to ensure easy digestion and acceptance.
- Monitor for digestive issues or behavioral changes and adjust ingredients accordingly to prevent adverse effects.
- Feed essential nutrients like calcium, fatty acids, and fiber to avoid deficiencies.
- Track water intake and urine color to ensure proper hydration, especially for dogs switching from kibble.
- Regularly check coat quality, digestion, energy levels, and weight to maintain overall well-being.

Get the most of what you have just learned:

- Fill out the template provided in this chapter to understand what your dog currently eats—protein sources, carbs, fats, and any supplements—to understand what to keep in their homemade meals.
- Check in with your vet to make sure your pup is healthy.
- Fill out the template given when choosing a transitioning method for your dog.
- List the ingredients for your first few recipes; the ingredients should be similar to what your dog already eats.

You've got the transition plan ready—now it's time for the fun part! The next chapter is packed with vet-approved homemade dog food recipes that are nutritious AND delicious. Whether you're looking for simple starter meals or well-balanced long-term options, you'll find plenty of easy-to-follow recipes to keep your pup happy and healthy. Let's get into cooking!

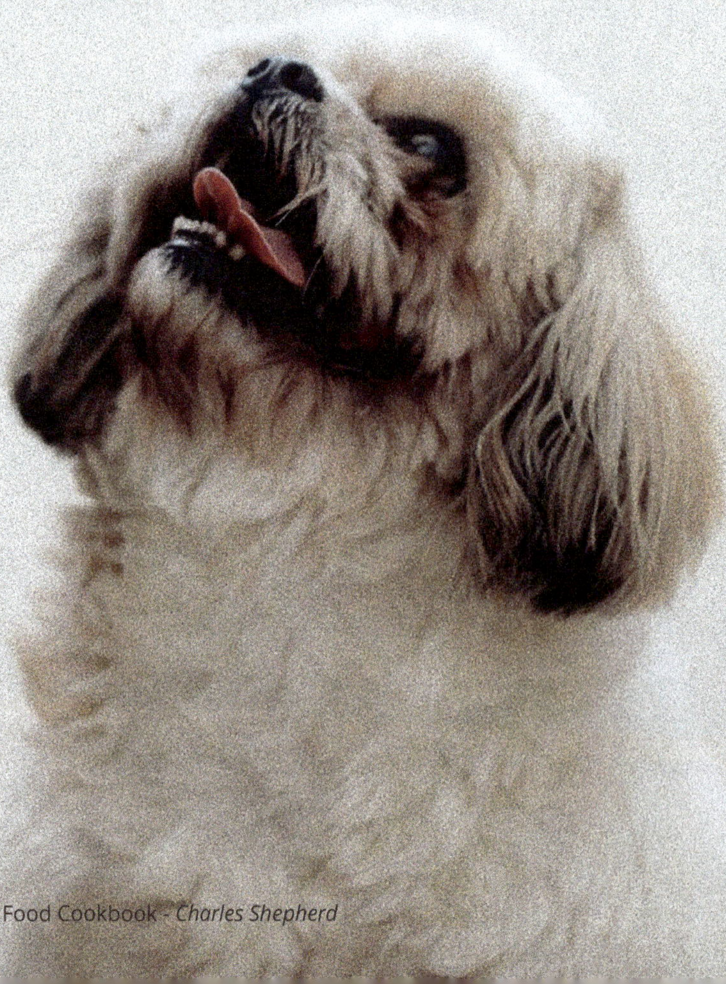

CHAPTER 3:

Vet-Approved Homemade Dog Food Recipes

"If you think making dog food at home is complicated, think again! These simple, balanced recipes will have your dog wagging their tail in no time."

Making healthy, homemade meals for your dog is easier than you think. All it takes are a few simple, balanced recipes and that's exactly what you'll find here. These vet-approved meals are easy to put together, with no special skills or complicated ingredients required.

However, keep in mind that dog owners should **adhere to the guidelines** when preparing their pet's meals. Dr. Amanda Ardente, a veterinarian with a PhD in animal nutrition, has spent years studying how diet affects animal health, from household pets to exotic species. She stresses that while selecting high-quality, nutritious ingredients is important, following the recipe is even more crucial (Ardente, 2020). Everything from portion sizes to cooking methods affects your dog's nutrition, so you have to prepare the recipe in the exact way it is provided. Cooking methods like boiling, roasting, or steaming can significantly change the amount of each nutrient in the food. Likewise, swapping ingredients—like using chicken instead of beef—might seem harmless, but it can throw off the balance and cause health problems. Unless mentioned in the recipe, do not replace an ingredient.

Moreover, the recipes below are the result of years of hands-on experience, research, and collaboration with veterinary nutrition experts. They are carefully designed to provide balanced nutrition for your dog to get all the nutrients they need. Every ingredient and portion has been tested and refined to create healthy and easy-to-prepare meals. So, to truly benefit your dog, stick to the recipe as written and trust the process. Believe me, it's simpler than it seems!

Balanced Meals for Every Life Stage

A dog's nutritional needs depends on many factors, but age matters the most. Puppies need foods that support their growth and development, while adult dogs require meals that fuel their active lifestyle. Meals for senior dogs should include ingredients that promote healthy joints and higher immunity. This section covers recipes for each life stage, so your dog stays strong, healthy, and full of energy.

Puppy-Specific Recipes

Here are my best growth-boosting meals for your pup that support strong bones and higher immunity. These recipes are soft-textured, so your little pup can easily digest food without upsetting their stomach.

1. Beef & Sweet Potato Power Meal for Puppies

(High-calorie, growth-boosting, packed for muscle & bone development)

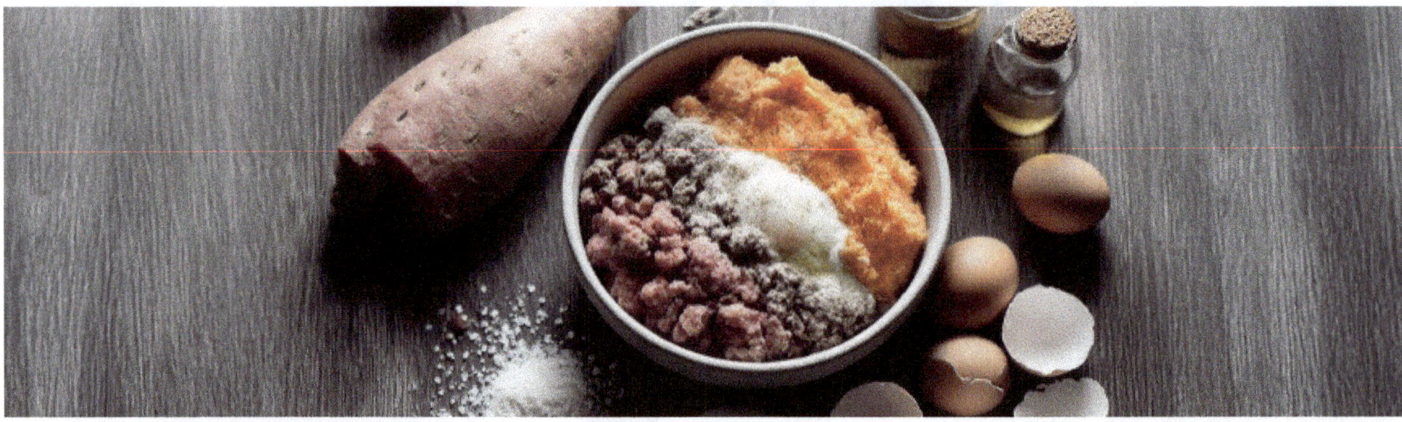

Ingredients:

- 1 lb. ground beef (85% lean)
- 1 cup cooked sweet potato (mashed)
- 1 boiled egg (mashed)
- 2 tsp fish oil (provides DHA & EPA for brain and vision development)
- 1 tsp ground eggshells OR 2 crushed calcium tablets (for optimal bone growth)
- ½ tsp iodized salt (for iodine & sodium balance)

Optional:

- 250 mg taurine (for heart and muscle health)
- 150 mg L-methionine (supports growth and muscle metabolism)

Instructions:

1. In a pan, cook the ground beef until browned (no added oil).
2. Add the mashed sweet potato and mashed boiled egg. Mix well.
3. Stir in fish oil, crushed calcium tablets (or eggshell powder), and iodized salt.
4. Cool before serving.

Ingredient Substitutions:

- Replace sweet potato with pumpkin.
- Use ground bison instead of beef.

Nutrition per 500g serving:

Final Weight	~500g
Calories	~650-700 kcal (high-energy for growing puppies)
Protein	~42-45g
Fat	~32g
Carbohydrates	~50g (from sweet potato)

2. Chicken & Rice Gentle Growth Meal for Puppies

(High-calorie, growth-boosting, packed for muscle & bone development)

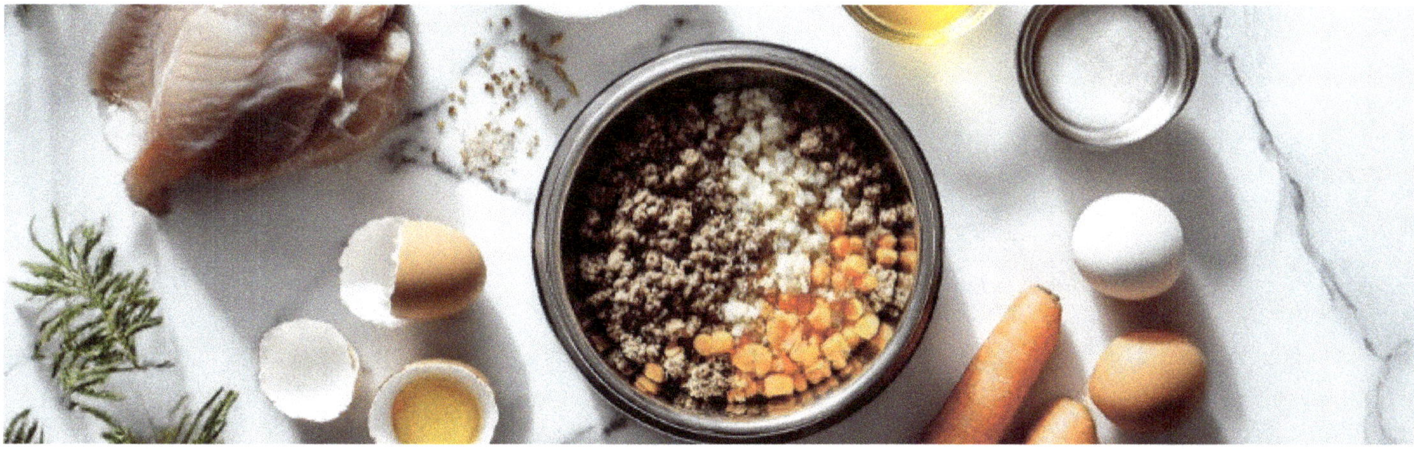

Ingredients:

- 1 lb. ground chicken (dark meat preferred)
- 1 cup cooked brown rice
- ½ cup finely chopped carrots
- 1 tsp coconut oil
- 1 tsp ground eggshell OR 2 crushed calcium tablets 1000mg (for balanced bone growth)
- ½ tsp iodized salt (iodine & sodium source)

Optional:

- 250 mg taurine (supports heart & eye health)
- 150 mg L-methionine (supports muscle & liver function)

Instructions:

1. In a pan, add the ground chicken and cook thoroughly (no added oil).
2. Add the cooked brown rice and finely chopped carrots. Mix well.
3. Stir in coconut oil, ground eggshells/calcium tablets, and iodized salt.
4. Let cool before serving.

Ingredient Substitutions:

- Swap brown rice for quinoa (high digestibility, protein boost).
- Use olive oil instead of coconut oil (good monounsaturated fats).
- Swap brown rice for quinoa.
- Use cooked ground turkey instead of chicken.

Nutrition per 500g serving:

Final Weight	~500g
Calories	550-600 kcal (gentle energy source for puppies)
Protein	~35g
Fat	~22g
Carbohydrates	~60g

3. Turkey & Pumpkin Growth Bowl

(Balanced high-protein bowl with omega-3s and essential minerals for healthy puppy growth)

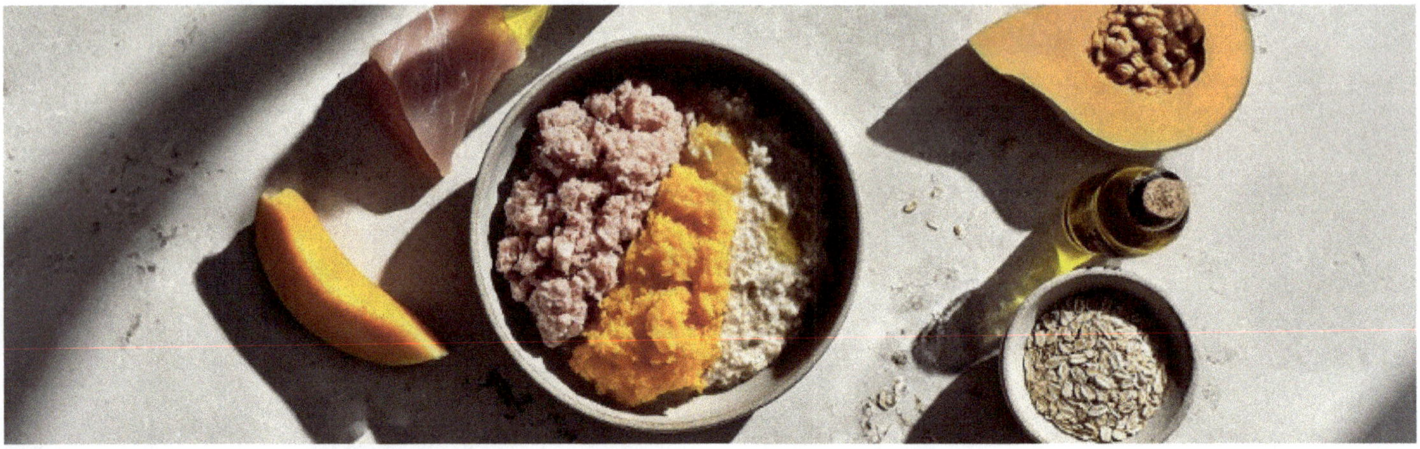

Ingredients:

- 1 lb. (450g) ground turkey (93% lean)
- 1 cup (245g) cooked pumpkin
- ½ cup (40g) cooked oats
- 1 tsp (4.5g) flaxseed oil
- 1 tsp fish oil (provides EPA & DHA)

Instructions:

1. Cook turkey in a pan until fully done (don't use any oil).
2. Add the pumpkin and cooked oats.
3. Mix in flaxseed oil and fish oil.
4. Allow to cool before serving.

Ingredient Substitutions:

- Swap oats for quinoa or brown rice.
- Replace turkey with lean pork or chicken breast (adjust fat content accordingly).
- Substitute fish oil with sardines in water (unsalted) for natural EPA/DHA.

Nutrition per 500g serving:

Final Weight	~500g
Calories	~580 kcal
Protein	~40g
Fat	~24g
Carbohydrates	~50g

4. Lamb & Peas Muscle Booster for Puppies

(High-fat, nutrient-dense bowl for puppies needing healthy weight gain and muscle support)

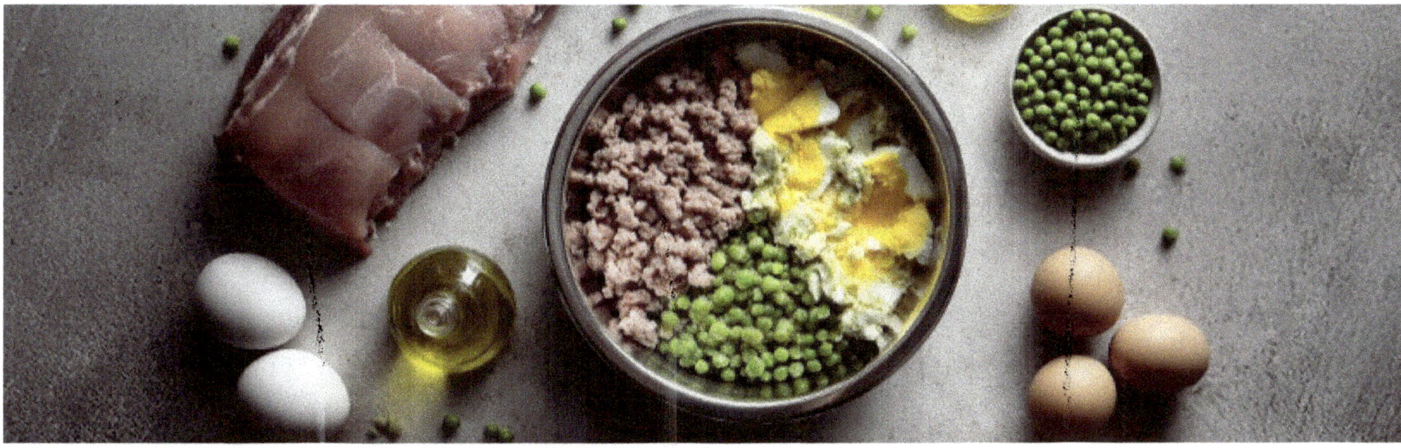

Ingredients:

- 1 lb. (450g) ground lamb
- 1 cup (160g) green peas (mashed)
- 1 boiled egg (mashed)
- 1 tsp (4.5g) olive oil
- 1 tsp fish oil (provides EPA & DHA)

Instructions:

1. Cook lamb in a pan without oil until fully done.
2. Stir in mashed peas and boiled egg.
3. Mix in olive oil and fish oil.
4. Cool before serving.

Ingredient Substitutions:

- Swap peas for green beans or finely chopped zucchini.
- Use avocado oil instead of olive oil.
- Replace lamb with lean beef or pork, adjusting fat content if needed.

Nutrition per 500g serving:

Final Weight	~500g
Calories	~650 kcal
Protein	~45g
Fat	~36g
Carbohydrates	~40g

5. Salmon & Quinoa Brain Booster

(A nutrient-dense meal packed with Omega-3 fatty acids, essential minerals, and vitamins for brain and coat health in growing puppies)

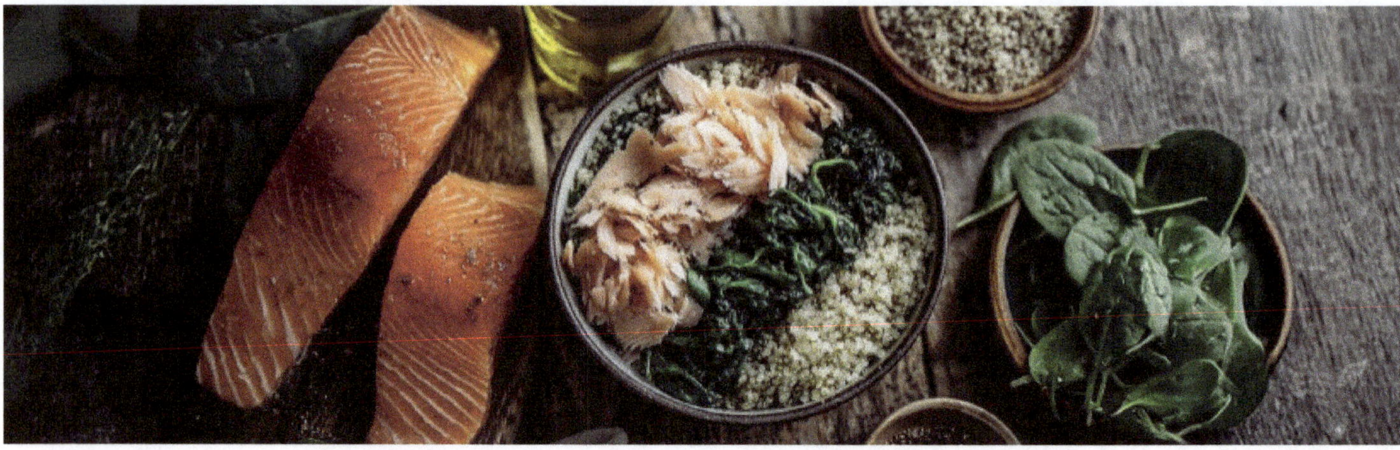

Ingredients:

- 1 lb. (450g) cooked boneless salmon
- 1 cup (185g) cooked quinoa
- ½ cup (90g) steamed spinach (chopped)
- 1 tsp (4.5g) fish oil

Instructions:

1. Flake the cooked salmon.
2. Mix with quinoa and steamed spinach.
3. Stir in fish oil.
4. Let cool before serving.

Ingredient Substitutions:

- Swap quinoa for brown rice or barley.
- Replace spinach with kale or chopped zucchini.
- Use sardines (boneless) instead of salmon for variety.

Nutrition per 500g serving:

Final Weight	~500g
Calories	~650 kcal
Protein	~46g
Fat	~28g
Carbohydrates	~48g

6. Duck & Butternut Squash Energy Mix

(High-calorie, iron-rich bowl to fuel active puppies, with essential nutrients for growth support)

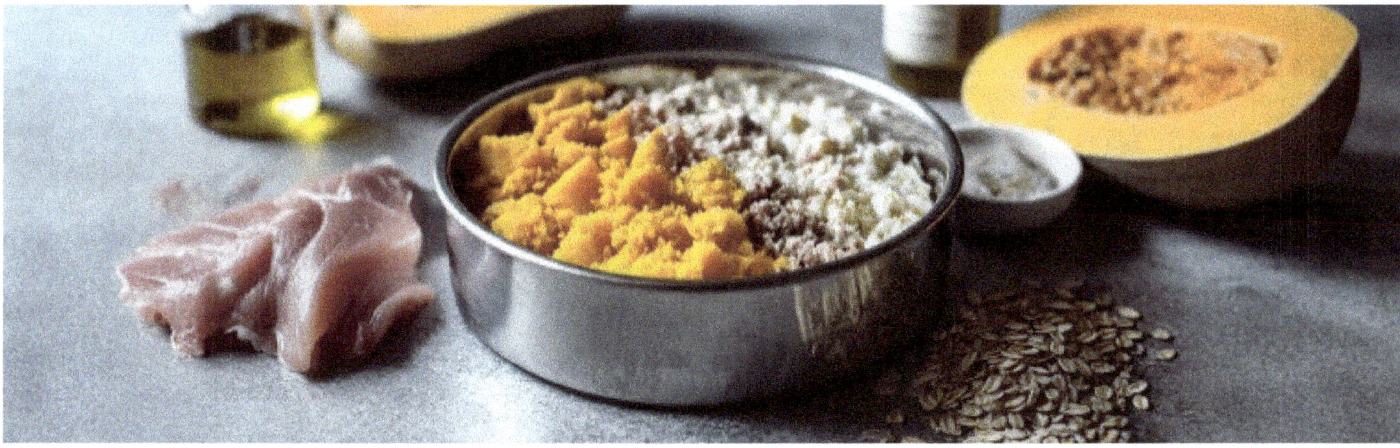

Ingredients:

- 1 lb. (450g) ground duck (skin removed to control excess fat)
- 1 cup (205g) cooked butternut squash (mashed)
- ½ cup (40g) cooked oats
- 1 tsp (4.5g) flaxseed oil
- 1 tsp fish oil (anchovy or salmon oil; provides EPA & DHA)

Instructions:

1. Cook ground duck thoroughly without using any oil.
2. Mash butternut squash and mix with cooked oats.
3. Stir in flaxseed oil and fish oil.
4. Cool before serving.

Ingredient Substitutions:

- Replace duck with chicken thighs (skinless, boneless).
- Use pumpkin or sweet potato instead of butternut squash.
- Substitute oats for quinoa or brown rice if desired.

Nutrition per 500g serving:

Final Weight	~500g
Calories	~620 kcal
Protein	~40g
Fat	~32g
Carbohydrates	~48g

7. Venison & Brown Rice Growth Formula

(Lean, hypoallergenic protein bowl rich in essential minerals and omega-3s to support growth and muscle development)

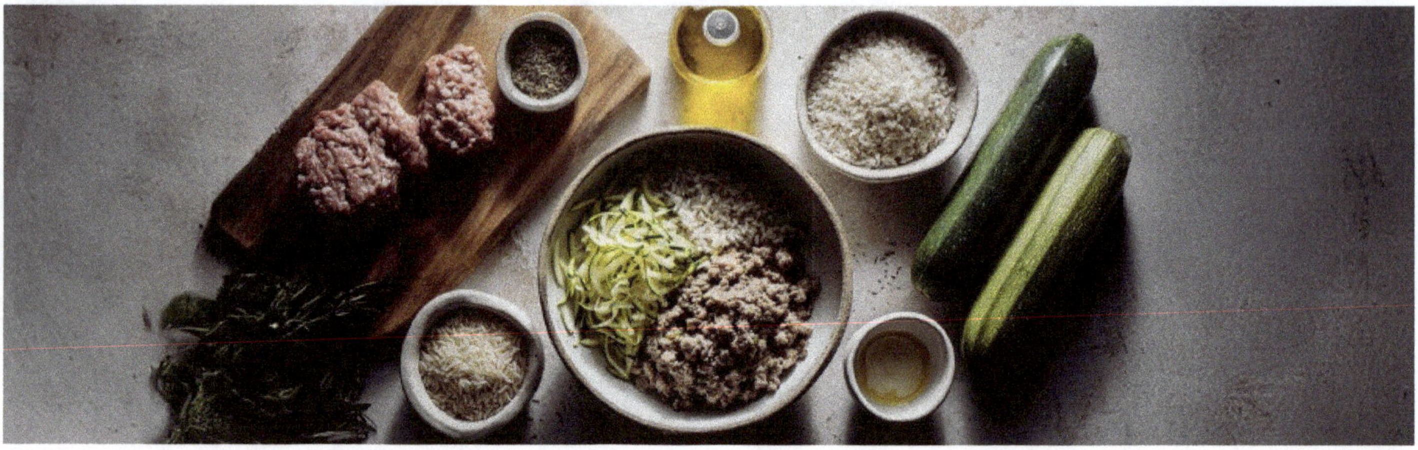

Ingredients:

- 1 lb. (450g) ground venison
- 1 cup (195g) cooked brown rice
- ½ cup (65g) shredded zucchini (lightly steamed)
- 1 tsp (4.5g) olive oil
- 1 tsp fish oil (anchovy/salmon oil; provides EPA & DHA)

Instructions:

1. Brown the venison in a pan without using any oil.
2. Mix in cooked brown rice and shredded zucchini.
3. Stir in olive oil and fish oil.
4. Let cool before serving.

Ingredient Substitutions:

- Swap brown rice for quinoa or barley.
- Replace venison with lean beef, turkey, or lamb (adjust fat content if needed).
- Substitute olive oil with avocado oil for variety.

Nutrition per 500g serving:

Final Weight	~500g
Calories	~580 kcal
Protein	~42g
Fat	~26g
Carbohydrates	~52g

8. Sardine & Sweet Potato Coat Booster

(Omega-3 powerhouse for brain development, skin, and coat health in growing puppies)

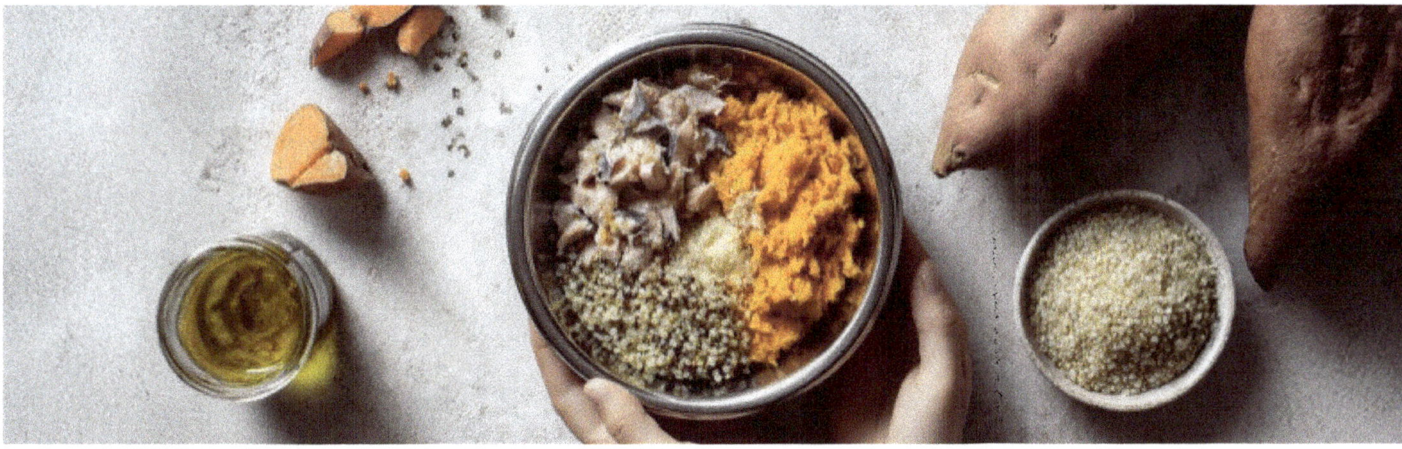

Ingredients:

- 1 can (3.75 oz/106g) sardines in water, no salt added, drained
- 1 cup (200g) cooked sweet potato (mashed)
- ½ cup (90g) cooked quinoa
- 1 tsp (4.5g) fish oil (for additional EPA/DHA)

Instructions:

1. Mash sardines and mix with mashed sweet potato.
2. Stir in cooked quinoa.
3. Add fish oil.
4. Allow to cool before serving.

Ingredient Substitutions:

- Swap quinoa for brown rice or barley.
- Replace sardines with cooked salmon, mackerel, or herring (ensure bones are removed and salt-free).

Nutrition per 500g serving:

Final Weight	~500g
Calories	~600 kcal
Protein	~44g
Fat	~28g
Carbohydrates	~48g

9. Rabbit & Carrot Growth Meal

(Lean, high-protein meal to promote muscle development and essential nutrient intake in growing puppies)

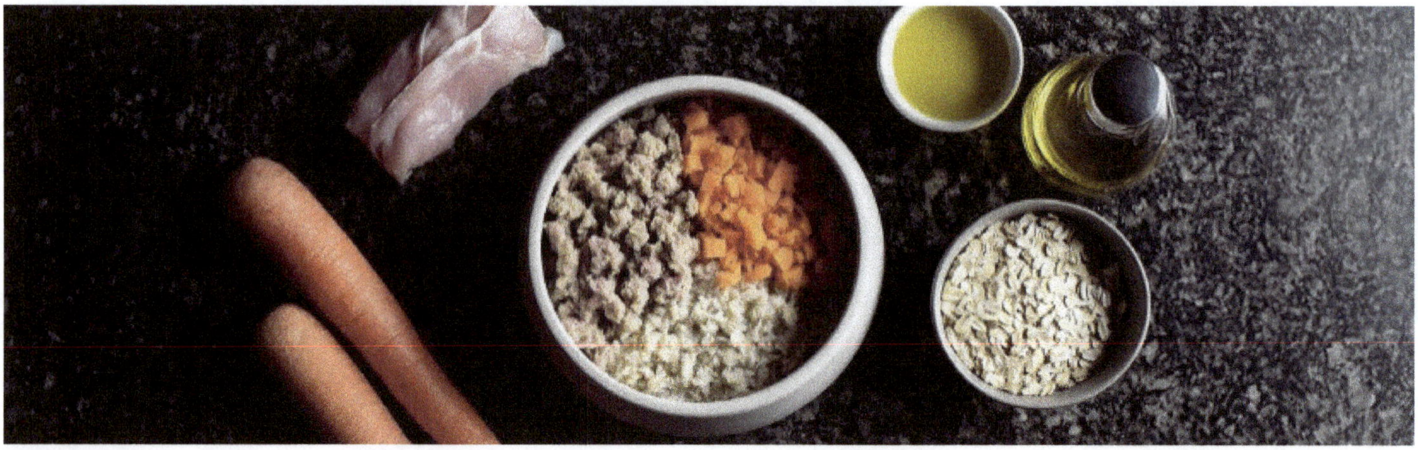

Ingredients:

- 1 lb. (450g) ground rabbit meat
- 1 cup (130g) cooked carrots (mashed)
- ½ cup (40g) cooked oatmeal
- 1 tsp (4.5g) coconut oil (or olive oil substitution)
- 1 tsp fish oil (anchovy/salmon oil; EPA & DHA source)

Instructions:

1. Brown the ground rabbit meat in a pan (without oil).
2. Mash cooked carrots and mix with cooked oatmeal.
3. Mix in coconut oil and fish oil.
4. Cool before serving.

Ingredient Substitutions:

- Replace rabbit meat with lean turkey or chicken breast (adjust fat content if needed).
- Use olive oil or flaxseed oil instead of coconut oil.
- Swap oatmeal for quinoa or brown rice.

Nutrition per 500g serving:

Final Weight	~500g
Calories	~560 kcal
Protein	~44g
Fat	~23g
Carbohydrates	~52g

10. High-Protein Plant-Based Puppy Meal

(Nutrient-dense, vegetarian bowl fortified for growth with essential amino acids, vitamins, and minerals)

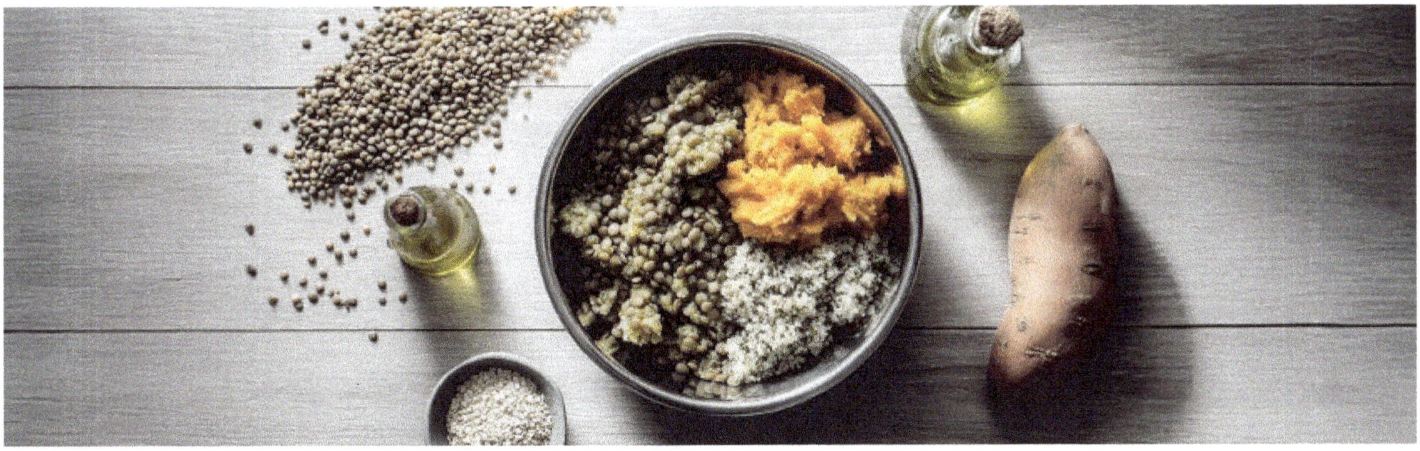

Ingredients:

- 1 cup (198g) cooked lentils
- 1 cup (200g) mashed sweet potato
- ½ cup (90g) cooked quinoa
- 1 tsp (4.5g) flaxseed oil
- 1 tsp algal oil (provides EPA & DHA)

Instructions:

1. Cook lentils thoroughly and mash in a bowl.
2. Mix mashed sweet potato and cooked quinoa with mashed lentils.
3. Stir in flaxseed oil and algal oil.
4. Let cool before serving.

Ingredient Substitutions:

- Swap quinoa for brown rice or millet.
- Replace lentils with chickpeas or black beans.
- Substitute flaxseed oil with avocado oil or hemp seed oil (still add algal oil for EPA/DHA).

Nutrition per 500g serving:

Final Weight	~500g
Calories	~580 kcal
Protein	~40g
Fat	~20g
Carbohydrates	~68g

11. Duck & Pumpkin Growth Delight for Puppies

(Rich in novel protein, omega-3s, gentle on digestive system)

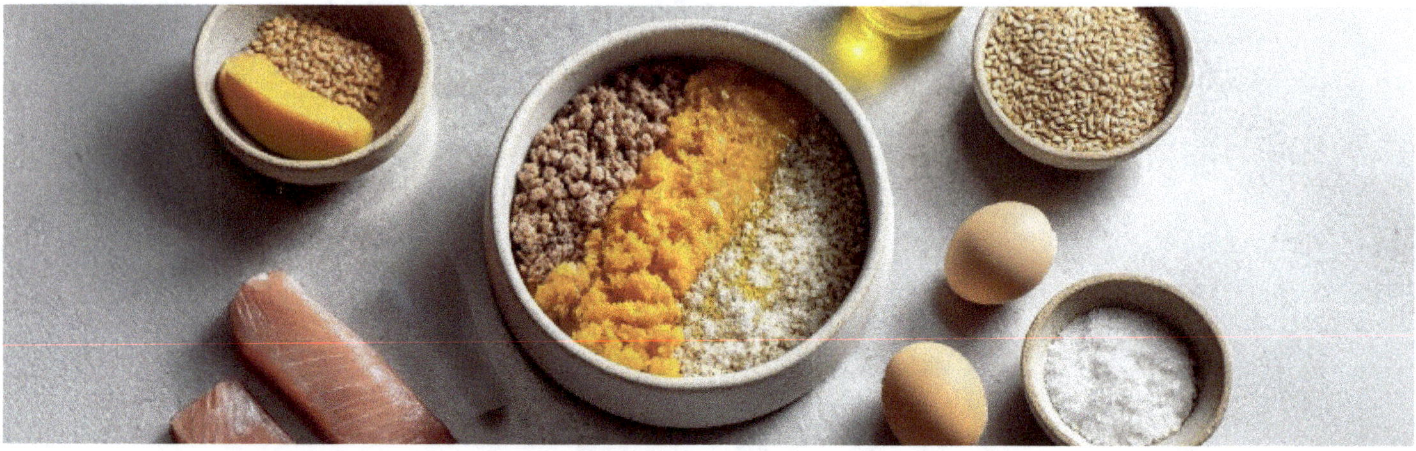

Ingredients:

- 1 lb. ground duck (skin removed)
- 1 cup cooked pumpkin (plain, mashed)
- ½ cup cooked quinoa
- 2 tsp fish oil (for DHA & EPA)
- 1 tsp ground eggshell powder OR 2 crushed calcium tablets (for bone development)
- ½ tsp iodized salt (iodine & sodium balance)

Instructions:

1. Cook ground duck thoroughly (no added oil).
2. Stir in cooked pumpkin and quinoa.
3. Mix in fish oil, calcium source, and iodized salt.
4. Let cool before serving.

Ingredient Substitutions:

- Replace pumpkin with sweet potato.
- Swap ground duck for ground turkey or rabbit.

Nutrition per 500g serving:

Final Weight	~500g
Calories	~620 kcal
Protein	~40g
Fat	~28g
Carbohydrates	~50g

12. Turkey & Cottage Cheese Growth Bowl for Puppies

(High-protein, calcium-rich, excellent for muscle & bone growth)

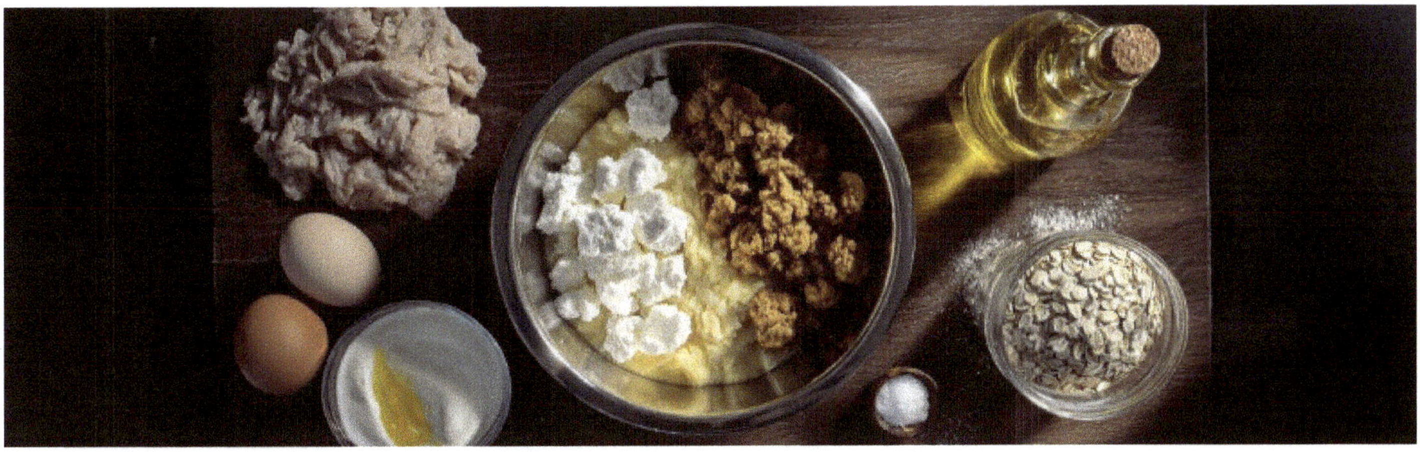

Ingredients:

- 1 lb. ground turkey (93% lean)
- ½ cup plain cottage cheese (high-calcium)
- ½ cup cooked oats
- 1 tsp fish oil (EPA/DHA)
- 1 tsp ground eggshell powder OR 2 crushed calcium tablets (for bone development)
- ½ tsp iodized salt

Instructions:

1. Cook turkey until browned.
2. Mix in cooked oats and cottage cheese.
3. Stir in fish oil, calcium, salt, and multivitamin/mineral.
4. Let cool before serving.

Ingredient Substitutions:

- Swap oats for brown rice.
- Replace turkey with chicken or lean beef.

Nutrition per 500g serving:

Final Weight	~500g
Calories	~630 kcal
Protein	~43g
Fat	~26g
Carbohydrates	~46g

Don't forget to get your free *Homemade Dog Treats Cookbook* to delight your dog with healthy, easy-to-make treats that boost nutrition, curb begging, and perfectly complement their new homemade meals.

SCAN THE QR CODE

High Calcium Recipes for Strong Bones

1. Beef & Bone Growth Booster (Higher Calcium Content)

(Beef-based, calcium-rich meal promoting strong bone development and muscle growth in puppies)

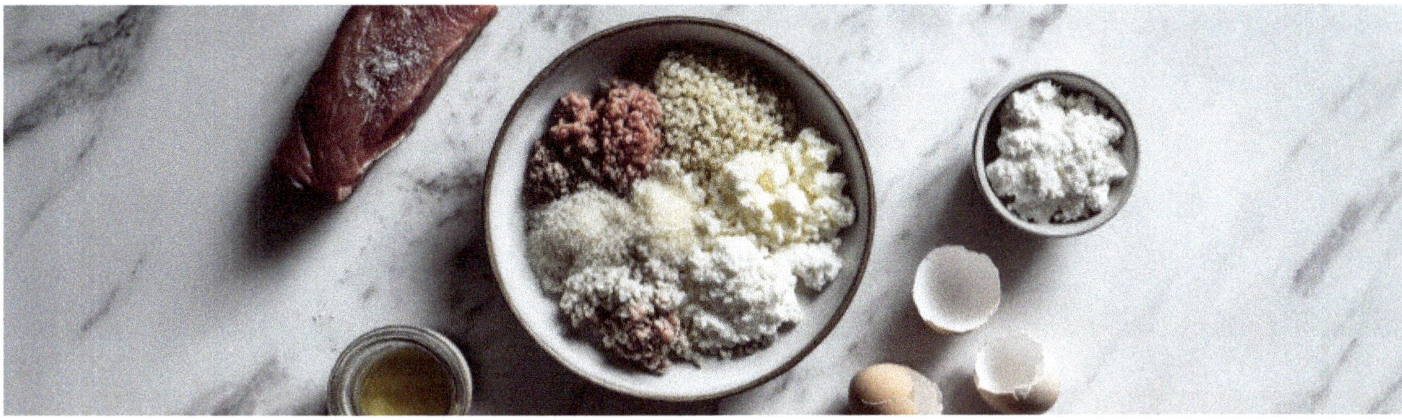

Ingredients:

- 1 lb. (450g) ground beef (80/20)
- ½ cup (113g) cottage cheese (high-calcium)
- ½ cup (90g) cooked quinoa
- 1 tsp ground eggshell powder (calcium source)
- 1 tsp fish oil (anchovy/salmon oil; source of EPA/DHA)

Optional:

- ¼ cup steamed green beans (chopped) for fiber boost

Instructions:

1. Cook ground beef thoroughly in a pan over medium heat (don't add any oil). Drain excess fat.
2. Cook quinoa as per package instructions.
3. Once beef and quinoa are cool, mix in cottage cheese, eggshell powder, and green beans if using.
4. Add fish oil and stir well before serving.

Ingredient Substitutions:

- Swap quinoa with cooked brown rice or barley.
- Replace cottage cheese with plain Greek yogurt (adjust calcium levels if necessary).
- Use bone meal powder instead of eggshell powder for an alternative calcium source.

Nutrition per 500g serving:

Final Weight	~500g
Calories	~975 kcal/500g (~195 kcal/100g)
Protein	~22g/100g
Fat	~13g/100g
Carbohydrates	~7g/100g

2. Chicken & Yogurt Puppy Meal (Higher Calcium Content)

(Chicken-based, calcium-rich meal supporting lean muscle development and healthy bones in growing puppies)

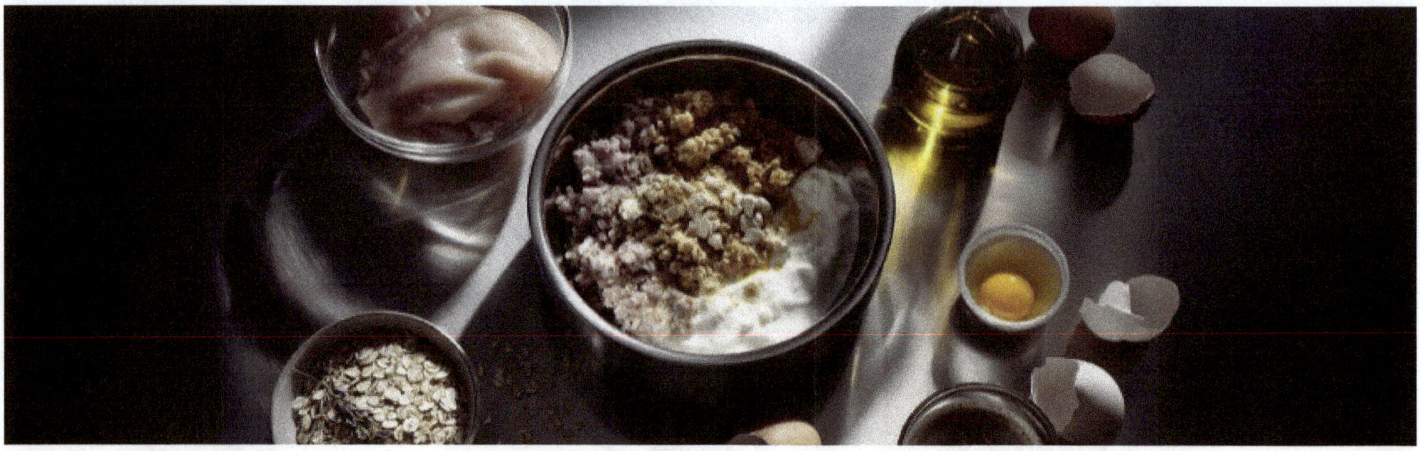

Ingredients:

- 1 lb. (450g) boneless, skinless chicken breast (option: replace ¼ lb. with chicken thigh for extra fat)
- ½ cup (113g) plain Greek yogurt (calcium-rich)
- ½ cup (40g) cooked oats
- 1 tsp ground eggshell powder (calcium source)
- 1 tsp flaxseed oil

Optional:

- ¼ cup steamed green beans or carrots (finely chopped) for added fiber

Instructions:

1. Boil chicken breast (and optional thigh) until fully cooked. Shred in a bowl.
2. Cook oats as per package instructions.
3. Let chicken and oats cool, then mix with Greek yogurt, eggshell powder, and green beans/ carrots if using.
4. Stir in flaxseed oil before serving.

Ingredient Substitutions:

- Swap oats with cooked brown rice or quinoa.
- Replace Greek yogurt with low-fat cottage cheese (adjust calcium if necessary).
- Use bone meal powder instead of eggshell powder (adjust quantity accordingly).

Nutrition per 500g serving:

Final Weight	~500g
Calories	~850 kcal
Protein	~43g
Fat	~15g
Carbohydrates	~50g

3. Goat & Millet Puppy Growth Boost

(Goat-based, balanced meal rich in protein, calcium, and nutrients for strong puppy development)

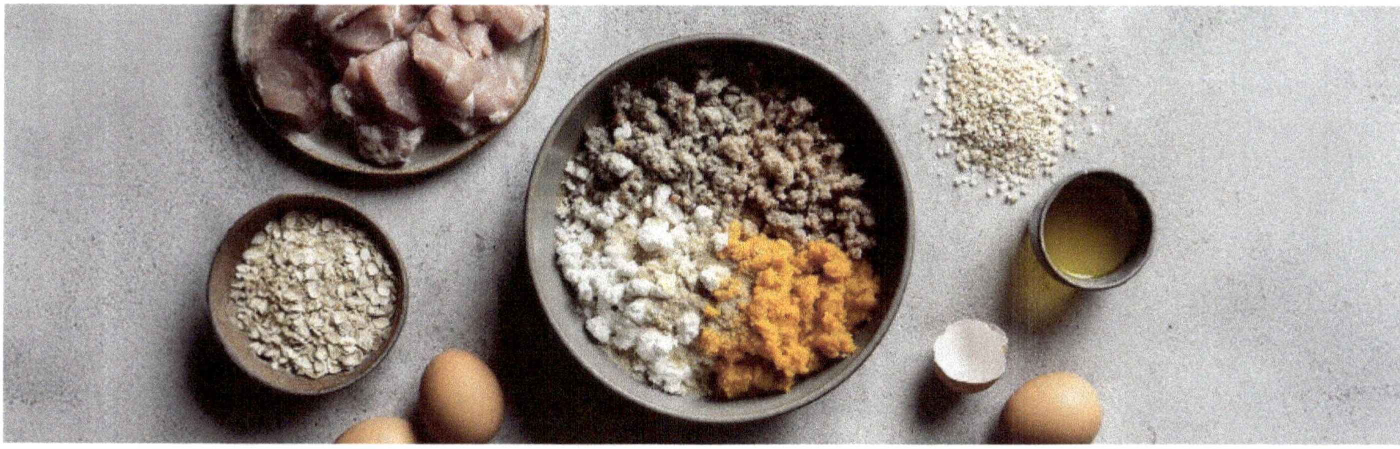

Ingredients:

- 1 lb. (450g) ground goat
- ½ cup (85g) millet
- ½ cup (125g) mashed butternut squash
- 1 tsp ground eggshell powder (calcium source for bone development)
- ½ tsp salmon oil (omega-3s and vitamin D for brain and skeletal growth)

Optional:

- ¼ cup steamed kale (chopped, for added vitamins and fiber)

Instructions:

1. In a non-stick pan, cook ground goat over medium heat until fully browned (no oil needed). Drain any excess fat.
2. Cook millet in a 1:2 water ratio (½ cup millet to 1 cup water) until soft, about 15 minutes.
3. Steam and mash butternut squash until smooth.
4. Let all cooked ingredients cool, then mix in ground eggshell powder and steamed kale (if using).
5. Stir in salmon oil evenly and serve appropriate portions based on puppy size/age.

Ingredient Substitutions:

- Replace goat with ground lamb or rabbit.
- Swap millet with buckwheat or amaranth.
- Use pumpkin puree instead of butternut squash.

Nutrition per 500g serving:

Final Weight	~500g
Calories	~925 kcal
Protein	~45g
Fat	~20g
Carbohydrates	~50g

4. Lamb & Kefir Bone Booster

(Mineral-rich lamb-based meal supporting strong bones, joint health, and digestive health in growing puppies)

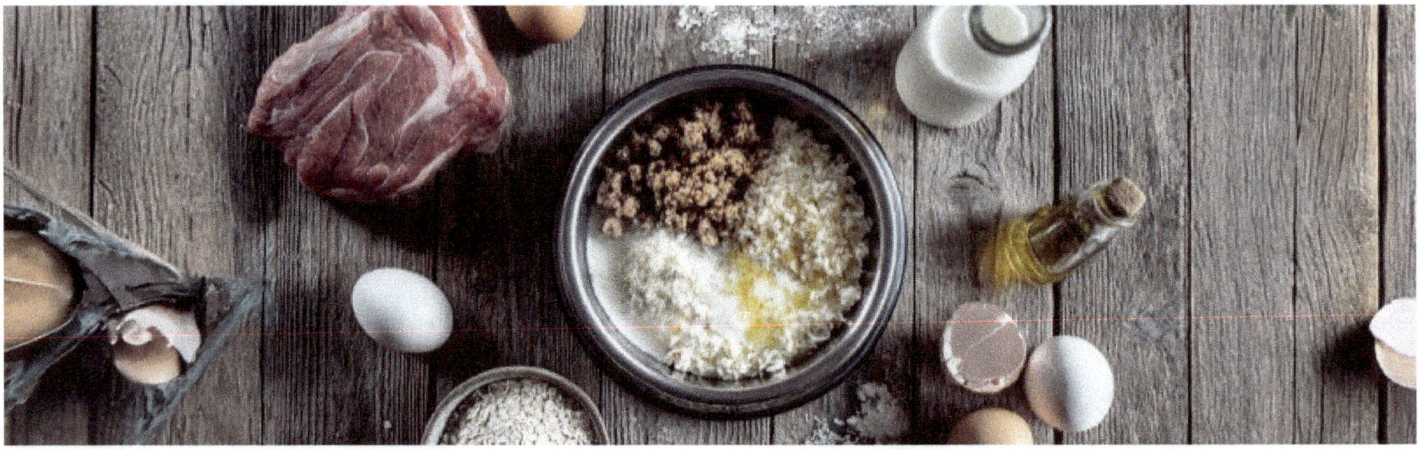

Ingredients:

- 1 lb. (450g) ground lamb (rich in iron & minerals)
- ½ cup (120g) plain kefir (high in calcium & probiotics)
- ½ cup (90g) cooked brown rice
- 1 tsp ground eggshell powder (calcium source)
- 1 tsp fish oil (anchovy/salmon oil; provides EPA/DHA & Vitamin D)

Optional:

- ¼ cup steamed carrots or spinach (chopped) for extra fiber

Instructions:

1. Cook ground lamb over medium heat until fully done (no oil needed). Drain excess fat.
2. Cook brown rice as per package instructions.
3. When lamb and rice are cooled, add to a bowl and mix.
4. Mix in kefir, ground eggshell powder, and optional veggies.
5. Stir in fish oil and serve.

Ingredient Substitutions:

- Replace kefir with plain yogurt.
- Swap brown rice with quinoa or barley.
- Use bone meal powder instead of eggshell powder (adjust quantity accordingly).

Nutrition per 500g serving:

Final Weight	~500g
Calories	~1000 kcal
Protein	~42g
Fat	~38g
Carbohydrates	~45g

5. Fish & Pumpkin Calcium Puppy Meal

(Balanced, omega-rich fish-based meal to support bone development, skin, and coat health in growing puppies)

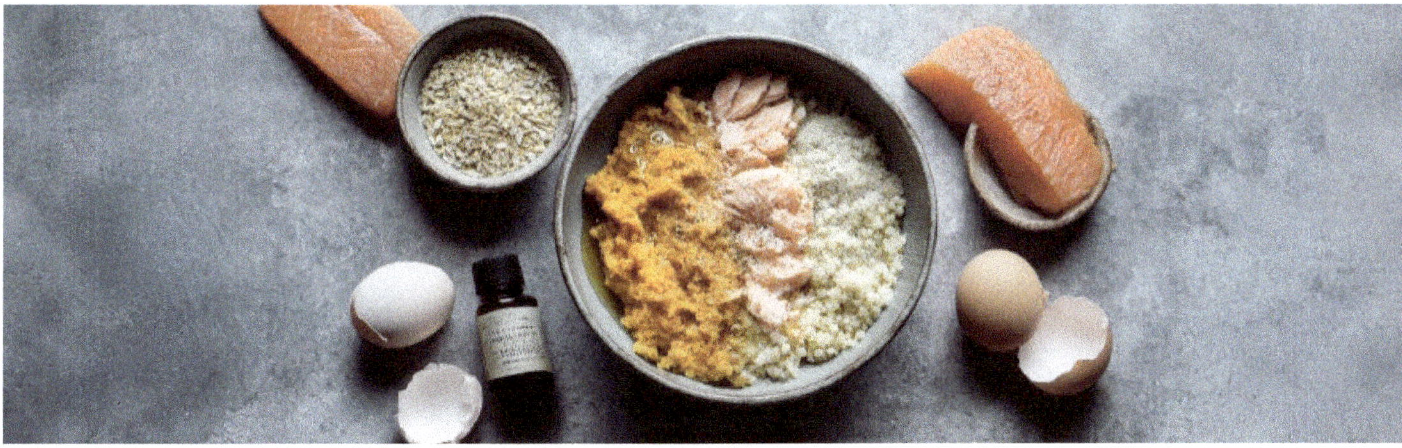

Ingredients:

- 1 lb. (450g) cooked boneless salmon (baked or steamed)
- ½ cup (120g) pumpkin puree
- ½ cup (90g) cooked millet
- 1 tsp ground eggshell powder (calcium source)
- 1 tsp fish oil (anchovy/salmon oil; provides EPA/DHA & Vitamin D)

Optional:

- ¼ cup steamed spinach or green beans (chopped) for added fiber

Instructions:

1. Bake or steam salmon until fully cooked, then flake it into small pieces.
2. Cook millet as per instructions.
3. Let all ingredients cool, then add to a bowl and mix.
4. Mix in pumpkin puree, eggshell powder, and optional veggies.
5. Stir in fish oil and serve.

Ingredient Substitutions:

- Replace pumpkin puree with mashed carrots.
- Swap millet with quinoa or brown rice.
- Use bone meal powder instead of eggshell powder (adjust quantity accordingly).

Nutrition per 500g serving:

Final Weight	~500g
Calories	~950 kcal
Protein	~45g
Fat	~22g
Carbohydrates	~45g

6. Egg & Spinach Calcium Booster

(Vegetarian, nutrient-dense meal promoting strong bones, iron support, and brain health in growing puppies)

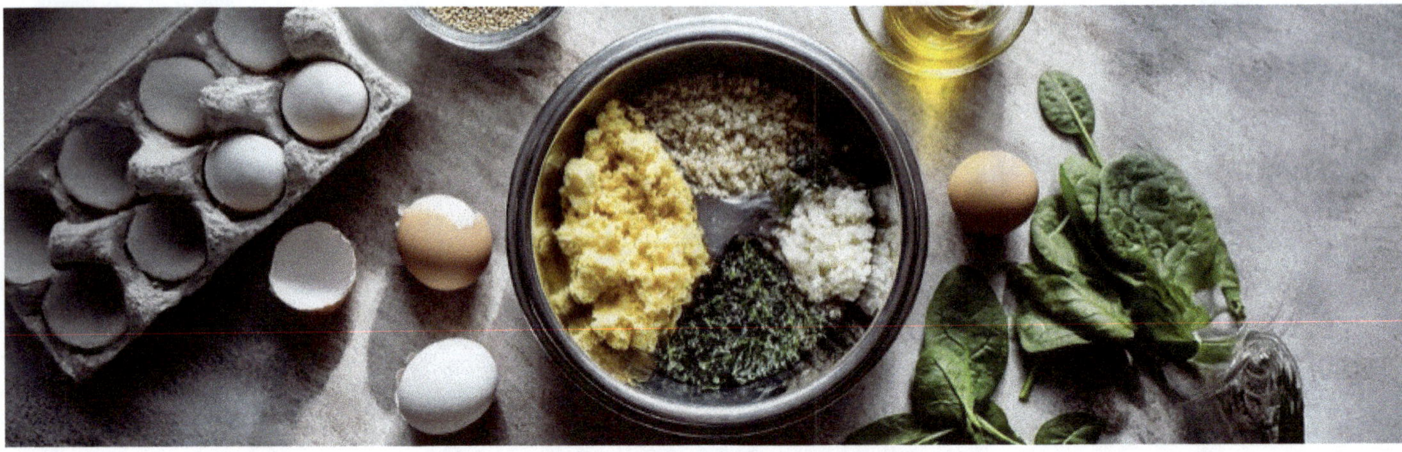

Ingredients:

- 3 large eggs (scrambled)
- ½ cup (113g) plain cottage cheese (high-calcium)
- ½ cup (90g) cooked quinoa
- ½ cup (90g) steamed spinach (finely chopped)
- 1 tsp ground eggshell powder (calcium source)
- 1 tsp algal oil (plant-based EPA/DHA source) or 1 tsp fish oil (if not strictly vegetarian)

Optional:

- ¼ cup steamed carrots or zucchini (chopped) for added fiber

Instructions:

1. Scramble the eggs over medium heat without any oil.
2. Steam spinach until soft and finely chop.
3. Cook quinoa as per package instructions.
4. Allow ingredients to cool, then mix eggs, spinach, quinoa, cottage cheese, eggshell powder, and optional veggies.
5. Stir in algal oil (or fish oil) and serve.

Ingredient Substitutions:

- Replace spinach with kale or bok choy.
- Swap quinoa with millet or brown rice.
- Use bone meal powder instead of eggshell powder (adjust quantity accordingly)

Nutrition per 500g serving:

Final Weight	~500g
Calories	~850 kcal
Protein	~38g
Fat	~25g
Carbohydrates	~35g

7. Sardine & Brown Rice Puppy Power Meal

(Omega-3 and calcium-rich fish-based meal supporting strong bones, brain development, and joint health in growing puppies)

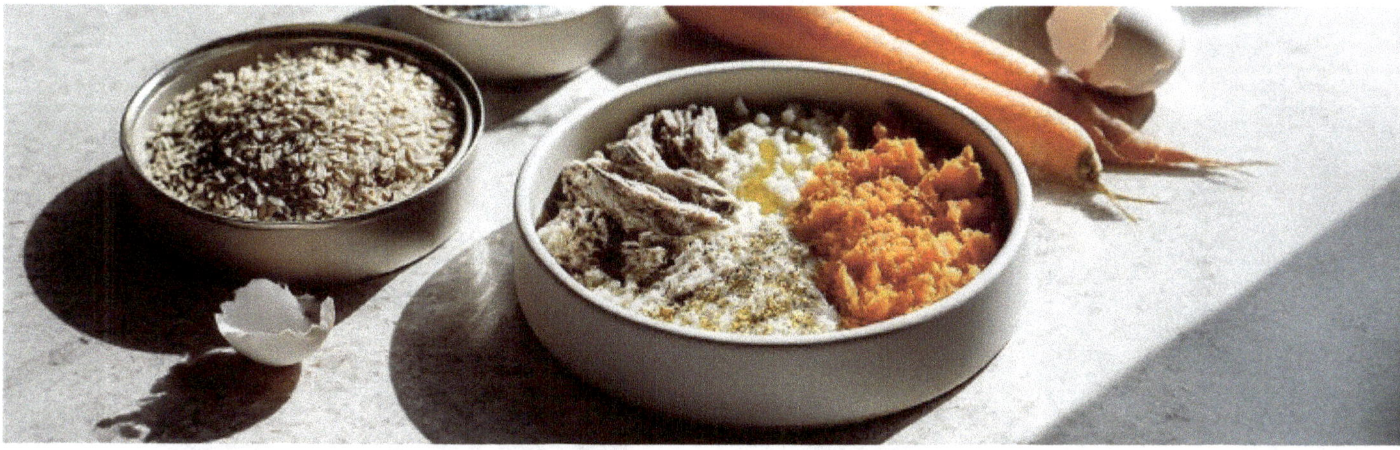

Ingredients:

- 1 can (3.75 oz/106g) sardines in water (with soft bones)
- ½ cup (90g) cooked brown rice
- ½ cup (90g) cooked carrots (mashed)
- 1 tsp ground eggshell powder (calcium source)
- 1 tsp fish oil (anchovy/salmon oil; for EPA/DHA & Vitamin D)

Optional:

- ¼ cup steamed spinach or green beans (chopped) for added fiber

Instructions:

1. Mash the sardines, including soft bones.
2. Cook brown rice and carrots until soft.
3. Let all ingredients cool, then add to a bowl and mix.
4. Add eggshell powder and optional veggies.
5. Stir in fish oil and serve.

Ingredient Substitutions:

- Swap brown rice with quinoa or millet.
- Replace sardines with cooked salmon or mackerel (ensure boneless if bones are too hard).
- Use bone meal powder instead of eggshell powder (adjust amount).

Nutrition per 500g serving:

Final Weight	~500g
Calories	~850 kcal
Protein	~42g
Fat	~25g
Carbohydrates	~35g

Soft-textured foods for Easy digestion

1. Beef & Pumpkin Puppy Mash (Easy Digestion)

(Soft-textured, gut-friendly, protein-packed meal with balanced minerals and essential vitamins for growing puppies)

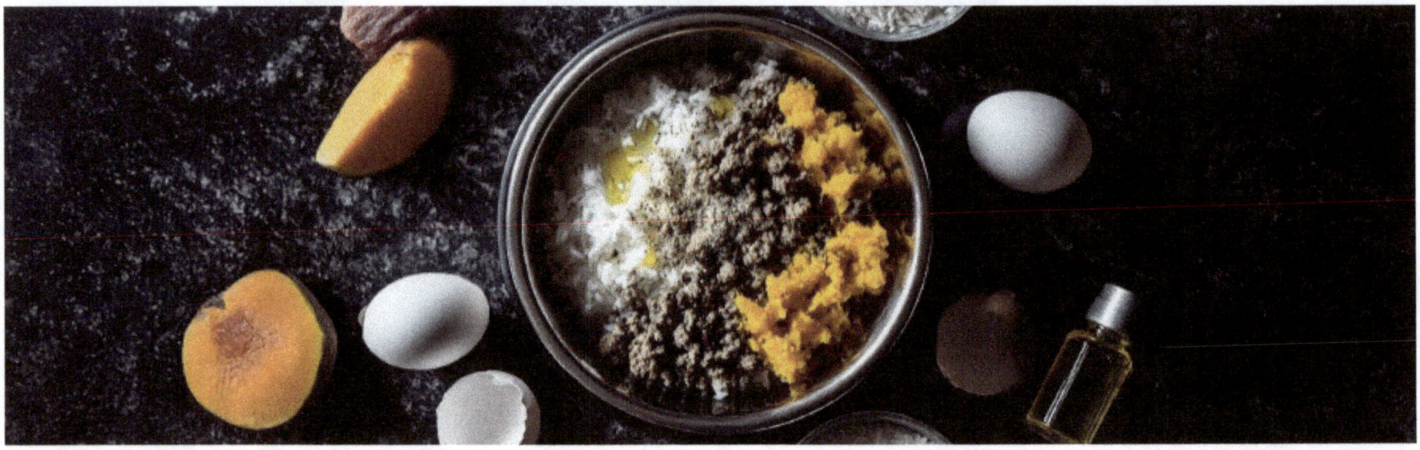

Ingredients:

- 1 lb. (450g) lean ground beef (90% lean)
- 1 cup (245g) cooked pumpkin (pureed)
- ½ cup (85g) cooked white rice (soft)
- 1 tsp fish oil (anchovy/salmon oil; Omega-3 source)
- 1 tsp ground eggshell powder (calcium source)

Optional:

- 1 tsp coconut oil (to slightly boost fat content)

Instructions:

1. In a pan, cook ground beef over medium heat until fully browned (no oil added).
2. Add cooked pumpkin and white rice. Mix gently.
3. Let cool slightly before mixing in fish oil, eggshell powder, and optional coconut oil.
4. Mash well for a soft texture. Serve at room temperature.

Ingredient Substitutions:

- Use lean turkey instead of beef for a lower-fat version.
- Substitute sweet potato for pumpkin for extra fiber.

Nutrition per 500g serving:

Final Weight	~500g
Calories	~750 kcal
Protein	~42g
Fat	~18g
Carbohydrates	~38g

2. Turkey & Carrot Stew (Easy Digestion)

(Soft, protein-packed stew loaded with antioxidants and balanced essential nutrients for growing puppies)

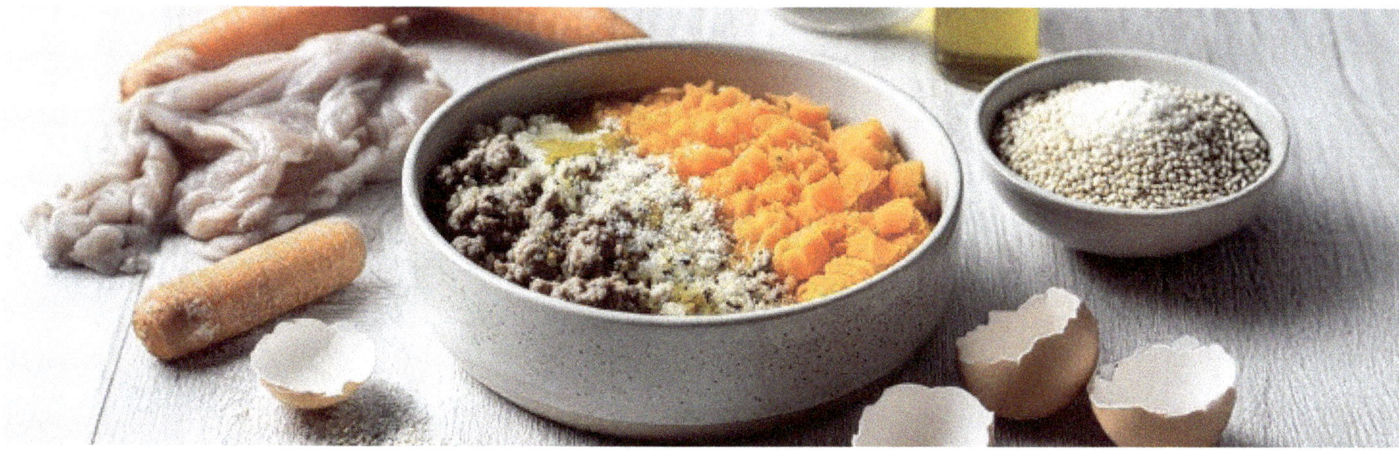

Ingredients:

- 1 lb. (450g) lean ground turkey
- ½ cup (120g) mashed carrots (steamed or boiled)
- ½ cup (90g) cooked quinoa
- 1 cup (240ml) low-sodium turkey broth
- 1 tsp ground eggshell powder (calcium source)
- 1 tsp fish oil (anchovy/salmon oil; Omega-3 EPA/DHA + Vitamin D)

Optional:

- 1 tsp coconut oil (to increase fat content further)
- ¼ cup steamed green beans or spinach (chopped) for fiber boost

Instructions:

1. Cook ground turkey in a pan over medium heat until fully done (no oil needed).
2. In another pot, cook quinoa with turkey broth until soft.
3. Mash the cooked carrots for a soft texture.
4. Mix turkey, quinoa, and mashed carrots together in a bowl.
5. Let cool slightly, then stir in eggshell powder, fish oil, and optional coconut oil and veggies.
6. Serve slightly warm.

Ingredient Substitutions:

- Replace quinoa with cooked brown rice.
- Swap olive oil with coconut oil (still ensure fish oil for EPA/DHA).

Nutrition per 500g serving:

Final Weight	~500g
Calories	~725 kcal
Protein	~40g
Fat	~18g
Carbohydrates	~35g

3. Chicken & Oatmeal Puppy Porridge (Easy Digestion)

(Gentle, protein-rich porridge perfect for sensitive stomachs, balanced with essential vitamins, minerals, and healthy fats for growth)

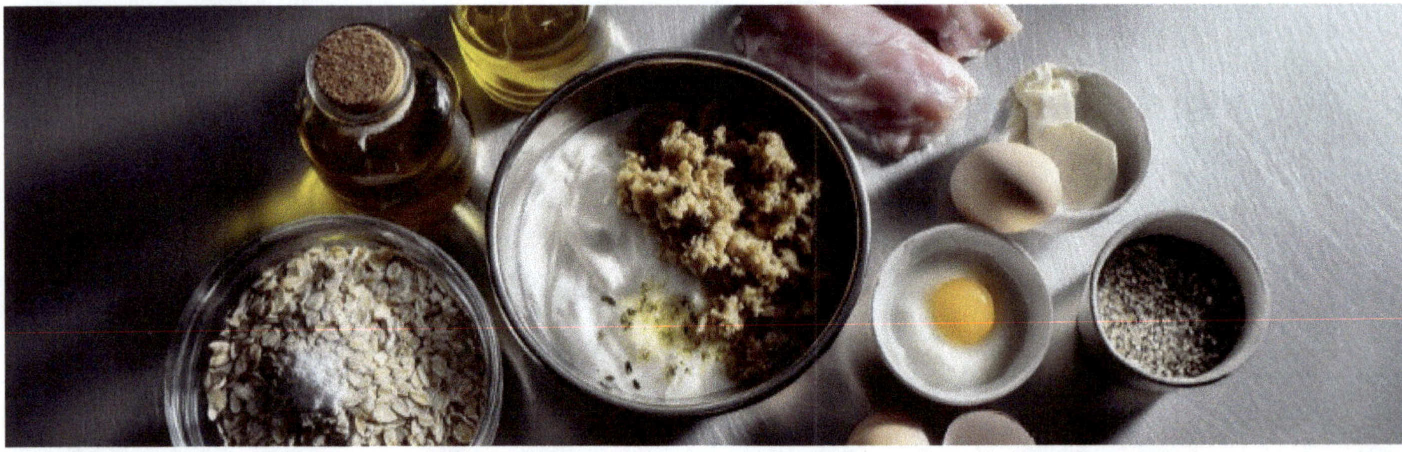

Ingredients:

- 1 lb. (450g) ground chicken (or minced; optionally swap in chicken thigh for more fat)
- ½ cup (45g) rolled oats (soft-cooked)
- 1 cup (240ml) low-sodium chicken broth
- 1 tbsp (20g) plain Greek yogurt
- 1 tsp ground eggshell powder (calcium source)
- 1 tsp fish oil (anchovy/salmon oil; provides EPA/DHA Omega-3s)

Optional:

- 1 tsp coconut oil (for fat boost)
- ¼ cup steamed carrots or zucchini (chopped) for added fiber

Instructions:

1. In a pan, cook ground chicken over medium heat until fully done (no oil needed).
2. In another pot, cook oats in chicken broth until soft and porridge-like.
3. Mix cooked chicken and oats together.
4. Let cool slightly, then stir in Greek yogurt, eggshell powder, fish oil, and optional coconut oil and veggies.
5. Serve warm for a soft, mushy texture.

Ingredient Substitutions:

- Replace chicken with turkey for variety.
- Swap Greek yogurt with goat's milk yogurt for better digestibility.

Nutrition per 500g serving:

Final Weight	~500g
Calories	~700 kcal
Protein	~38g
Fat	~18g
Carbohydrates	~35g

4. Lamb & Black Bean Puppy Growth Mash

(Lamb-based, nutrient-dense meal for picky eaters, rich in protein, vitamins, and minerals for growth)

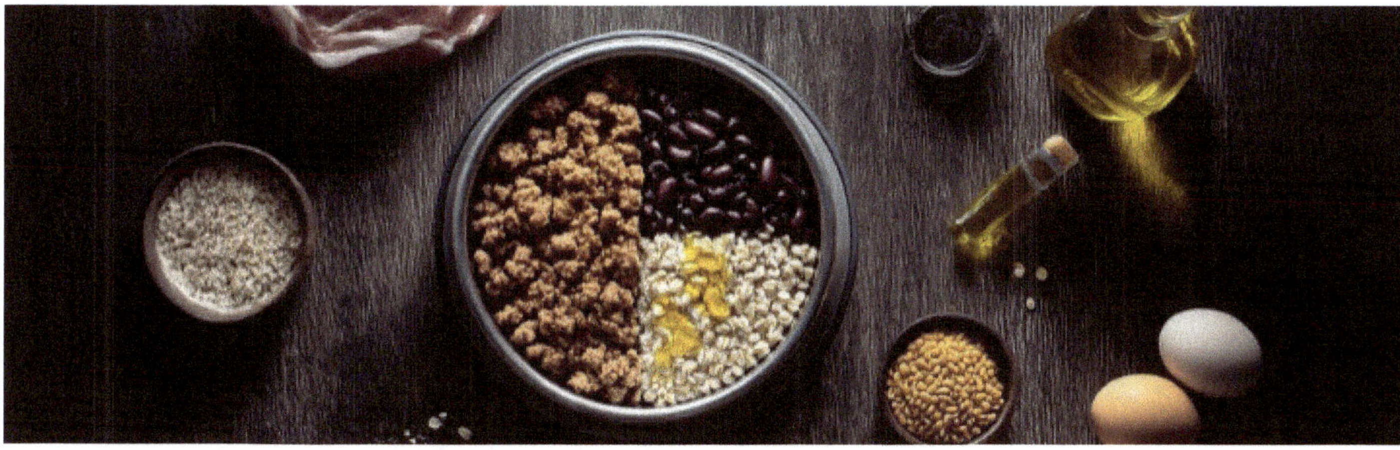

Ingredients:

- 1 lb. (450g) ground lamb
- ½ cup (100g) cooked black beans
- ½ cup (100g) cooked barley
- 1 tsp sunflower oil
- 1 tsp fish oil
- 1 tsp ground eggshell powder

Optional:

- 1 tsp coconut oil (extra fat for energy)
- ¼ cup steamed Swiss chard (chopped, for vitamins and fiber)

Instructions:

1. Cook ground lamb in a pan over medium heat until browned (no oil needed), drain excess fat.
2. Cook black beans (soak overnight, boil until soft) and mash; cook barley (1:2 water ratio) until tender.
3. Once cooled, mix lamb, black beans, and barley together.
4. Stir in sunflower oil, fish oil, eggshell powder, and optional coconut oil/Swiss chard.
5. Serve warm, portioned for puppy size.

Ingredient Substitutions:

- Replace black beans with pinto beans or chickpeas.
- Swap barley with millet or couscous.
- Use lean beef or ground turkey instead of lamb.

Nutrition per 500g serving:

Final Weight	~500g
Calories	~1300 kcal
Protein	~80g
Fat	~20g
Carbohydrates	~45g

5. Salmon & Rice Puppy Pudding

(A soft, omega-3-rich pudding designed for optimal brain development and balanced growth in puppies)

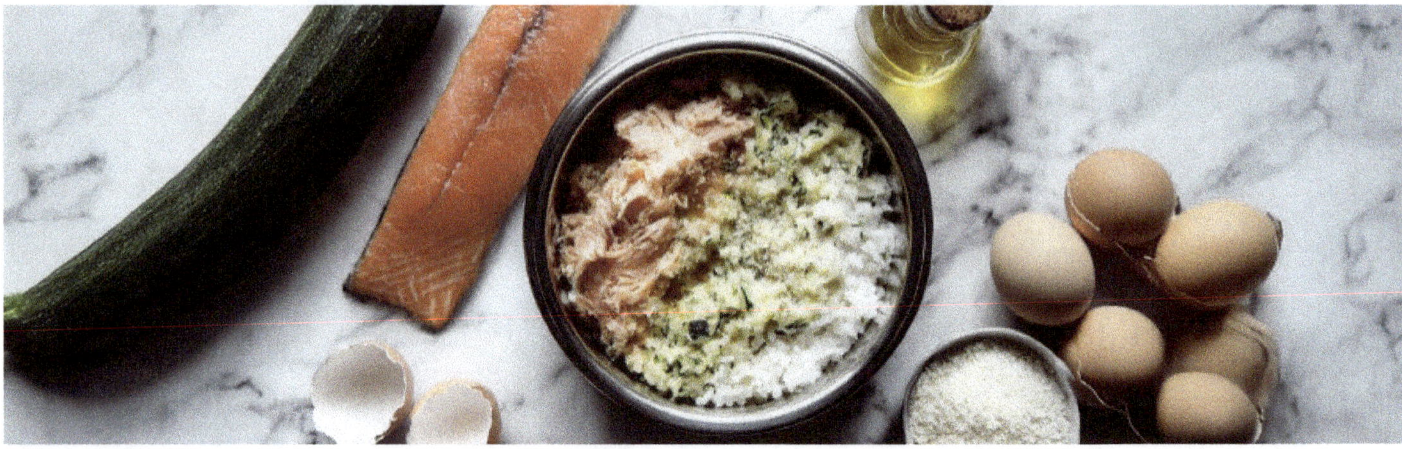

Ingredients:

- 1 cup (170g) cooked boneless salmon (flaked)
- ½ cup (85g) cooked white rice
- ½ cup (90g) steamed zucchini (mashed)
- 1 tsp fish oil (anchovy/salmon oil; rich in EPA/DHA + Vitamin D)
- 1 tsp ground eggshell powder (calcium source)

Optional:

- 1 tsp coconut oil (to increase fat content)
- ¼ cup steamed carrots or green beans (chopped) for extra fiber

Instructions:

1. Cook salmon and flake it into small pieces.
2. Steam zucchini and mash well.
3. Mix salmon, rice, and zucchini together in a bowl.
4. Stir in fish oil, eggshell powder, and optional coconut oil and veggies.
5. Serve warm for a soft pudding-like texture.

Ingredient Substitutions:

- Replace salmon with cooked tilapia or cod (note: fat and Omega-3 content will drop, so adjust fish oil accordingly).
- Swap zucchini with cooked carrots for extra Vitamin A.

Nutrition per 500g serving:

Final Weight	~500g
Calories	~750 kcal
Protein	~40g
Fat	~18g
Carbohydrates	~35g

6. Whitefish & Sweet Potato Brain Booster for Puppies

(Low-fat, omega-3 enriched, perfect for coat and cognitive development)

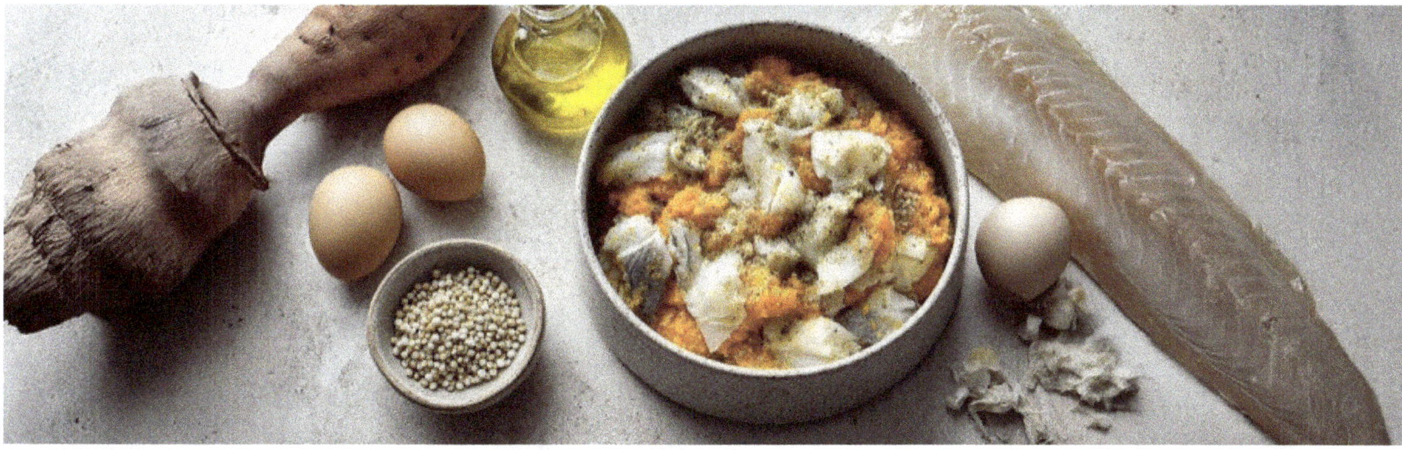

Ingredients:

- 1 lb. boneless whitefish (cod or tilapia, steamed)
- 1 cup cooked sweet potato (mashed)
- ½ cup cooked millet
- 2 tsp fish oil (extra DHA & EPA)
- 1 tsp ground eggshell powder OR 2 crushed calcium tablets

Instructions:

1. Steam fish until fully cooked, flake into small pieces.
2. Mix with mashed sweet potato and cooked millet.
3. Stir in fish oil and calcium source.
4. Let cool before serving.

Ingredient Substitutions:

- Swap sweet potato for pumpkin.
- Replace millet with quinoa.

Nutrition per 500g serving:

Final Weight	~500g
Calories	~580 kcal
Protein	~40g
Fat	~22g
Carbohydrates	~50g

Adult Dog Recipes

Everyday Energy Meals

These everyday meals for your big furry friend are packed with nutrients that promote healthy skin and fur, boost energy levels, and support overall well-being. These recipes also include balanced portions to maintain healthy weight.

1. Beef & Sweet Potato Power Bowl

(High-energy, iron-rich, omega-3-packed bowl designed for adult maintenance with balanced vitamins and minerals)

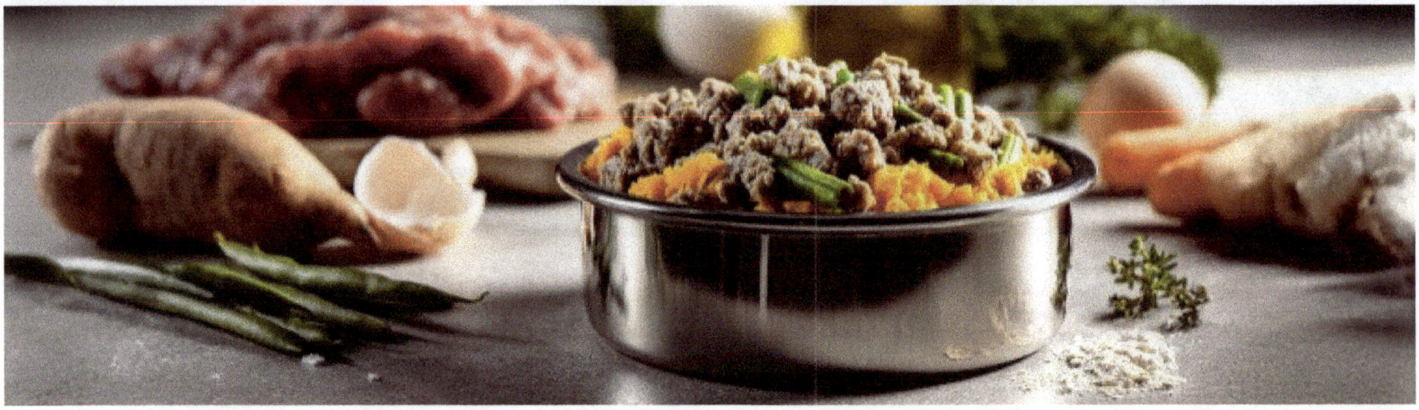

Ingredients:

- 1 lb. (450g) lean ground beef (90% lean)
- 1 cup (200g) cooked sweet potato (mashed)
- ½ cup (75g) steamed green beans (chopped)
- 1 tsp fish oil (anchovy/salmon oil; for Omega-3 & Vitamin D)
- ½ tsp ground eggshell powder (or 500 mg calcium carbonate powder; for calcium)

Ingredient Substitutions:

- Substitute lean turkey for beef if desired.
- Replace sweet potato with pumpkin puree.
- Use chopped spinach instead of green beans for more iron.

Instructions:

1. Cook the ground beef over medium heat until fully browned (without using any oil). Drain excess fat.
2. Steam or bake the sweet potato until soft, then mash in a bowl.
3. Lightly steam green beans and chop into bite-sized pieces.
4. Combine beef, sweet potato, green beans, fish oil, and eggshell powder.
5. Allow to cool before serving.

Nutrition per 500g serving:

Final Weight	~500g
Calories	~925 kcal
Protein	~45g
Fat	~20g
Carbohydrates	~60g

2. Bison & Barley Energy Bowl

(High-energy, iron-rich, omega-3-packed bowl designed for adult maintenance with balanced vitamins and minerals)

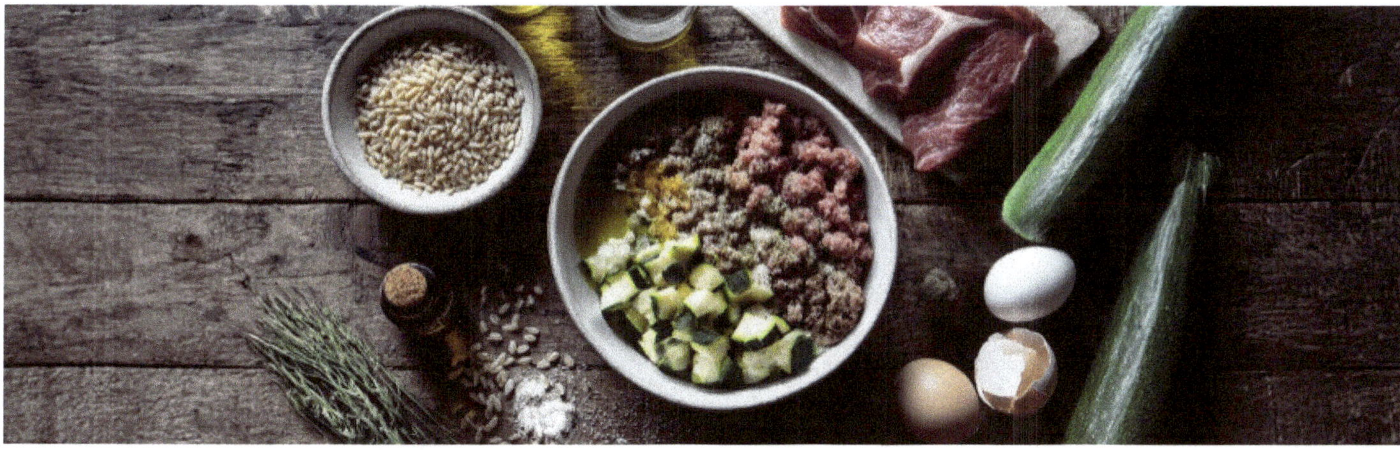

Ingredients:

- 1 lb. (450g) ground bison
- 1 cup (200g) cooked barley
- ½ cup (75g) steamed zucchin
- 1 tsp fish oil
- ½ tsp ground eggshell powder

Optional

- ¼ cup steamed spinach, green beans, or pumpkin puree for extra fiber

Instructions:

1. Brown ground bison in pan.
2. Cook barley in a 1:2 water ratio.
3. Lightly steam zucchini and chop into bite-sized pieces.
4. Combine and allow to cool before serving.

Ingredient Substitutions:

- Substitute bison with ground elk or venison for variety.
- Replace barley with millet or couscous.
- Use steamed asparagus or Swiss chard instead of zucchini for different nutrients.

Nutrition per 500g serving:

Final Weight	~500g
Calories	~1200 kcal
Protein	~90g
Fat	~20g
Carbohydrates	~55g

3. Turkey & Pumpkin Power Mix

(High-fiber, protein-packed mix that supports digestive health, balanced energy, and complete nutrition for adult dogs)

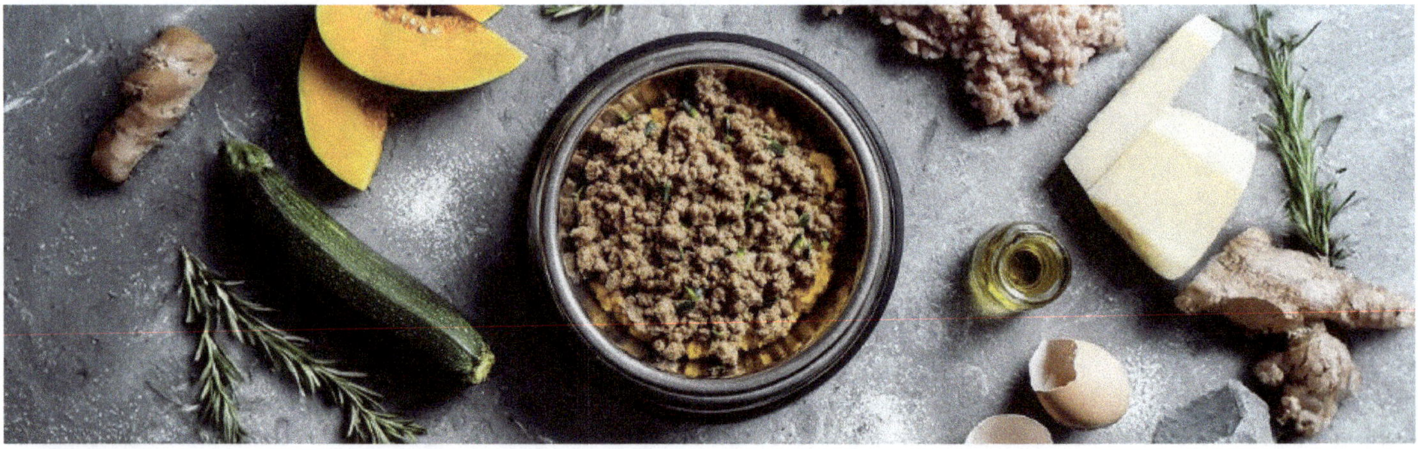

Ingredients:

- 1 lb. (450g) lean ground turkey (93%)
- 1 cup (245g) cooked pumpkin (plain, unsweetened)
- ½ cup (90g) steamed zucchini (chopped)
- 1 tsp fish oil (anchovy/salmon oil; for Omega-3 EPA/DHA + Vitamin D)
- ½ tsp ground eggshell powder (or 500 mg calcium carbonate powder)

Optional

- 1 tsp flaxseed oil (for Omega-6 & ALA balance)
- ¼ cup steamed spinach or green beans (chopped) for extra fiber & iron

Instructions:

1. Cook the ground turkey over medium heat until fully browned (don't add any oil). Drain excess fat.
2. Steam or cook pumpkin until soft and mash.
3. Lightly steam zucchini and chop into small pieces.
4. Mix turkey, pumpkin, zucchini, eggshell powder, fish oil, and optional flaxseed oil & veggies.
5. Allow to cool before serving.

Ingredient Substitutions:

- Use lean chicken instead of turkey.
- Swap pumpkin for butternut squash for flavor variety.
- Add spinach instead of zucchini for extra iron.

Nutrition per 500g serving:

Final Weight	~500g
Calories	~800 kcal
Protein	~42g
Fat	~18g
Carbohydrates	~30g

4. Lamb & Brown Rice Strength Meal

(Iron-rich, fatty acid-packed strength meal designed for active adult dogs, supporting muscle, skin, and coat health)

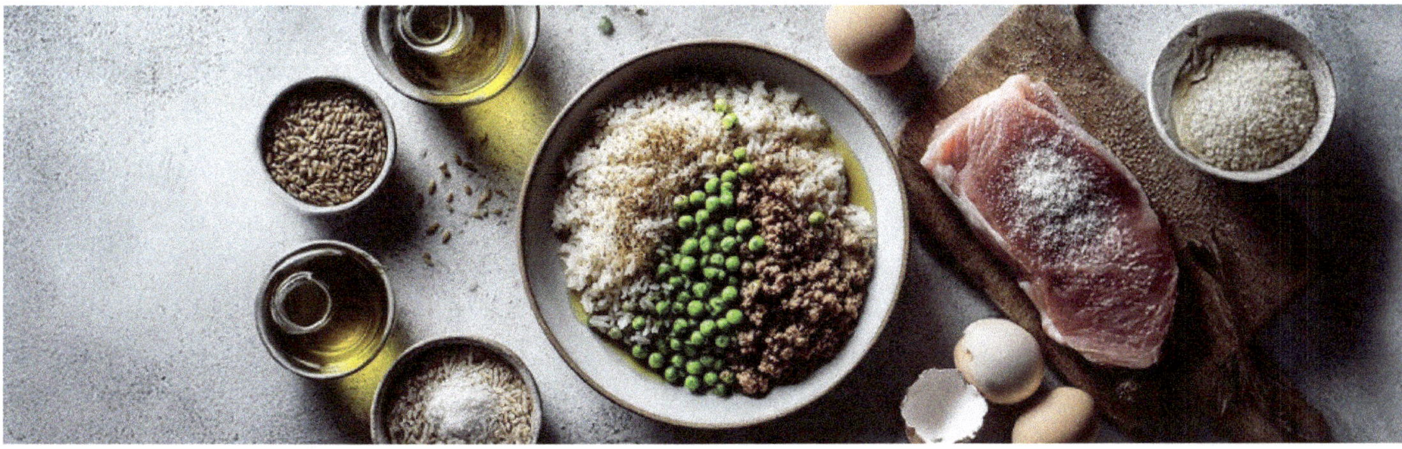

Ingredients:

- 1 lb. (450g) ground lamb (85% lean)
- 1 cup (195g) cooked brown rice
- ½ cup (80g) steamed peas
- 1 tsp olive oil (Omega-6 source)
- ½ tsp ground eggshell powder (or 500 mg calcium carbonate powder; for calcium balance)

Optional

- ¼ cup steamed spinach or zucchini (chopped) for fiber boost

Instructions:

1. In a pan, cook ground lamb over medium heat until fully browned (no oil needed). Drain excess fat.
2. In another pan, cook brown rice as per package instructions.
3. Steam peas until soft.
4. Combine lamb, brown rice, peas, olive oil, eggshell powder, and optional veggies.
5. Serve when cooled.

Ingredient Substitutions:

- Substitute ground beef for lamb if needed.
- Use quinoa instead of brown rice for extra protein.
- Replace peas with green beans for a low-carb option.

Nutrition per 500g serving:

Final Weight	~500g
Calories	~950 kcal
Protein	~40g
Fat	~24g
Carbohydrates	~50g

5. Beef & Brown Rice Power Bowl

(Protein-packed, great for daily energy and muscle maintenance)

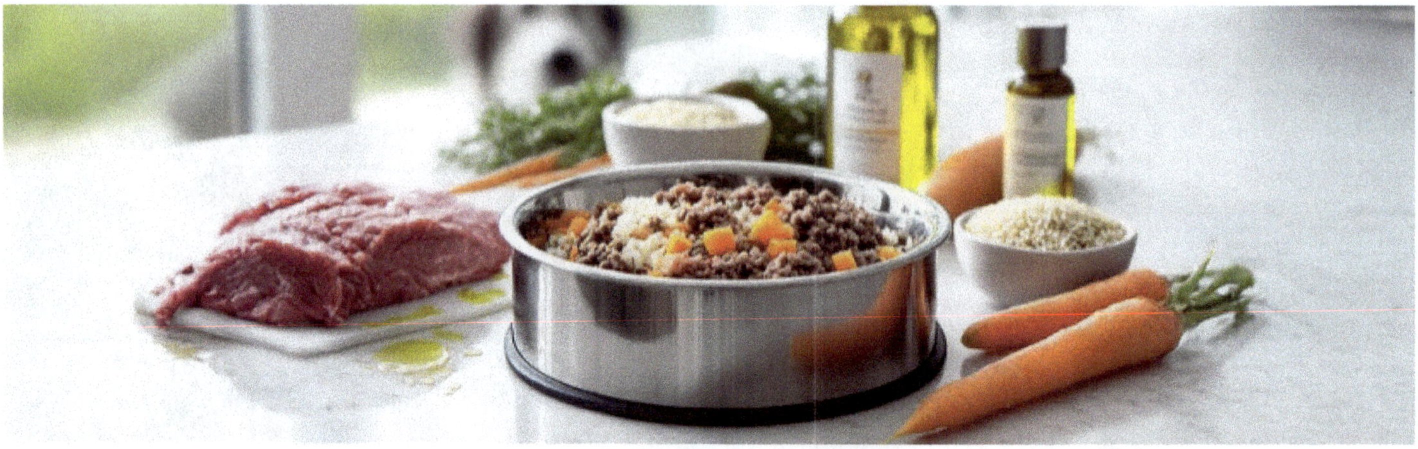

Ingredients:

- 1 lb. lean ground beef (90% lean)
- 1 cup cooked brown rice
- ½ cup steamed carrots (chopped)
- 1 tsp fish oil (EPA/DHA)
- 1 tsp olive oil

Instructions:

1. Brown beef thoroughly.
2. Mix in cooked brown rice and steamed carrots.
3. Stir in oils.
4. Let cool before serving.

Ingredient Substitutions:

- Replace brown rice with quinoa.
- Swap beef for turkey or lamb.

Nutrition per 500g serving:

Final Weight	~500g
Calories	~620 kcal
Protein	~40g
Fat	~28g
Carbohydrates	~42g

6. Duck & Couscous Daily Energy Bowl

(Lean protein + complex carbs for sustained energy in adult dogs)

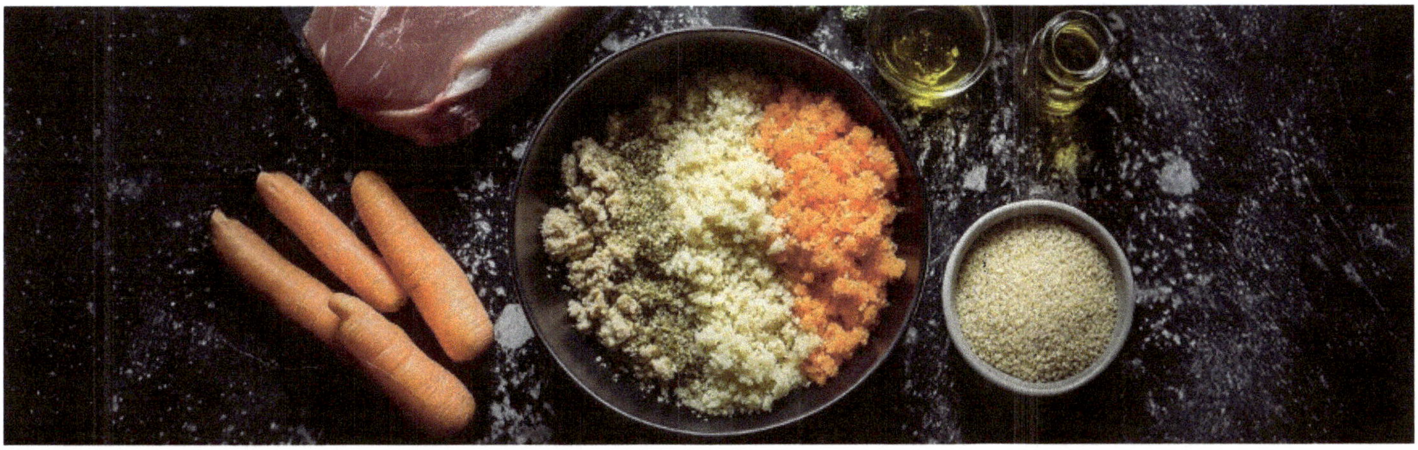

Ingredients:

- 1 lb. (450g) ground duck
- 1 cup (175g) cooked couscous
- ½ cup (75g) steamed carrots
- 1 tsp fish oil
- 1 tsp flaxseed oil

Instructions:

1. Brown ground duck.
2. Prepare couscous by boiling 1 cup water.
3. Lightly steam carrots and chop into small pieces.
4. Mix cooked duck, couscous, and carrots in a bowl.
5. then stir in fish oil and flaxseed oil.
6. Let cool before serving appropriate portions based on dog size.

Ingredient Substitutions:

- Swap oats for brown rice.
- Replace chicken with turkey.

Nutrition per 500g serving:

Final Weight	~500g
Calories	~590 kcal
Protein	~38g
Fat	~22g
Carbohydrates	~40g

7. Salmon & Quinoa Vitality Meal

(Omega-3 rich, supports skin, coat, and overall energy)

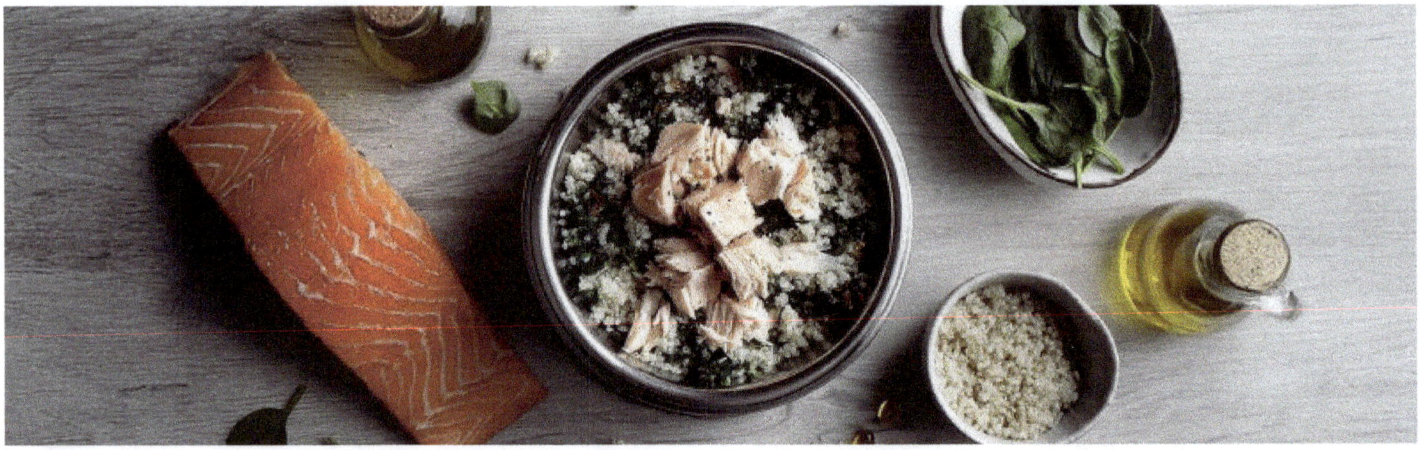

Ingredients:

- 1 lb. boneless salmon (steamed)
- 1 cup cooked quinoa
- ½ cup steamed spinach (chopped)
- 1 tsp fish oil
- 1 tsp olive oil

Instructions:

1. Steam salmon, flake into pieces.
2. Mix with quinoa and spinach.
3. Stir in oils.
4. Let cool before serving.

Ingredient Substitutions:

- Replace quinoa with brown rice.
- Swap spinach for broccoli.

Nutrition per 500g serving:

Final Weight	~500g
Calories	~610 kcal
Protein	~42g
Fat	~26g
Carbohydrates	~38g

8. Turkey & Barley Energy Booster

(Lean, filling, and ideal for weight management + energy)

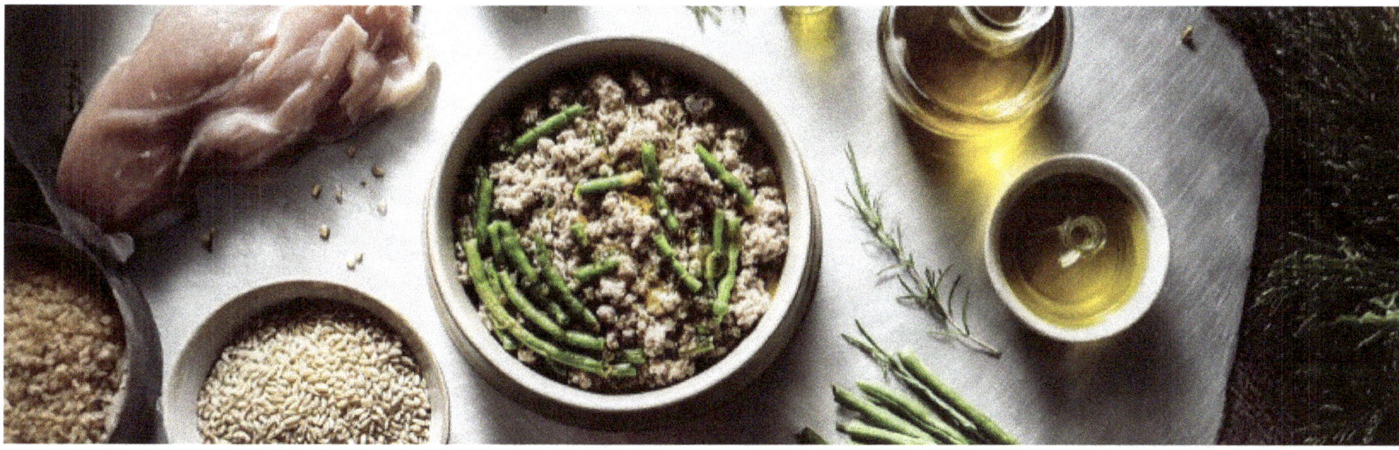

Ingredients:

- 1 lb. ground turkey (93% lean)
- 1 cup cooked barley
- ½ cup steamed green beans (chopped)
- 1 tsp flaxseed oil
- 1 tsp olive oil

Instructions:

1. Cook turkey thoroughly.
2. Mix in cooked barley and green beans.
3. Stir in oils.
4. Let cool before serving.

Ingredient Substitutions:

- Replace barley with oats.
- Swap turkey for chicken or lean beef.

Nutrition per 500g serving:

Final Weight	~500g
Calories	~580 kcal
Protein	~38g
Fat	~22g
Carbohydrates	~42g

9. Lamb & Pumpkin Daily Energy Meal

(Rich in essential minerals, supports stamina and digestion)

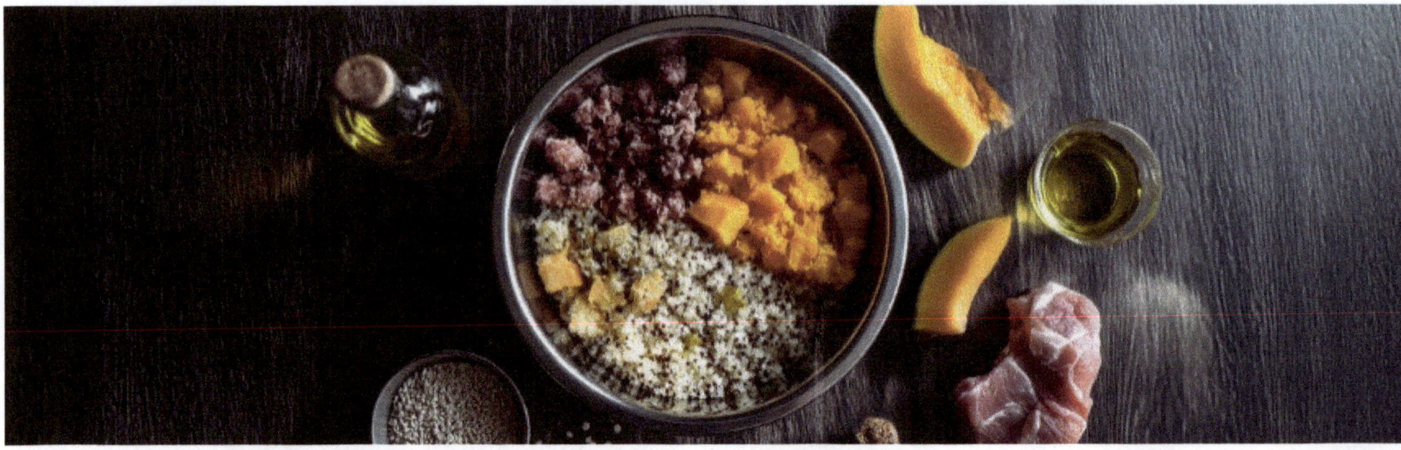

Ingredients:

- 1 lb. ground lamb (85% lean)
- 1 cup mashed pumpkin
- ½ cup cooked quinoa
- 1 tsp flaxseed oil
- 1 tsp fish oil

Instructions:

1. Brown lamb thoroughly.
2. Stir in mashed pumpkin and quinoa.
3. Mix in oils.
4. Let cool before serving.

Ingredient Substitutions:

- Replace quinoa with brown rice.
- Swap pumpkin with sweet potato.

Nutrition per 500g serving:

Final Weight	~500g
Calories	~640 kcal
Protein	~40g
Fat	~28g
Carbohydrates	~42g

10. Whitefish & Millet Energy Boost Bowl

(Low-fat, ideal for sensitive stomachs while providing steady energy)

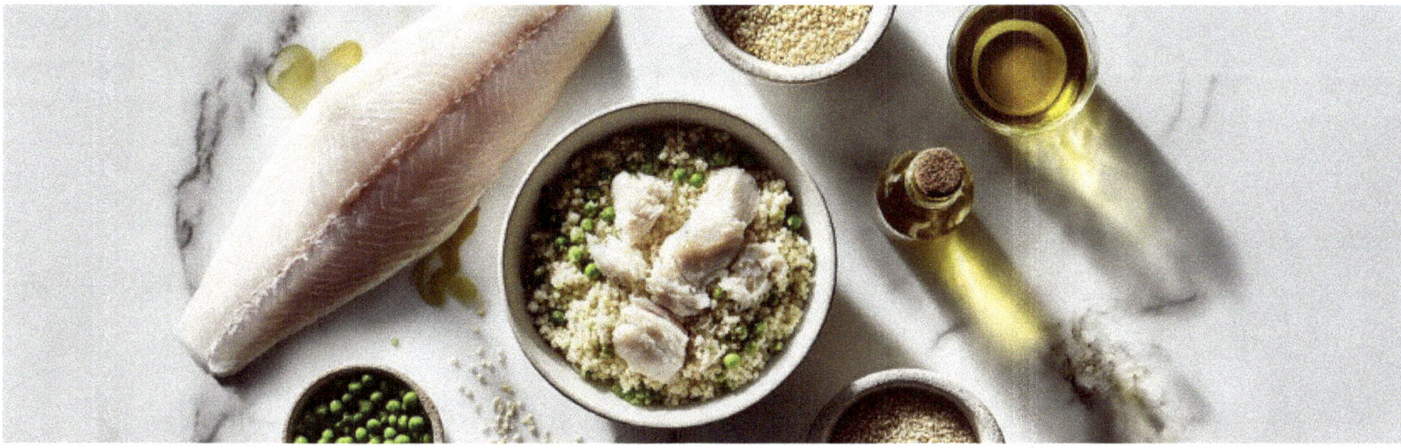

Ingredients:

- 1 lb. boneless whitefish (steamed)
- 1 cup cooked millet
- ½ cup steamed peas
- 1 tsp fish oil
- 1 tsp olive oil

Instructions:

1. Steam fish until fully cooked, flake.
2. Mix in millet and peas.
3. Stir in oils.
4. Let cool before serving.

Ingredient Substitutions:

- Replace millet with oats.
- Swap peas for green beans.

Nutrition per 500g serving:

Final Weight	~500g
Calories	~580 kcal
Protein	~38g
Fat	~20g
Carbohydrates	~44g

11. Egg & Brown Rice Protein Bowl

(High-protein, soft-textured, nutrient-rich)

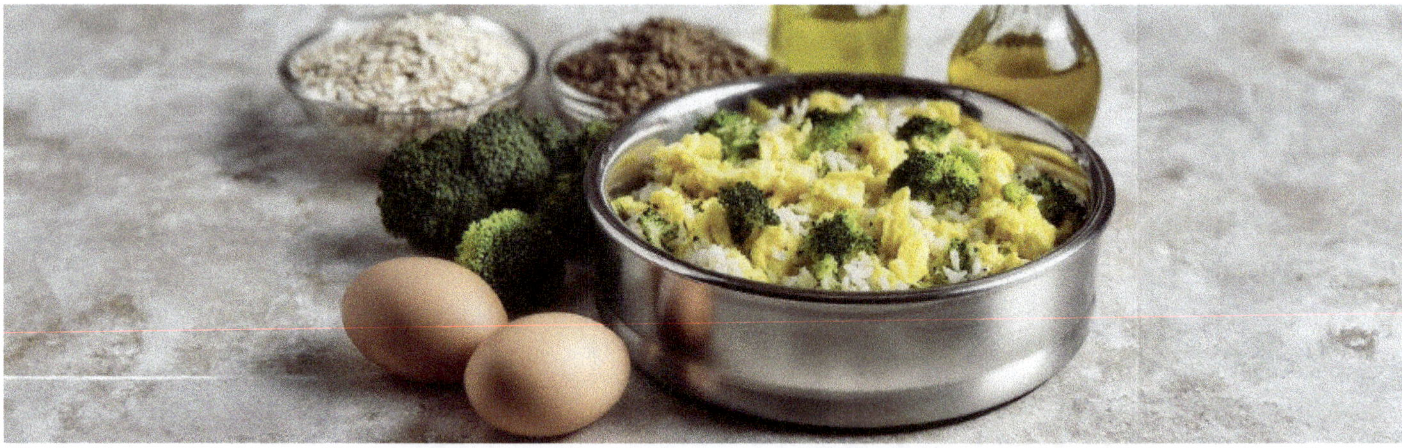

Ingredients:

- 4 large scrambled eggs
- 1 cup cooked brown rice
- ½ cup steamed broccoli (chopped)
- 1 tsp olive oil
- 1 tsp flaxseed oil

Instructions:

1. Scramble eggs gently.
2. Mix in brown rice and broccoli.
3. Stir in oils.
4. Let cool before serving.

Ingredient Substitutions:

- Swap brown rice with quinoa.
- Replace broccoli with spinach.

Nutrition per 500g serving:

Final Weight	~500g
Calories	~600 kcal
Protein	~36g
Fat	~26g
Carbohydrates	~36g

12. Beef & Lentil Energy Meal

(Fiber-rich, iron-packed, provides lasting energy)

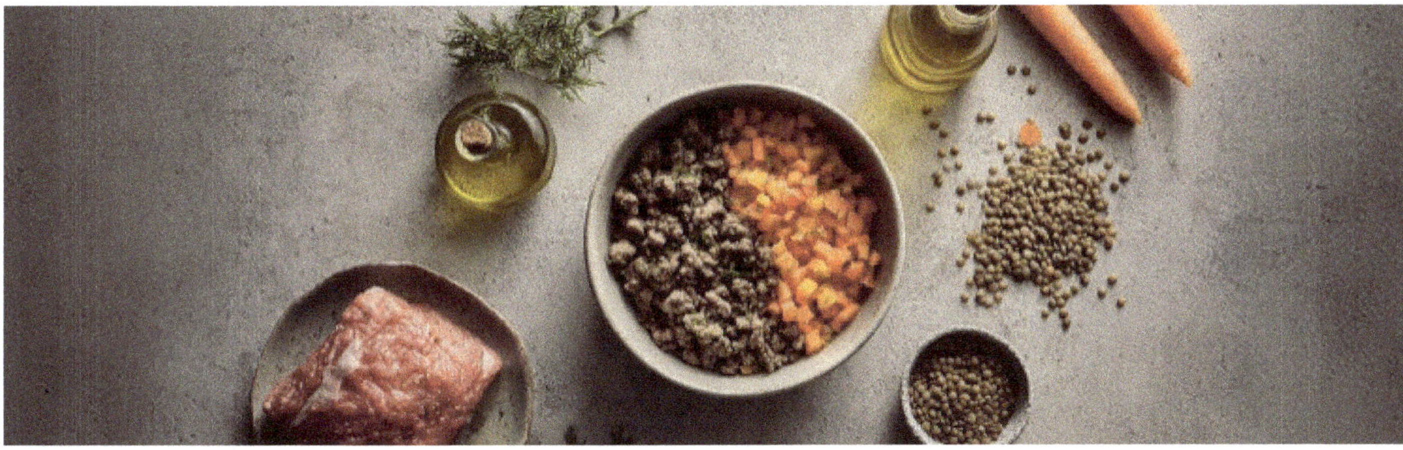

Ingredients:

- 1 lb. lean ground beef (90%)
- 1 cup cooked lentils
- ½ cup steamed carrots (chopped)
- 1 tsp flaxseed oil
- 1 tsp olive oil

Instructions:

1. Brown beef thoroughly.
2. Stir in cooked lentils and carrots.
3. Mix in oils.
4. Let cool before serving.

Ingredient Substitutions:

- Replace lentils with chickpeas.
- Swap beef for turkey.

Nutrition per 500g serving:

Final Weight	~500g
Calories	~630 kcal
Protein	~40g
Fat	~26g
Carbohydrates	~42g

13. Chicken & Barley Stamina Bowl

(Balanced meal for sustained energy and muscle maintenance)

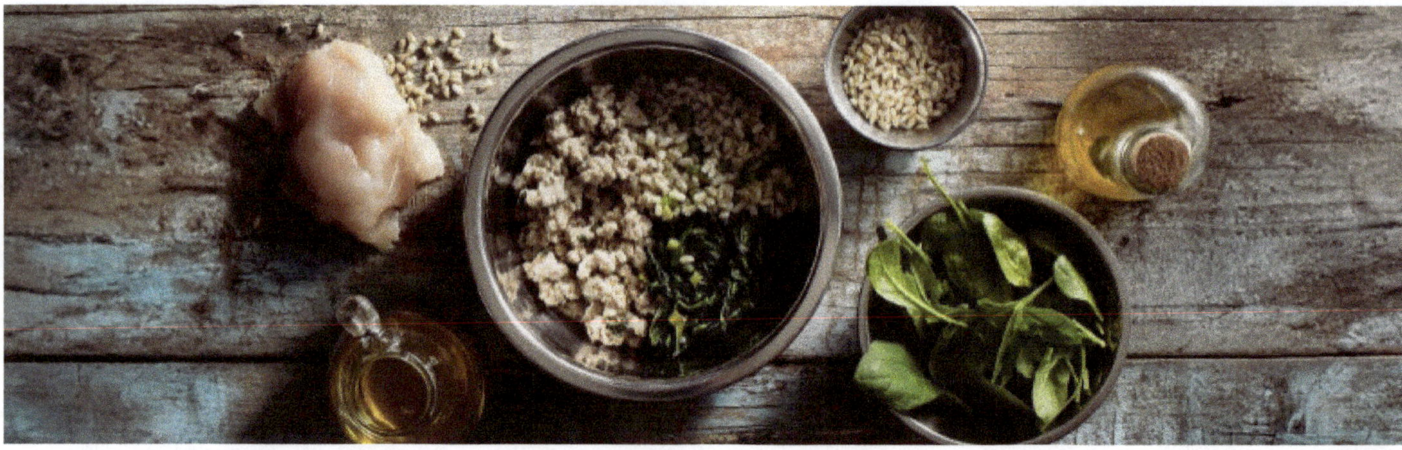

Ingredients:

- 1 lb. ground chicken (93% lean)
- 1 cup cooked barley
- ½ cup steamed spinach (chopped)
- 1 tsp fish oil
- 1 tsp olive oil

Instructions:

1. Cook chicken thoroughly.
2. Stir in cooked barley and spinach.
3. Mix in oils.
4. Let cool before serving.

Ingredient Substitutions:

- Replace barley with oats.
- Swap chicken with turkey.

Nutrition per 500g serving:

Final Weight	~500g
Calories	~590 kcal
Protein	~38g
Fat	~22g
Carbohydrates	~40g

14. Turkey & Sweet Potato Power Meal

(Easily digestible, protein & carb balanced for daily energy)

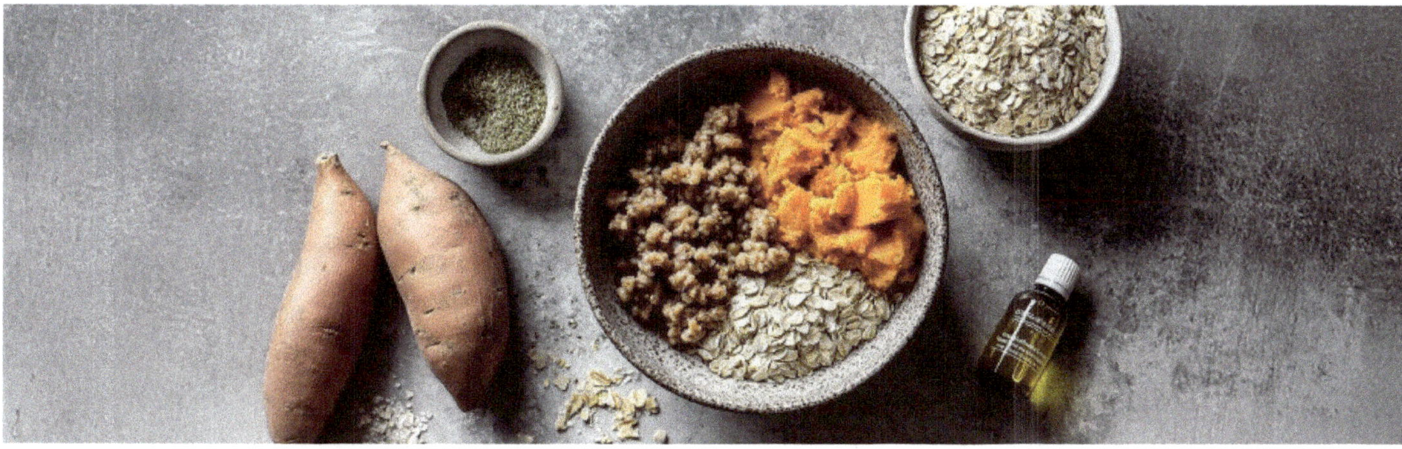

Ingredients:

- 1 lb. ground turkey (93% lean)
- 1 cup mashed sweet potato
- ½ cup oats
- 1 tsp flaxseed oil
- 1 tsp fish oil

Instructions:

1. Cook turkey thoroughly.
2. Mix in mashed sweet potato and oats.
3. Stir in oils.
4. Let cool before serving.

Ingredient Substitutions:

- Replace oats with brown rice.
- Swap sweet potato with pumpkin.

Nutrition per 500g serving:

Final Weight	~500g
Calories	~600 kcal
Protein	~40g
Fat	~24g
Carbohydrates	~42g

15. Beef & Oatmeal Muscle Fuel

(High-protein, fiber-rich recipe tailored for active adult dogs, supporting muscle maintenance, energy, digestion, and coat health)

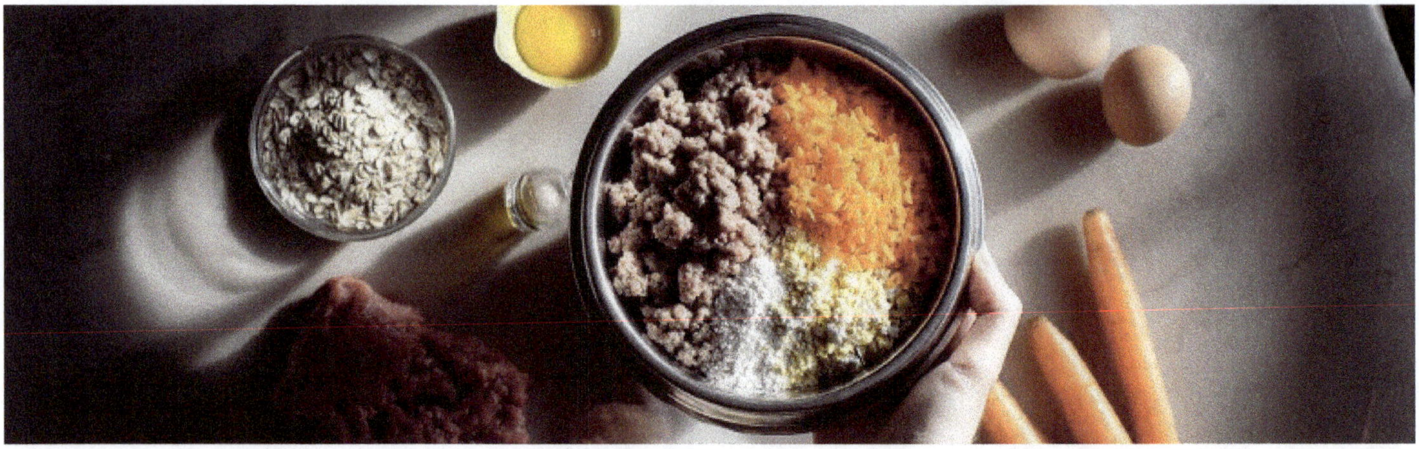

Ingredients:

- 1 lb. (450g) lean ground beef (90% lean)
- 1 cup (80g) cooked oatmeal (plain, unsweetened)
- ½ cup (80g) steamed carrots (chopped)
- 1 tsp fish oil
- ½ tsp ground eggshell powder (or 500 mg calcium carbonate powder)

Optional:

- ¼ cup steamed spinach or green beans (chopped) for fiber boost

Instructions:

1. Cook ground beef over medium heat until fully browned. Drain excess fat.
2. Prepare oatmeal according to package instructions, using only water.
3. Steam carrots until soft, then chop.
4. Mix beef, oatmeal, carrots, fish oil, eggshell powder, and optional veggies together.
5. Let cool before serving.

Ingredient Substitutions:

- Swap beef for turkey or chicken.
- Use quinoa instead of oatmeal for a grain-free option.
- Replace carrots with pumpkin for digestive support.

Nutrition per 500g serving:

Final Weight	~500g
Calories	~900 kcal
Protein	~45g
Fat	~20g
Carbohydrates	~40g

16. Pork & Millet Strength Mix

(Protein-rich, endurance-fueling, and joint-supporting meal tailored for adult dogs)

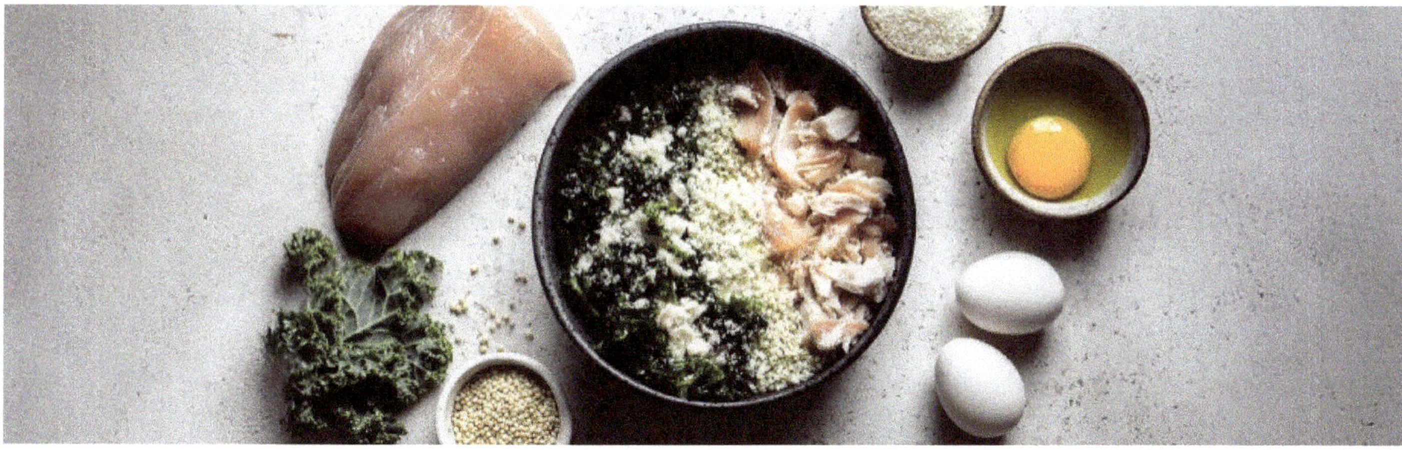

Ingredients:

- 1 lb. (450g) ground pork loin (cooked and shredded)
- 1 cup (200g) cooked millet
- ½ cup (90g) steamed kale (chopped)
- 1 tsp coconut oil
- 1 tsp fish oil
- ½ tsp ground eggshell powder (or 500 mg calcium carbonate powder)

Optional

- ¼ cup steamed peas or carrots (chopped) for extra fiber & hydration

Instructions:

1. Cook pork loin until fully done, then shred.
2. Cook millet according to package instructions.
3. Steam kale until soft and chop.
4. Mix all ingredients together, adding coconut oil, fish oil, eggshell powder, and optional veggies.
5. Let cool before serving

Ingredient Substitutions:

- Use lean beef instead of pork.
- Swap millet for couscous for a lighter meal.
- Replace kale with Swiss chard for extra hydration.

Nutrition per 500g serving:

Final Weight	~500g
Calories	~1250 kcal
Protein	~80
Fat	~20g
Carbohydrates	~50g

17. Turkey & Green Bean Lean Meal

(A low-fat, high-protein recipe designed to maintain lean muscle while supporting overall health in adult dogs)

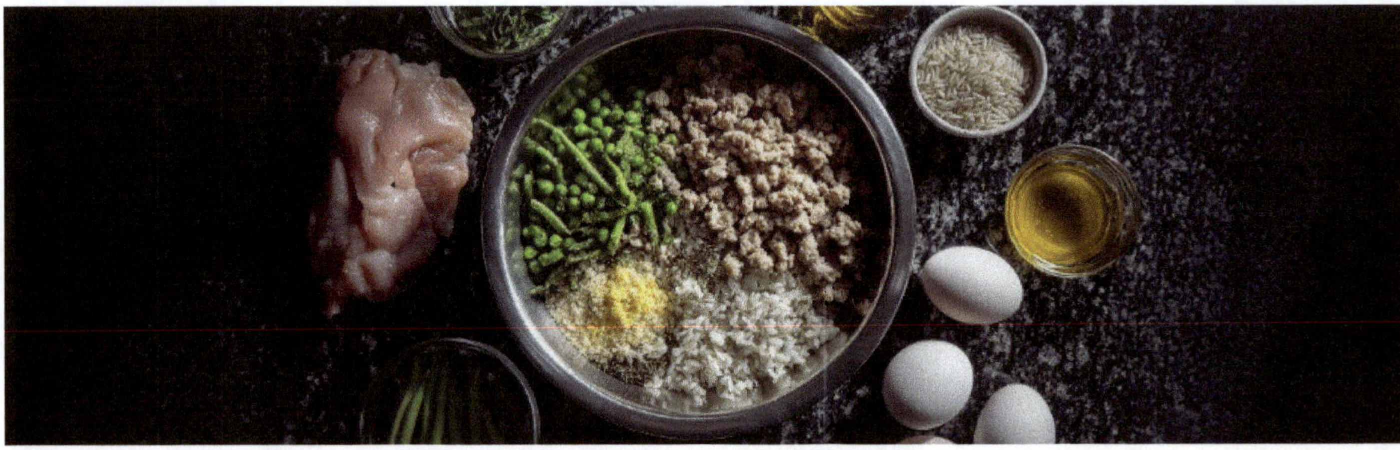

Ingredients:

- 1 lb. (450g) ground turkey (lean, 93%)
- 1 cup (195g) cooked brown rice
- ½ cup (75g) steamed green beans (chopped)
- 1 tsp fish oil
- ½ tsp flaxseed oil
- ½ tsp ground eggshell powder (or 500 mg calcium carbonate powder)

Optional:

- ¼ cup steamed broccoli, spinach, or carrots for extra fiber

Instructions:

1. Cook ground turkey in a pan over medium heat until fully browned. Drain excess fat.
2. Cook brown rice according to package instructions.
3. Lightly steam green beans, then chop finely.
4. Combine all ingredients, including fish oil, flaxseed oil (optional), eggshell powder, and optional veggies.
5. Let cool before serving.

Ingredient Substitutions:

- Replace turkey with lean chicken or fish.
- Use quinoa instead of brown rice for higher protein.
- Swap green beans with broccoli for extra antioxidants.

Nutrition per 500g serving:

Final Weight	~500g
Calories	~800 kcal
Protein	~42g
Fat	~16g
Carbohydrates	~30g

18. Lamb & Sweet Potato Endurance Meal

(A high-energy, nutrient-dense meal supporting muscle recovery, immune function, and coat health in active adult dogs)

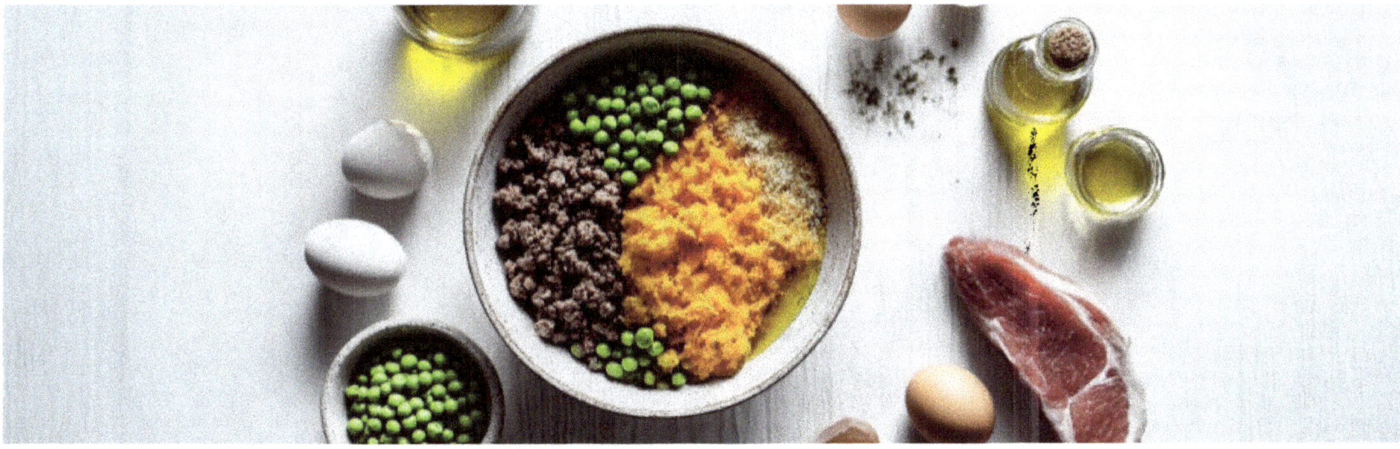

Ingredients:

- 1 lb. (450g) ground lamb (85% lean)
- 1 cup (245g) cooked sweet potato (mashed)
- ½ cup (80g) steamed peas
- 1 tsp olive oil
- 1 tsp fish oil
- ½ tsp ground eggshell powder

Optional

- ¼ cup steamed spinach or green beans (chopped)

Instructions:

1. Cook ground lamb over medium heat until fully browned. Drain excess fat.
2. Cook sweet potatoes until soft, mash.
3. Steam peas until tender.
4. Mix lamb, sweet potato, peas, olive oil, fish oil, eggshell powder, and optional veggies.
5. Let cool before serving.

Ingredient Substitutions:

- Swap lamb for beef if needed.
- Replace sweet potatoes with pumpkin or butternut squash.
- Use carrots instead of peas for an alternative fiber source.

Nutrition per 500g serving:

Final Weight	~500g
Calories	~1250 kcal
Protein	~80
Fat	~20g
Carbohydrates	~50g

19. Fish & Brown Rice Omega Meal

(Brain-boosting, skin-supportive recipe packed with Omega-3s, complete protein, and essential vitamins & minerals)

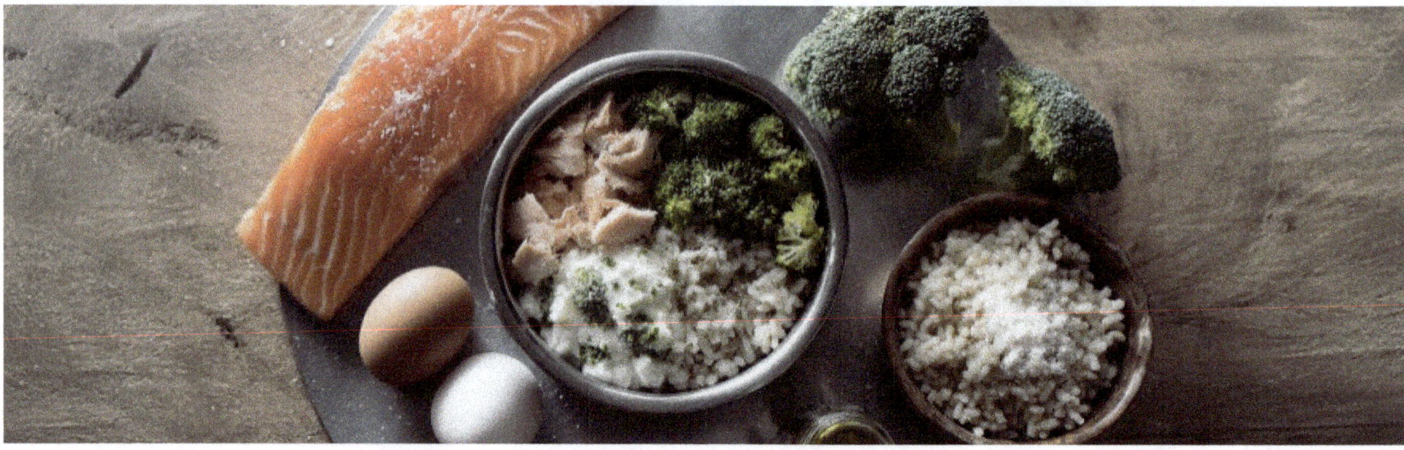

Ingredients:

- 1 lb. (450g) cooked salmon (or white fish like cod, flaked boneless)
- 1 cup (195g) cooked brown rice
- ½ cup (90g) steamed broccoli (chopped)
- 1 tsp fish oil
- ½ tsp ground eggshell powder (or 500 mg calcium carbonate powder)

Optional:

- ¼ cup steamed zucchini or green beans (chopped) for fiber

Instructions:

1. Bake or steam salmon (or cod) until fully cooked, flake into small pieces.
2. Cook brown rice according to package instructions.
3. Steam broccoli, chop finely.
4. Mix fish, brown rice, broccoli, fish oil, eggshell powder, and optional veggies.
5. Let cool before serving.

Ingredient Substitutions:

- Swap salmon for sardines or mackerel (increase Omega-3s naturally).
- Use quinoa instead of brown rice for a grain-free alternative.
- Replace broccoli with zucchini for a lighter meal.

Nutrition per 500g serving:

Final Weight	~500g
Calories	~900 kcal
Protein	~42g
Fat	~20g
Carbohydrates	~40g

Skin and Coat-Enhancing Recipes

1. Turkey & Green Bean Trim Mix (Skin & Coat Health)

(A high-protein, low-fat recipe designed for lean muscle maintenance and weight control, fully balanced for adult dogs)

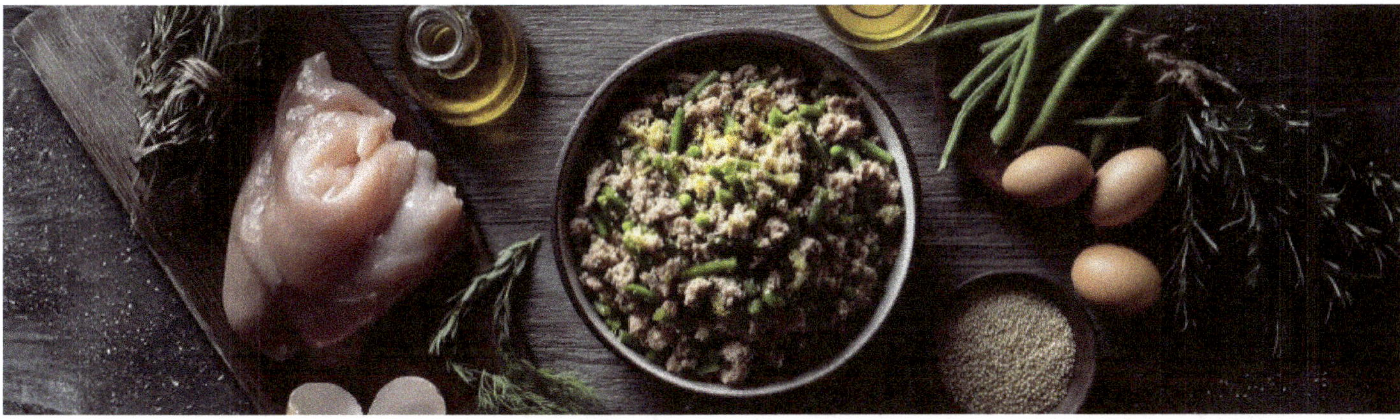

Ingredients:

- 1 lb. (450g) ground turkey (lean, 93%)
- 1 cup (185g) cooked quinoa
- ½ cup (75g) steamed green beans (chopped)
- 1 tsp olive oil
- 1 tsp fish oil
- ½ tsp ground eggshell powder (or 500 mg calcium carbonate powder)

Optional

- ¼ cup steamed broccoli or spinach (chopped) for fiber & added micronutrients

Instructions:

1. Cook ground turkey in a pan over medium heat until fully browned (don't use any oil). Drain excess fat.
2. Cook quinoa according to package instructions.
3. Lightly steam green beans, then chop.
4. Mix all ingredients including olive oil, fish oil, eggshell powder, and optional veggies.
5. Cool before serving.

Ingredient Substitutions:

- Use lean chicken instead of turkey.
- Swap quinoa for brown rice if preferred.
- Replace green beans with broccoli for extra fiber.

Nutrition per 500g serving:

Final Weight	~500g
Calories	~725 kcal
Protein	~42g
Fat	~16g
Carbohydrates	~35g

2. Lean Chicken & Pumpkin Slim Meal (Skin & Coat Health)

(Low-calorie, high-fiber, and nutrient-dense meal designed for healthy weight management and digestive support in adult dogs)

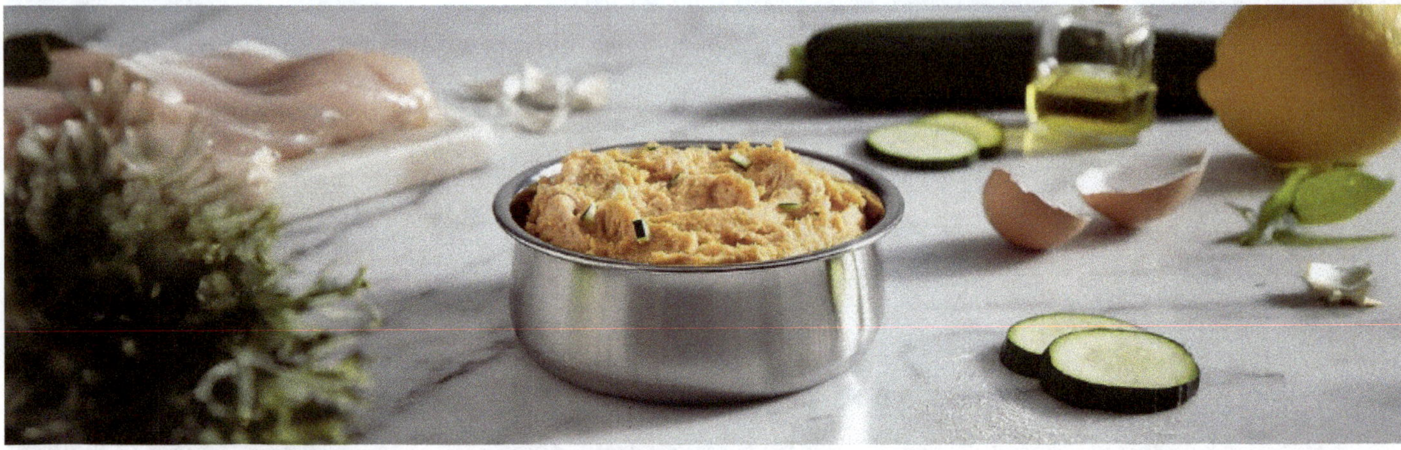

Ingredients:

- 1 lb. (450g) boneless, skinless chicken breast (cooked and shredded)
- 1 cup (245g) cooked pumpkin (plain, unsweetened)
- ½ cup (90g) steamed zucchini (chopped)
- 1 tsp fish oil
- ½ tsp ground eggshell powder (or 500 mg calcium carbonate powder)

Optional:

- ¼ cup steamed spinach or green beans (chopped) for extra fiber & micronutrients

Instructions:

1. In a pan, cook chicken breast until fully done (without oil). Shred in a bowl.
2. Cook pumpkin until soft, then mash.
3. Steam zucchini until tender, then chop.
4. Mix all ingredients, including fish oil, eggshell powder, and optional veggies.
5. Let cool before serving.

Ingredient Substitutions:

- Swap chicken for lean turkey or white fish.
- Replace pumpkin with butternut squash for variety.
- Use steamed spinach instead of zucchini for added iron.

Nutrition per 500g serving:

Final Weight	~500g
Calories	~750 kcal
Protein	~48g
Fat	~12g
Carbohydrates	~25g

3. Fish & Spinach Metabolism Booster (Skin & Coat Health)

(Low-fat, Omega-3 rich meal designed to support metabolism, lean muscle, and inflammation control in adult dogs)

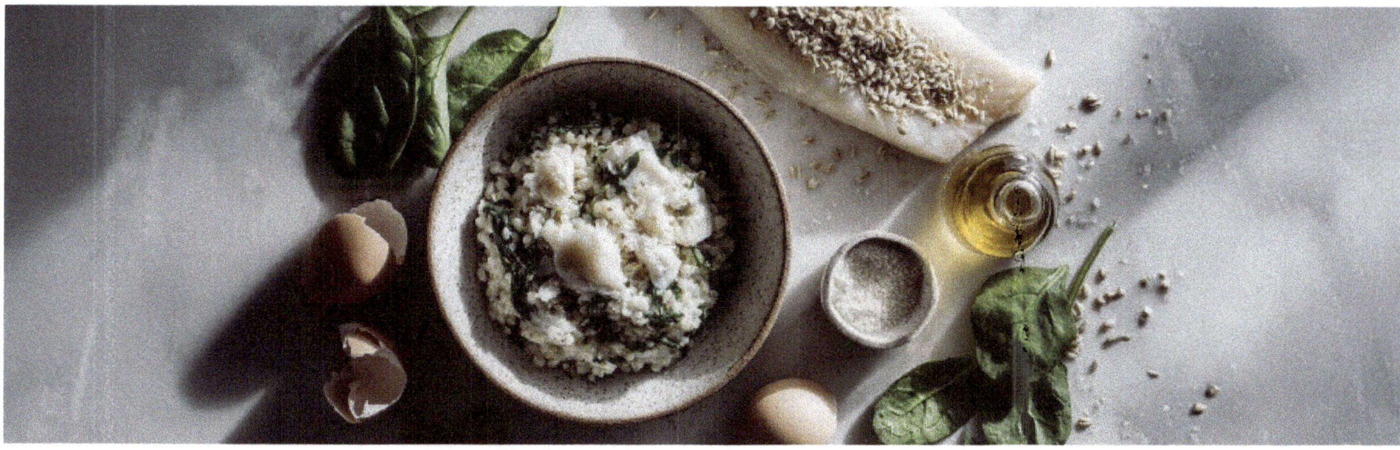

Ingredients:

- 1 lb. (450g) cooked cod (or white fish; flaked, boneless)
- 1 cup (200g) cooked barley
- ½ cup (90g) steamed spinach (chopped)
- 1 tsp fish oil
- ½ tsp ground eggshell powder (or 500 mg calcium carbonate powder)

Optional

- ¼ cup steamed zucchini, green beans, or carrots (chopped) for fiber boost

Instructions:

1. Bake or steam cod until fully cooked, then flake.
2. Cook barley according to package instructions.
3. Steam spinach, then chop finely.
4. Mix fish, barley, spinach, fish oil, eggshell powder, and optional veggies together.
5. Let cool before serving.

Ingredient Substitutions:

- Use salmon instead of cod for a stronger Omega-3 boost.
- Swap barley for quinoa for a gluten-free option.
- Replace spinach with zucchini for a lighter meal.

Nutrition per 500g serving:

Final Weight	~500g
Calories	~700 kcal
Protein	~40g
Fat	~14g
Carbohydrates	~35g

4. Lamb & Oatmeal Hydration Mix

(Zinc and Omega-6-rich recipe designed to relieve dry skin, promote coat health, and ensure balanced nutrition for adult dogs)

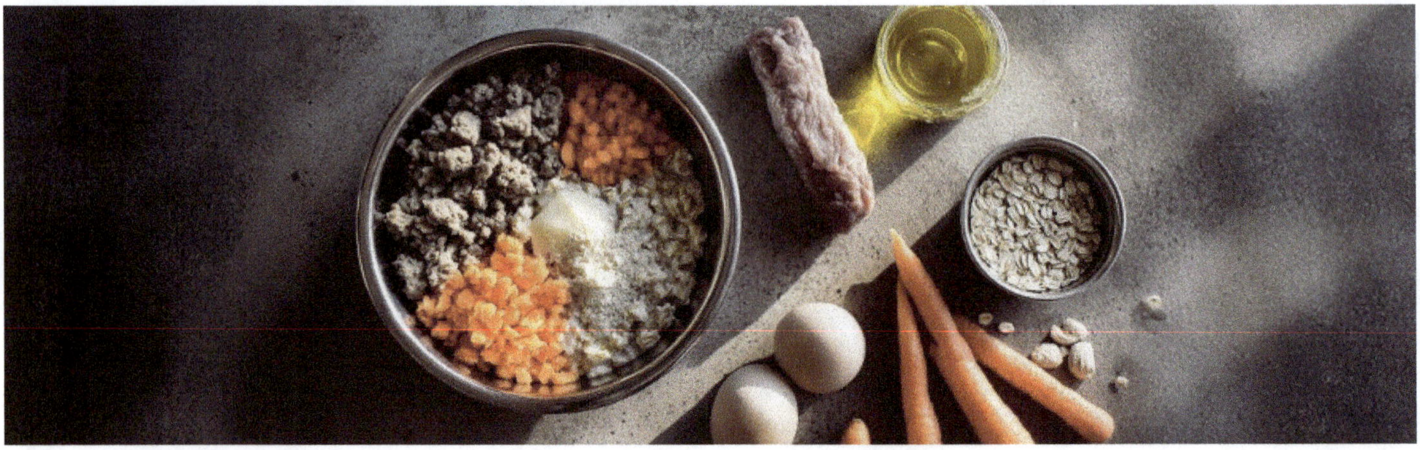

Ingredients:

- 1 lb. (450g) ground lamb (85% lean)
- 1 cup (80g) cooked oatmeal (plain, unsweetened)
- ½ cup (80g) steamed carrots (chopped)
- 1 tsp fish oil
- ½ tsp ground eggshell powder (or 500 mg calcium carbonate powder)

Optional:

- ¼ cup steamed pumpkin, spinach, or green beans for fiber & micronutrient boost

Instructions:

1. Cook ground lamb over medium heat until fully browned (no oil required). Drain excess fat.
2. In another pan, cook oatmeal using only water (no sugar or milk).
3. Steam carrots, then chop finely.
4. Mix all ingredients together, adding fish oil, eggshell powder, and optional veggies.
5. Let cool before serving.

Ingredient Substitutions:

- Swap lamb for lean beef or turkey.
- Use brown rice instead of oatmeal for grain variation.
- Replace carrots with pumpkin puree for extra fiber.

Nutrition per 500g serving:

Final Weight	~500g
Calories	~850 kcal
Protein	~40g
Fat	~20g
Carbohydrates	~35g

5. Mackerel & Green Bean Coat Care Recipe

(DHA/EPA-rich, antioxidant-packed meal designed to promote healthy skin, reduce inflammation, and enhance coat shine in adult dogs)

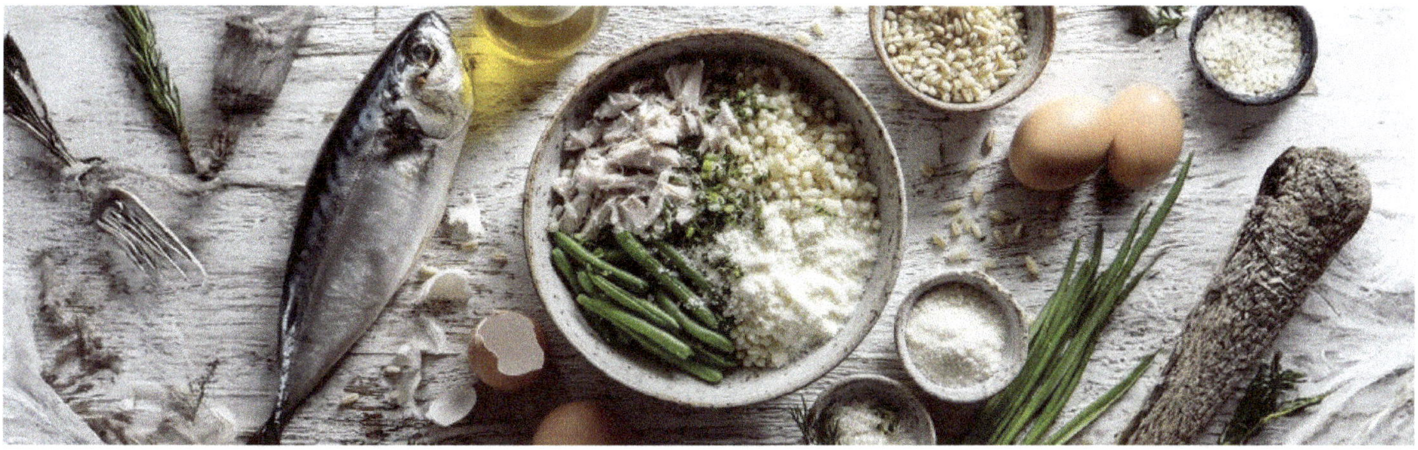

Ingredients:

- 1 lb. (450g) cooked mackerel (or sardines; flaked, boneless)
- 1 cup (200g) cooked barley
- ½ cup (90g) steamed green beans (chopped)
- 1 tsp fish oil
- ½ tsp ground eggshell powder (or 500 mg calcium carbonate powder)

Optional

- ¼ cup steamed zucchini, spinach, or carrots for fiber & antioxidants

Instructions:

1. Bake or steam mackerel until fully cooked, then flake into small pieces.
2. Cook barley according to package instructions.
3. Lightly steam green beans, then chop.
4. Combine fish, barley, green beans, fish oil, eggshell powder, and optional veggies.
5. Let cool before serving.

Ingredient Substitutions:

- Swap mackerel for salmon or sardines.
- Use quinoa instead of barley for higher protein.
- Replace green beans with zucchini for lower carbs.

Nutrition per 500g serving:

Final Weight	~500g
Calories	~850 kcal
Protein	~42g
Fat	~20g
Carbohydrates	~35g

6. Salmon & Oats Shine Meal

(Omega-3 rich, supports skin hydration and coat glossiness)

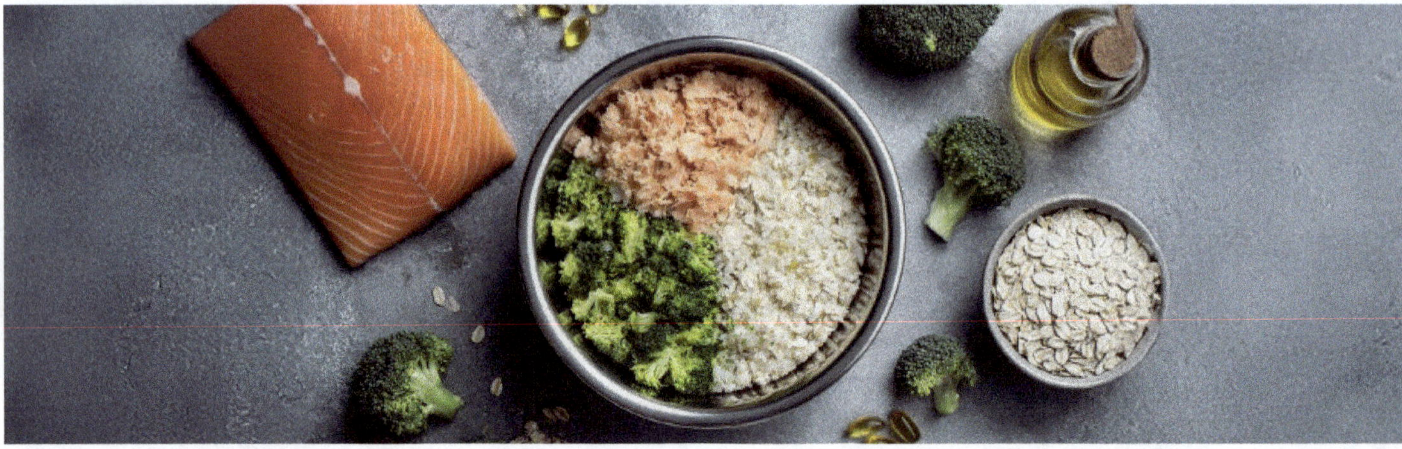

Ingredients:

- 1 lb. boneless salmon (steamed)
- 1 cup cooked oats
- ½ cup steamed broccoli (chopped)
- 1 tsp fish oil
- 1 tsp flaxseed oil

Instructions:

1. Steam salmon until fully cooked, flake into small pieces.
2. Mix with cooked oats and broccoli.
3. Stir in oils.
4. Let cool before serving.

Ingredient Substitutions:

- Replace oats with quinoa.
- Swap broccoli with spinach.

Nutrition per 500g serving:

Final Weight	~500g
Calories	~610 kcal
Protein	~42g
Fat	~26g
Carbohydrates	~36g

7. Trout & Pinto Bean Shine Meal

(Light, omega-packed, gentle on digestion, promotes healthy skin)

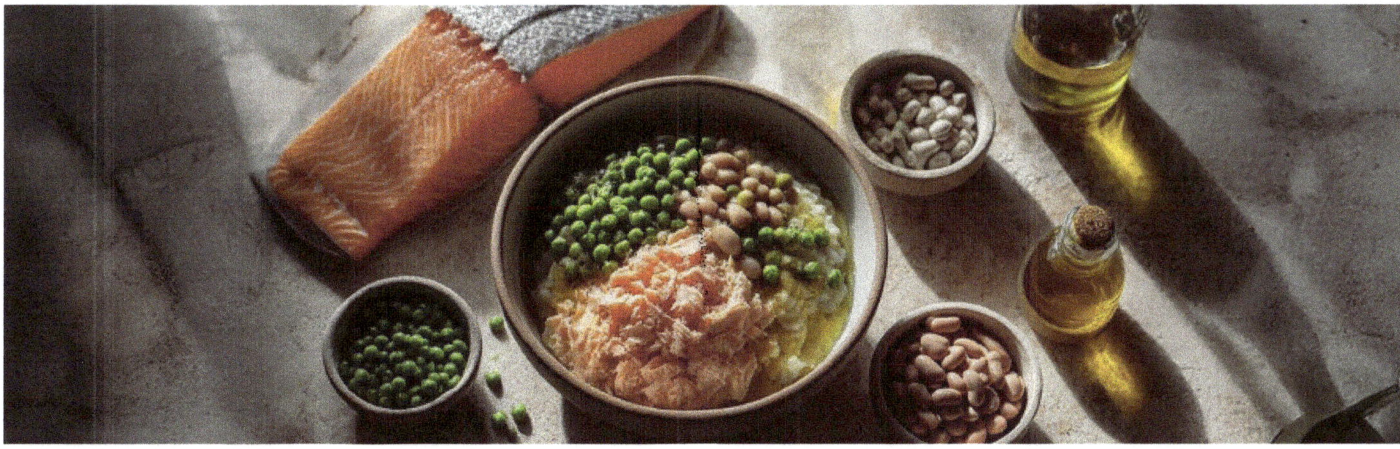

Ingredients:

- 1 lb. (450g) boneless trout (steamed)
- 1 cup (200g) cooked pinto beans (mashed)
- ½ cup (75g) steamed peas (chopped)
- 1 tsp fish oil
- 1 tsp olive oil

Instructions:

1. Steam trout until cooked, flake.
2. Mix in mashed pinto beans and peas.
3. Stir in oils.
4. Let cool before serving.

Ingredient Substitutions:

- Replace pinto beans with chickpeas.
- Swap peas with steamed carrots.

Nutrition per 500g serving:

Final Weight	~500g
Calories	~580 kcal
Protein	~38g
Fat	~22g
Carbohydrates	~40g

8. Turkey & Quinoa Skin Health Bowl

(Lean, rich in zinc and healthy fats, ideal for dry skin)

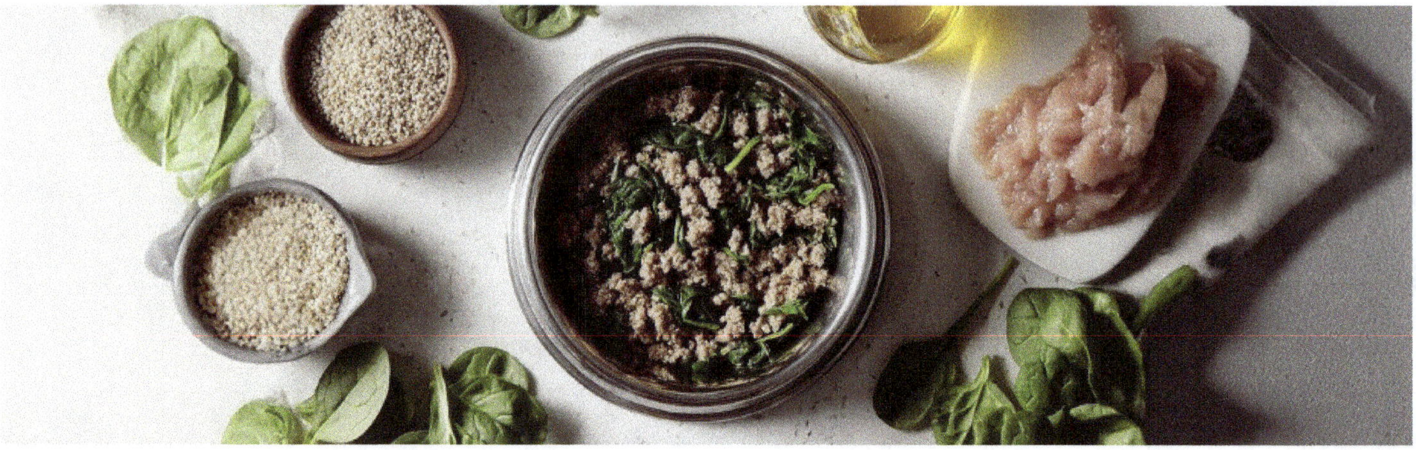

Ingredients:

- 1 lb. ground turkey (93% lean)
- 1 cup cooked quinoa
- ½ cup steamed spinach (chopped)
- 1 tsp flaxseed oil
- 1 tsp olive oil

Instructions:

1. Cook turkey thoroughly.
2. Stir in cooked quinoa and spinach.
3. Mix in oils.
4. Let cool before serving.

Ingredient Substitutions:

- Replace quinoa with brown rice.
- Swap spinach with broccoli.

Nutrition per 500g serving:

Final Weight	~500g
Calories	~580 kcal
Protein	~38g
Fat	~22g
Carbohydrates	~42g

9. Egg & Cottage Cheese Shine Boost Meal

(High-protein, calcium-rich, great for skin & coat nourishment)

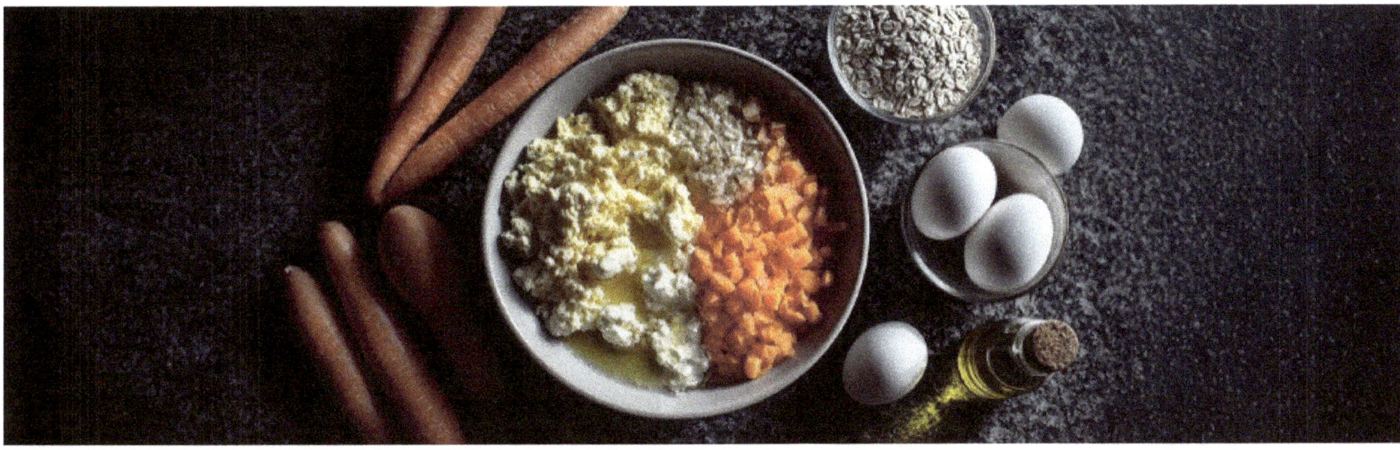

Ingredients:

- 3 large scrambled eggs
- ½ cup plain cottage cheese
- 1 cup cooked oats
- ½ cup steamed carrots (chopped)
- 1 tsp flaxseed oil
- 1 tsp olive oil

Instructions:

1. Scramble eggs gently.
2. Stir in cottage cheese, cooked oats, and carrots.
3. Add oils and mix thoroughly.
4. Let cool before serving.

Ingredient Substitutions:

- Replace oats with brown rice.
- Swap cottage cheese with plain Greek yogurt.

Nutrition per 500g serving:

Final Weight	~500g
Calories	~600 kcal
Protein	~36g
Fat	~24g
Carbohydrates	~40g

10. Salmon & Black Bean Coat Glow Bowl

(Mineral-rich salmon with balanced fats for coat shine)

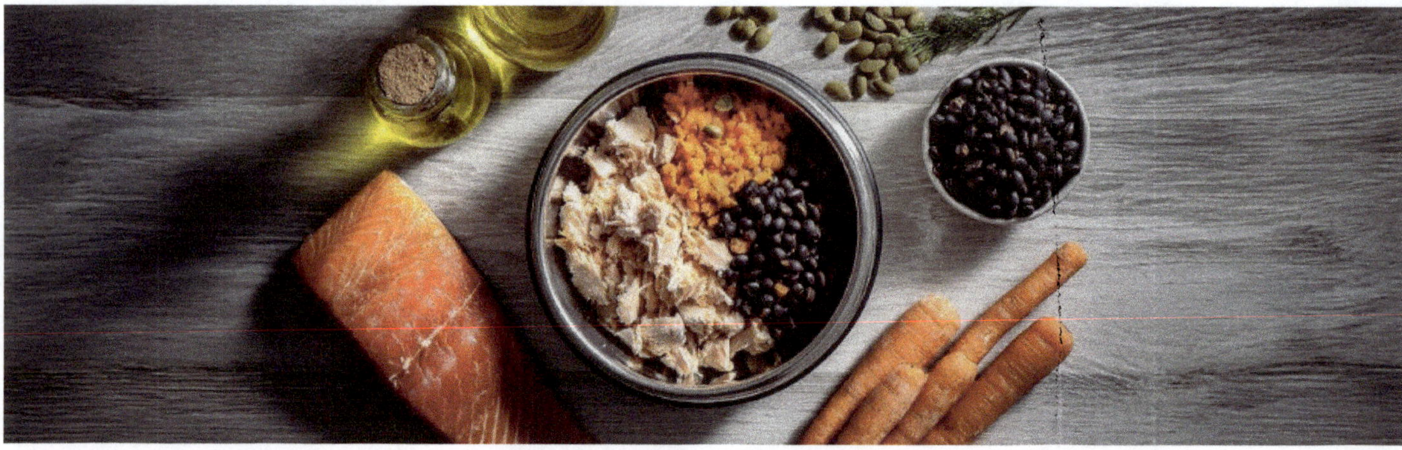

Ingredients:

- 1 lb. (450g) salmon (cooked, flaked, skin-on for extra fats)
- 1 cup (200g) cooked black beans (mashed)
- ½ cup (75g) steamed carrots (chopped)
- 1 tsp flaxseed oil
- 1 tsp fish oil

Instructions:

1. Cook salmon thoroughly
2. Stir in cooked beans and carrot.
3. Mix in oils.
4. Let cool before serving.

Ingredient Substitutions:

- Replace carrots with steamed zucchini.
- Swap black beans with pinto beans.

Nutrition per 500g serving:

Final Weight	~500g
Calories	~1250 kcal
Protein	~80g
Fat	~30g
Carbohydrates	~50g

Weight Management Recipes

1. Turkey & Green Bean Lean Meal

(High-protein, low-fat, keeps dogs full without excess calories)

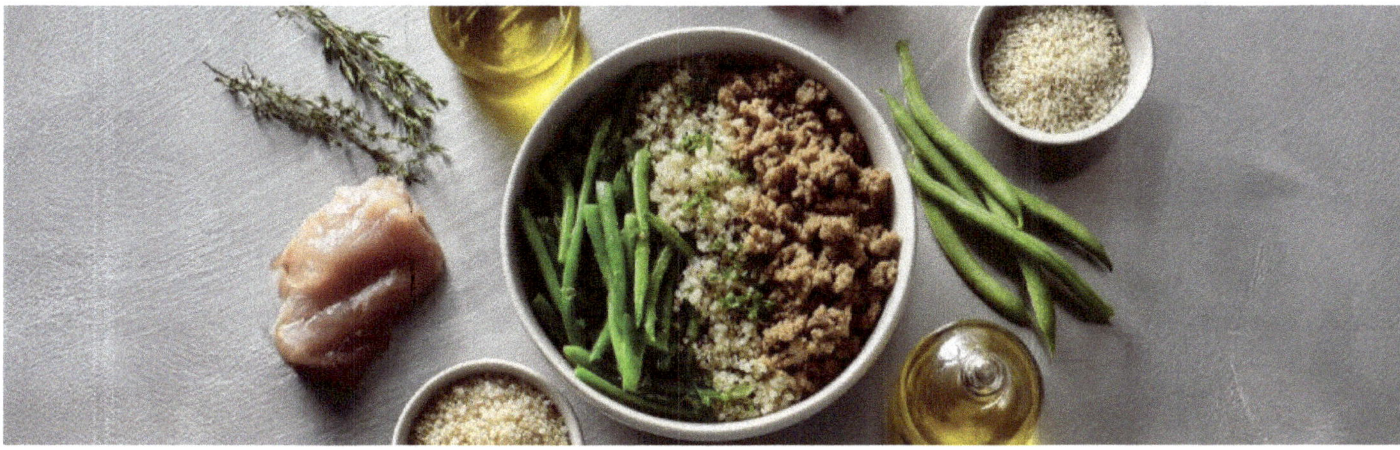

Ingredients:

- 1 lb. ground turkey (93% lean)
- 1 cup steamed green beans (chopped)
- ½ cup cooked quinoa
- 1 tsp flaxseed oil
- 1 tsp olive oil

Instructions:

1. Cook turkey thoroughly.
2. Stir in steamed green beans and quinoa.
3. Mix in oils.
4. Let cool before serving.

Ingredient Substitutions:

- Replace quinoa with oats.
- Swap green beans with broccoli.

Nutrition per 500g serving:

Final Weight	~500g
Calories	~520 kcal
Protein	~40g
Fat	~18g
Carbohydrates	~28g

2. Tilapia & Potato Lean Bowl

(Low-fat, light, and rich in omega-3s for lean body condition)

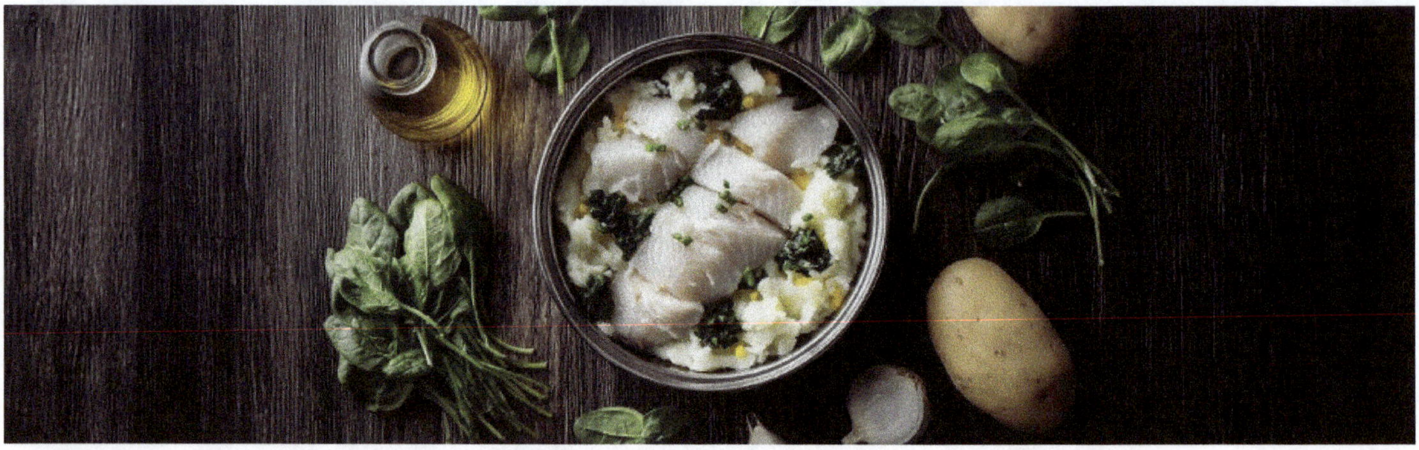

Ingredients:

- 1 lb. (450g) boneless tilapia (steamed)
- 1 cup (200g) steamed potato (mashed, white)
- ½ cup (75g) steamed spinach (chopped)
- 1 tsp fish oil
- 1 tsp olive oil

Instructions:

1. Steam tilapia thoroughly, flake.
2. Mix in steamed potato and spinach.
3. Stir in oils.
4. Let cool before serving.

Ingredient Substitutions:

- Replace potato with mashed tapioca.
- Swap spinach with steamed peas.

Nutrition per 500g serving:

Final Weight	~500g
Calories	~800 kcal
Protein	~68g
Fat	~18g
Carbohydrates	~46g

3. Chicken & Broccoli Light Meal

(Lean, fiber-rich, perfect for calorie control and satiety)

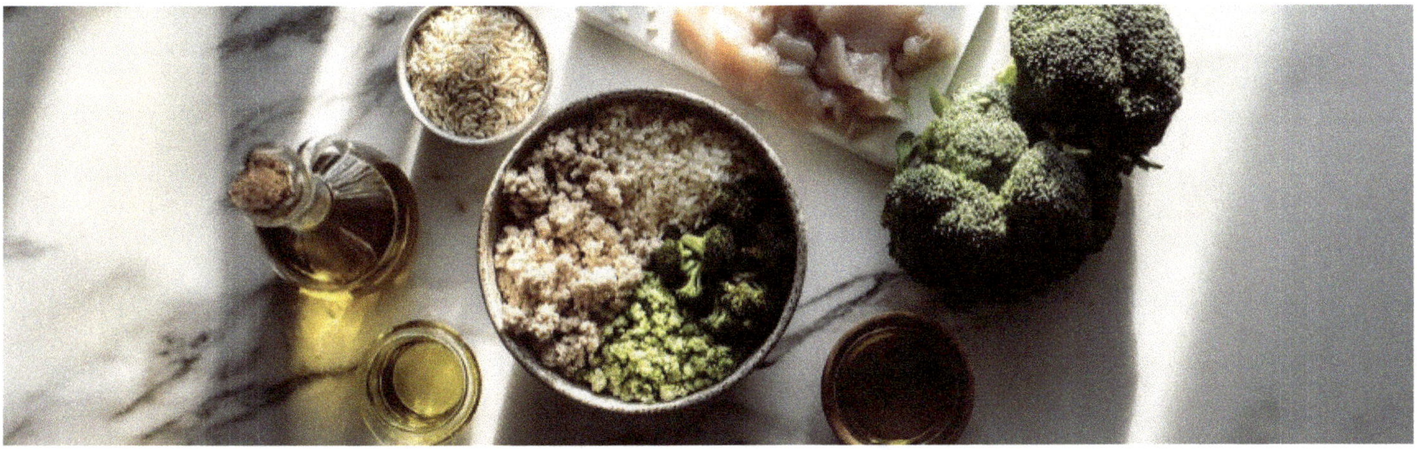

Ingredients:

- 1 lb. ground chicken (93% lean)
- 1 cup steamed broccoli (chopped)
- ½ cup cooked brown rice
- 1 tsp flaxseed oil
- 1 tsp olive oil

Instructions:

1. Cook chicken thoroughly.
2. Stir in broccoli and brown rice.
3. Mix in oils.
4. Let cool before serving.

Ingredient Substitutions:

- Replace brown rice with quinoa.
- Swap broccoli with green beans.

Nutrition per 500g serving:

Final Weight	~500g
Calories	~530 kcal
Protein	~38g
Fat	~20g
Carbohydrates	~30g

4. Beef & Spinach Weight Control Bowl

(Lean beef with nutrient-dense greens for fullness and energy balance)

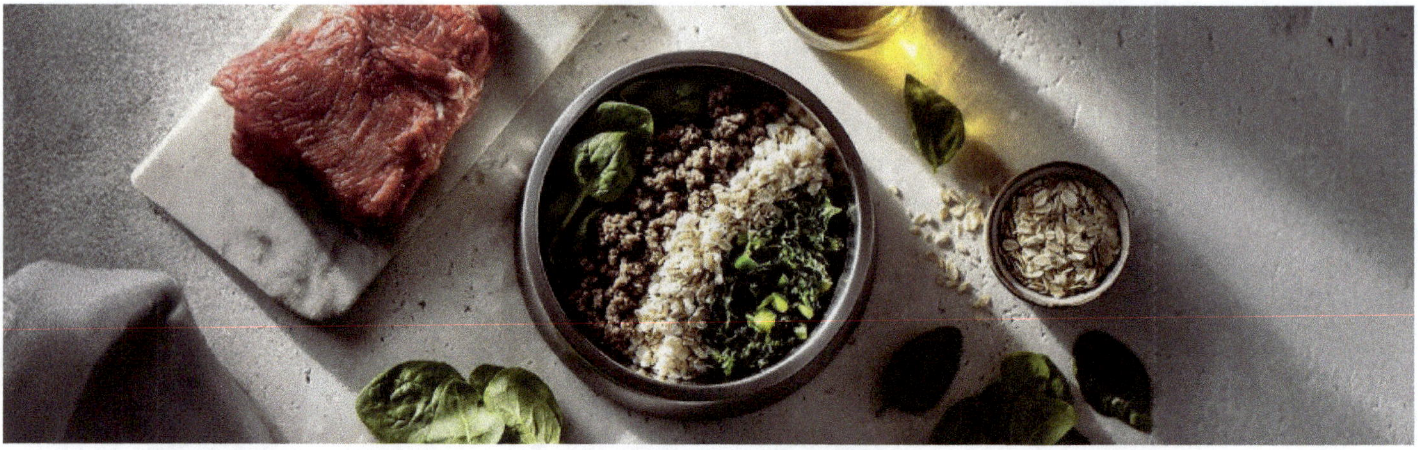

Ingredients:

- 1 lb. lean ground beef (90% lean)
- 1 cup steamed spinach (chopped)
- ½ cup cooked oats
- 1 tsp flaxseed oil
- 1 tsp olive oil

Instructions:

1. Brown beef thoroughly.
2. Stir in spinach and oats.
3. Mix in oils.
4. Let cool before serving.

Ingredient Substitutions:

- Replace oats with brown rice.
- Swap spinach with broccoli.

Nutrition per 500g serving:

Final Weight	~500g
Calories	~540 kcal
Protein	~40g
Fat	~22g
Carbohydrates	~30g

5. Egg & Pumpkin Slim Meal

(Low-calorie, high-fiber, gentle on digestion, ideal for weight loss)

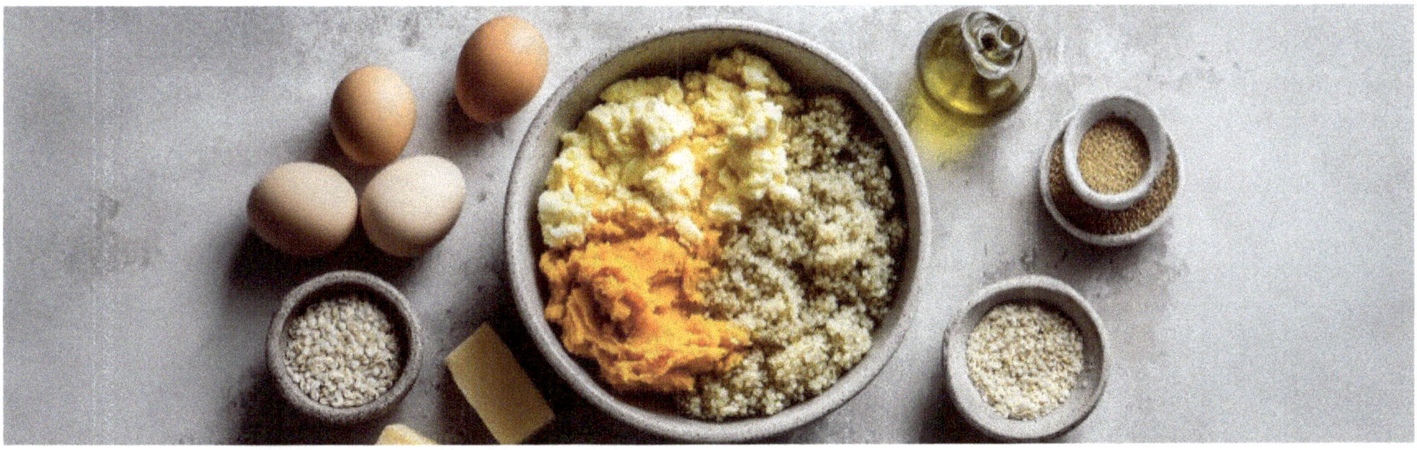

Ingredients:

- 3 large scrambled eggs
- 1 cup mashed pumpkin
- ½ cup cooked quinoa
- 1 tsp flaxseed oil
- 1 tsp olive oil

Instructions:

1. Scramble eggs gently.
2. Stir in mashed pumpkin and quinoa.
3. Mix in oils.
4. Let cool before serving.

Ingredient Substitutions:

- Replace quinoa with oats.
- Swap pumpkin with sweet potato (if needed for variety).

Nutrition per 500g serving:

Final Weight	~500g
Calories	~520 kcal
Protein	~36g
Fat	~20g
Carbohydrates	~28g

6. Turkey & Flaxseed Skin Booster (Weight Management)

(Linoleic acid-rich, vitamin-packed meal formulated to enhance skin health, soft fur, and support overall coat quality in adult dogs)

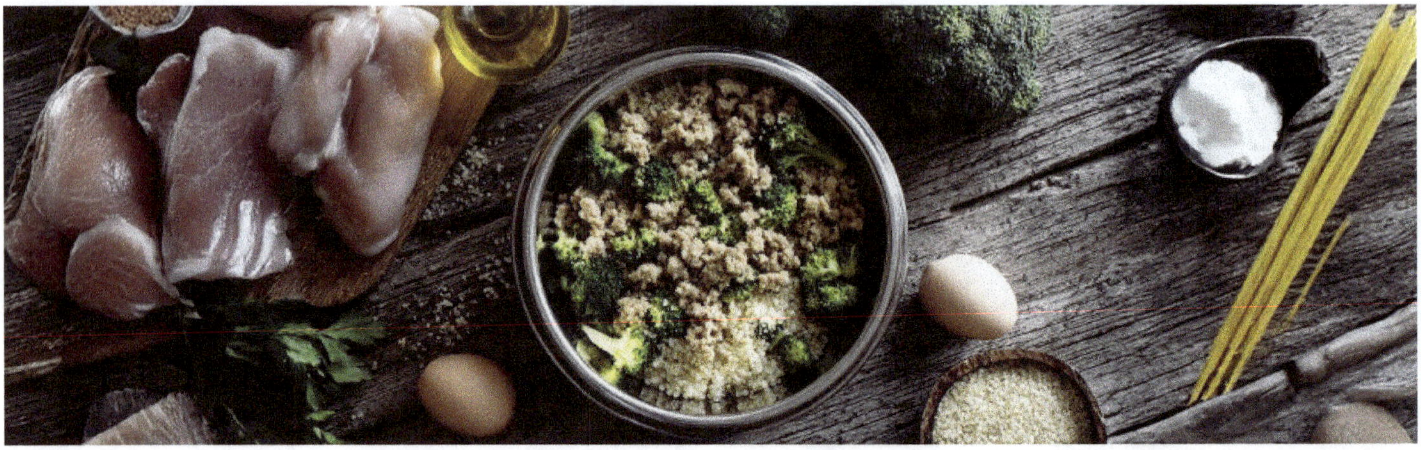

Ingredients:

- 1 lb. (450g) ground turkey (lean, 93%)
- 1 cup (185g) cooked quinoa
- ½ cup (90g) steamed broccoli (chopped)
- 1 tsp fish oil (anchovy/salmon oil; Omega-3 EPA/DHA + Vitamin D)
- ½ tsp ground eggshell powder (or 500 mg calcium carbonate powder; for calcium balance)

Optional:

- ¼ cup steamed kale, green beans, or spinach for fiber & antioxidants

Instructions:

1. Cook ground turkey over medium heat until fully browned (no oil). Drain excess fat.
2. Cook quinoa according to package instructions.
3. Steam broccoli, then chop finely.
4. Mix all ingredients, including fish oil, eggshell powder, and optional veggies.
5. Let cool before serving.

Ingredient Substitutions:

- Replace turkey with chicken or lean beef.
- Swap quinoa for oatmeal.
- Use steamed kale instead of broccoli for added antioxidants.

Nutrition per 500g serving:

Final Weight	~500g
Calories	~800 kcal
Protein	~42g
Fat	~18g
Carbohydrates	~35g

7. Salmon & Sweet Potato Glow Bowl (Weight management)

(Omega-3 powerhouse recipe designed to promote a glossy coat, healthy skin, and reduce inflammation in adult dogs)

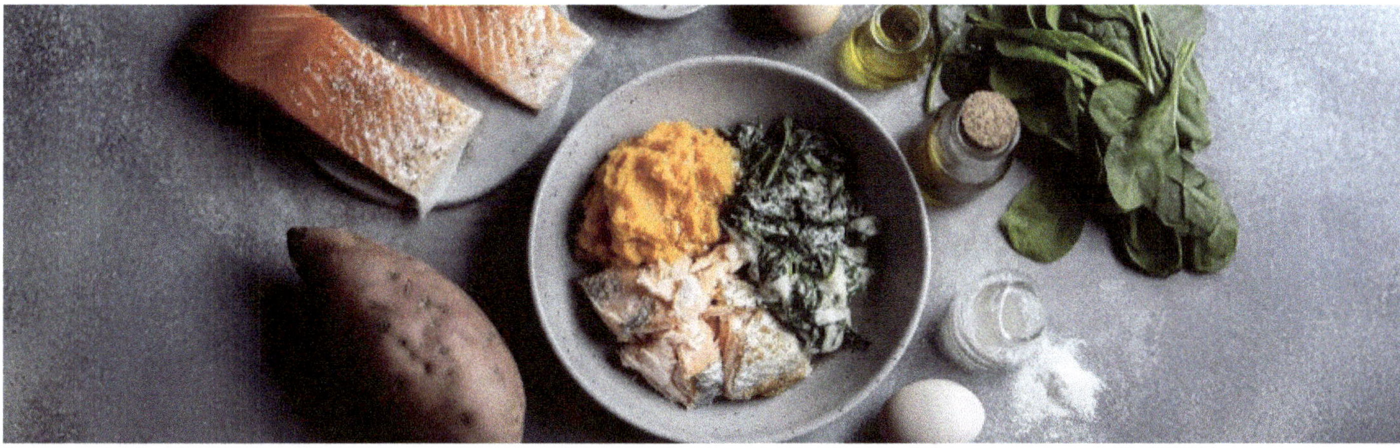

Ingredients:

- 1 lb. (450g) cooked salmon (or sardines/ mackerel; flaked, boneless)
- 1 cup (245g) cooked sweet potato (mashed)
- ½ cup (90g) steamed spinach (chopped)
- 1 tsp flaxseed oil (ALA source)
- 1 tsp fish oil (anchovy/salmon oil; rich in EPA/ DHA & Vitamin D)
- ½ tsp ground eggshell powder (or 500 mg calcium carbonate powder; for calcium balance)

Optional:

- ¼ cup steamed kale, green beans, or carrots for added fiber and antioxidants

Instructions:

1. Bake or steam salmon (or sardines) until fully cooked, flake into small pieces.
2. Cook sweet potato until soft, then mash it.
3. Steam spinach, then chop finely.
4. Combine all ingredients, including flaxseed oil, fish oil, eggshell powder, and optional veggies.
5. Let cool before serving.

Ingredient Substitutions:

- Swap salmon for mackerel or sardines for even more omega-3s.
- Replace sweet potato with pumpkin puree for extra fiber.
- Use kale instead of spinach for higher Vitamin C content.

Nutrition per 500g serving:

Final Weight	~500g
Calories	~900 kcal
Protein	~42g
Fat	~24g
Carbohydrates	~30g

8. Sardine & Brown Rice Shine Meal (Weight Management)

(Omega-rich, selenium-packed meal designed to promote skin hydration, antioxidant protection, and coat shine in adult dogs)

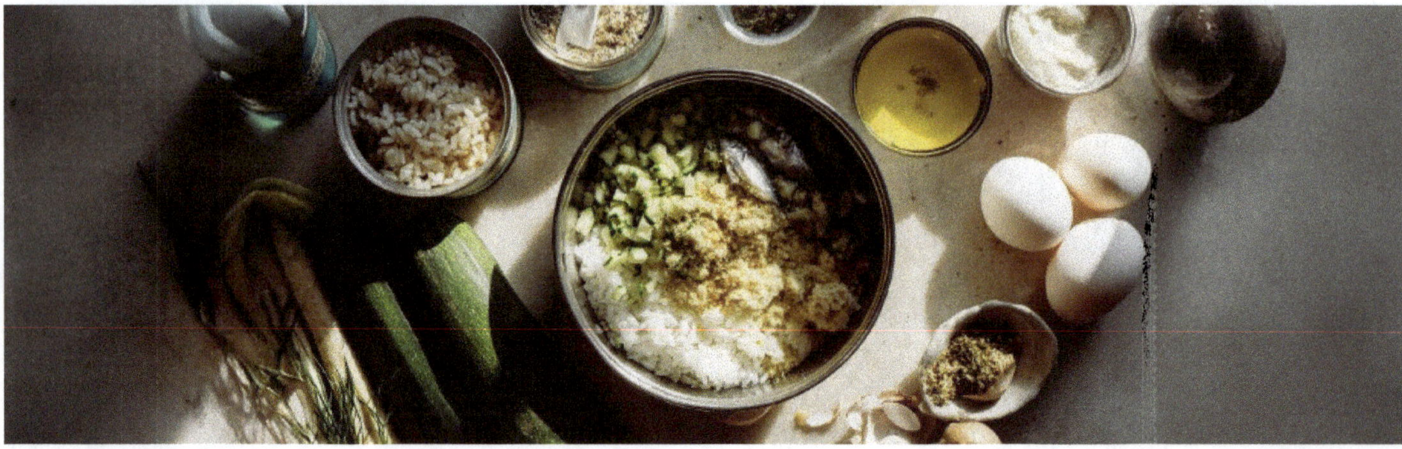

Ingredients:

- 1 lb. (450g) canned sardines in water (no salt, with soft bones mashed)
- 1 cup (195g) cooked brown rice
- ½ cup (90g) steamed zucchini (chopped)
- 1 tsp coconut oil (provides MCTs & skin moisture)
- ½ tsp ground eggshell powder (adjust carefully; ~500 mg calcium carbonate powder equivalent)

Optional:

- ¼ cup steamed carrots, green beans, or spinach for extra fiber & vitamins

Instructions:

1. Mash sardines in a bowl (ensure soft bones are mixed thoroughly).
2. Cook brown rice according to package instructions.
3. Steam zucchini, then chop finely.
4. Combine sardines, rice, zucchini, coconut oil, eggshell powder, and optional veggies.
5. Let cool before serving.

Ingredient Substitutions:

- Swap sardines for salmon or tuna (note: check mercury levels with tuna).
- Replace brown rice with quinoa for added protein.
- Use steamed carrots instead of zucchini for more Vitamin A.

Nutrition per 500g serving:

Final Weight	~500g
Calories	~850 kcal
Protein	~42g
Fat	~20g
Carbohydrates	~35g

9. Beef & Cauliflower Fat-Burn Mix

(A low-carb, high-protein, nutrient-dense meal ideal for active dogs focused on fat metabolism, muscle maintenance, and weight control)

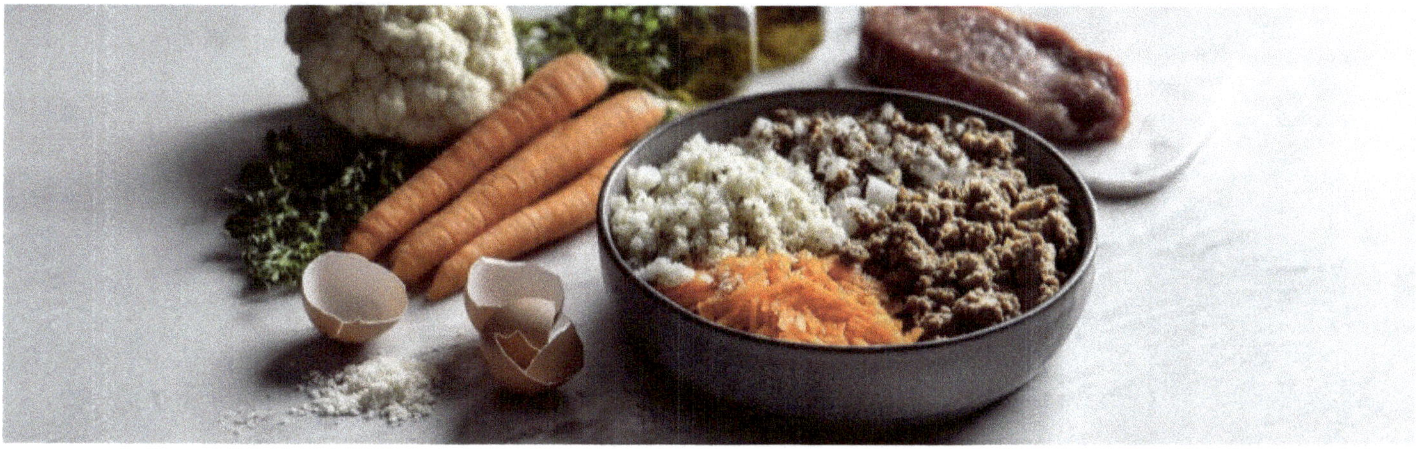

Ingredients:

- 1 lb. (450g) lean ground beef (90% lean)
- 1 cup (125g) cooked cauliflower rice
- ½ cup (80g) steamed carrots (chopped)
- 1 tsp fish oil (anchovy/salmon oil; source of Omega-3 EPA/DHA + Vitamin D)
- ½ tsp ground eggshell powder (or 500 mg calcium carbonate powder; for calcium balance)

Optional:

- ¼ cup steamed spinach, green beans, or broccoli for added fiber & micronutrients

Instructions:

1. Cook ground beef in a pan over medium heat until fully browned (no oil required). Drain excess fat.
2. In another pan, steam cauliflower rice until soft.
3. Likewise, steam carrots, then chop into small chunks.
4. Mix all ingredients, including fish oil, eggshell powder, and optional veggies.
5. Let cool before serving.

Ingredient Substitutions:

- Swap beef for turkey or chicken.
- Use broccoli rice instead of cauliflower rice.
- Replace carrots with pumpkin puree for extra fiber.

Nutrition per 500g serving:

Final Weight	~500g
Calories	~800 kcal
Protein	~42g
Fat	~18g
Carbohydrates	~25g

10. Lamb & Cabbage Weight Control Meal

(Lean, antioxidant-rich meal designed to support muscle retention and weight management in adult dogs)

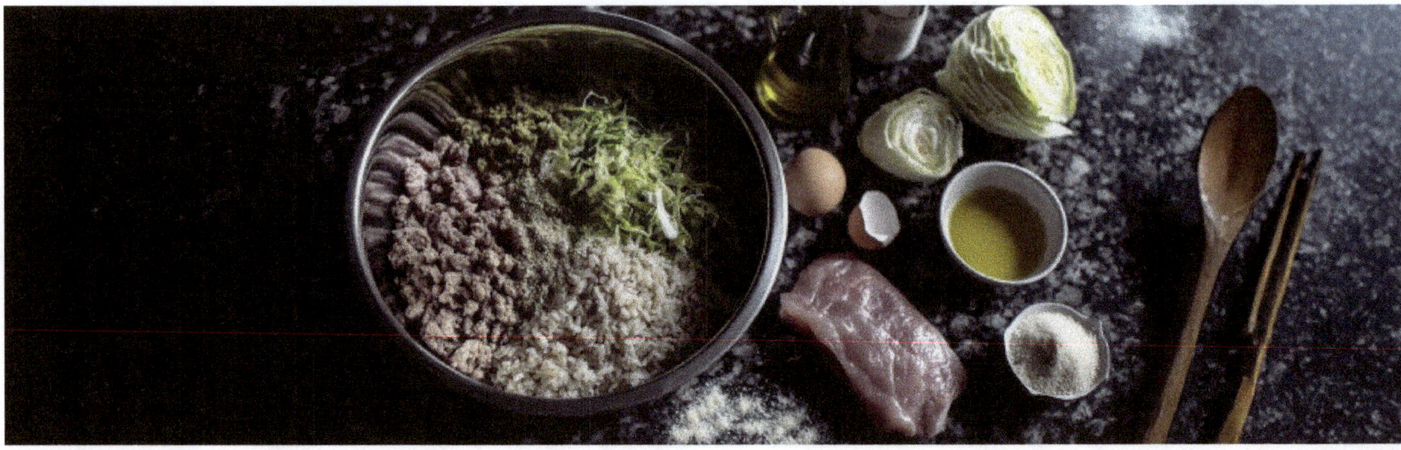

Ingredients:

- 1 lb. (450g) ground lamb (85% lean)
- 1 cup (195g) cooked brown rice
- ½ cup (75g) steamed cabbage (chopped)
- 1 tsp olive oil (Omega-6 source)
- 1 tsp fish oil (anchovy/salmon oil; Omega-3 EPA/DHA + Vitamin D)
- ½ tsp ground eggshell powder (or 500 mg calcium carbonate powder; for calcium balance)

Optional:

- ¼ cup steamed bok choy or spinach for fiber boost

Instructions:

1. Without using any oil, cook ground lamb in a pan over medium heat until fully browned. Drain excess fat.
2. Cook brown rice according to package instructions.
3. Steam cabbage, chop into small pieces.
4. Combine all ingredients, adding olive oil, fish oil, eggshell powder, and optional veggies.
5. Serve when cooled.

Ingredient Substitutions:

- Swap lamb for lean turkey or beef.
- Replace brown rice with quinoa for higher protein.
- Use bok choy instead of cabbage for extra crunch.

Nutrition per 500g serving:

Final Weight	~500g
Calories	~825 kcal
Protein	~40g
Fat	~18g
Carbohydrates	~35g

Senior Dog Recipes

Your senior furry friend needs extra care, which means meals that ease joint pain, boost immunity, and are easy to digest. These recipes are designed to do just that.

Joint Supporting Recipes

1. Salmon & Pumpkin Joint Care Meal

(Omega-3-rich, senior-friendly recipe designed to support joint lubrication, reduce inflammation, and maintain mobility in older dogs)

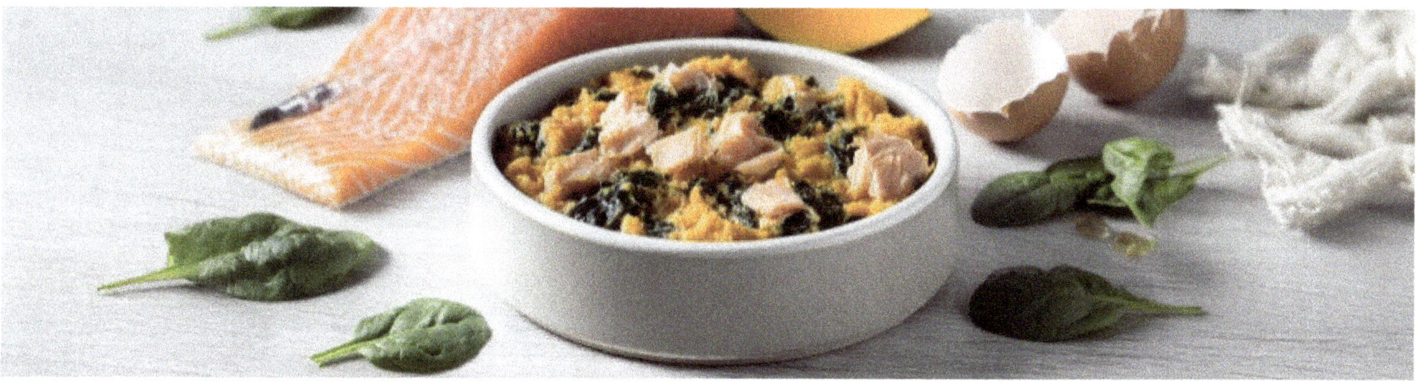

Ingredients:

- 1 lb. (450g) cooked salmon (or sardines/mackerel; flaked, boneless)
- 1 cup (245g) cooked pumpkin (plain, unsweetened)
- ½ cup (90g) steamed spinach (chopped)
- 1 tsp fish oil (anchovy/salmon oil; source of extra EPA/DHA + Vitamin D)
- ½ tsp ground eggshell powder (or 500 mg calcium carbonate powder; for calcium balance)

Optional:

- ¼ tsp turmeric powder or green-lipped mussel powder (for added joint support)

Instructions:

1. Bake or steam salmon until fully cooked, then flake into small pieces.
2. Cook pumpkin until soft, mash.
3. Steam spinach, chop finely.
4. Combine all ingredients, adding fish oil, eggshell powder, and optional joint supplements.
5. Let cool before serving.

Ingredient Substitutions:

- Swap salmon for mackerel or sardines for even higher DHA.
- Use sweet potato instead of pumpkin for extra fiber.
- Replace spinach with kale for added antioxidants.

Nutrition per 500g serving:

Final Weight	~500g
Calories	~520 kcal
Protein	~36g
Fat	~20g
Carbohydrates	~28g

2. Turkey & Quinoa Mobility Meal

(Protein-packed, glucosamine-rich recipe designed to protect cartilage, reduce inflammation, and support senior dogs' mobility)

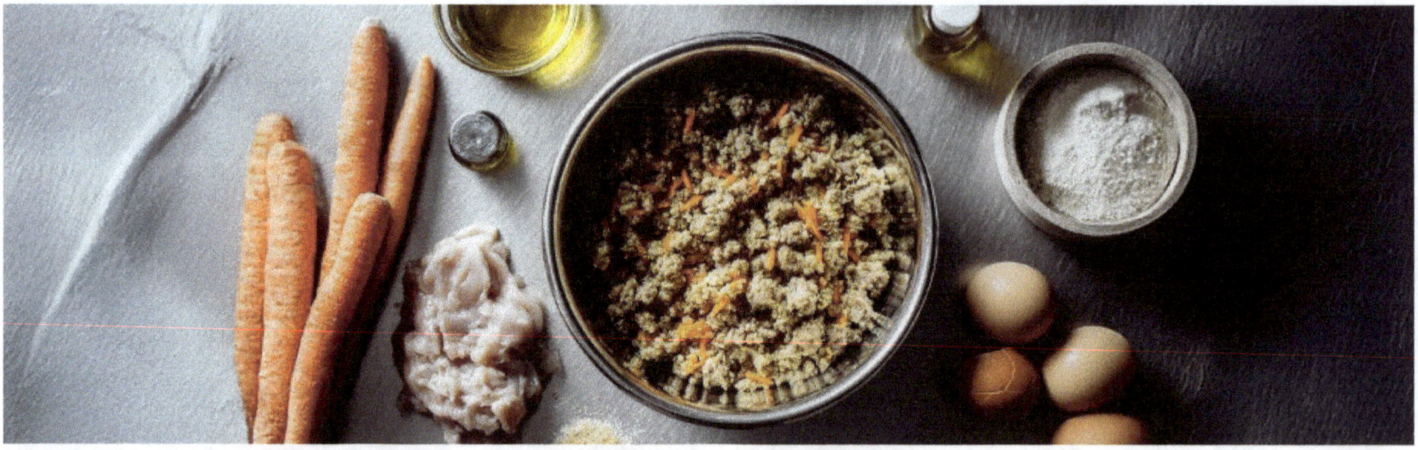

Ingredients:

- 1 lb. (450g) ground turkey (lean, 93%)
- 1 cup (185g) cooked quinoa
- ½ cup (80g) steamed carrots (chopped)
- 1 tsp flaxseed oil (ALA source, anti-inflammatory)
- 1 tsp fish oil (anchovy/salmon oil; EPA/DHA + Vitamin D)
- ½ tsp ground eggshell powder (or 500 mg calcium carbonate powder; for calcium balance)

Optional:

- ¼ tsp turmeric powder or ¼ tsp green-lipped mussel powder for joint health
- ¼ cup steamed spinach or green beans for extra fiber & nutrients

Instructions:

1. Cook ground turkey over medium heat until fully browned (no oil required). Drain excess fat.
2. Cook quinoa according to package instructions.
3. Steam carrots, then chop finely.
4. Combine all ingredients, including flaxseed oil, fish oil, eggshell powder, and optional joint boosters.
5. Allow to cool before serving.

Ingredient Substitutions:

- Use chicken instead of turkey.
- Swap quinoa for brown rice for a lighter meal.
- Replace carrots with zucchini for added hydration.

Nutrition per 500g serving:

Final Weight	~500g
Calories	~800 kcal
Protein	~42g
Fat	~18g
Carbohydrates	~35g

3. Lamb & Green Bean Joint Relief Meal

(Rich in collagen and zinc, this senior-friendly meal supports joint repair, tissue strength, and mobility)

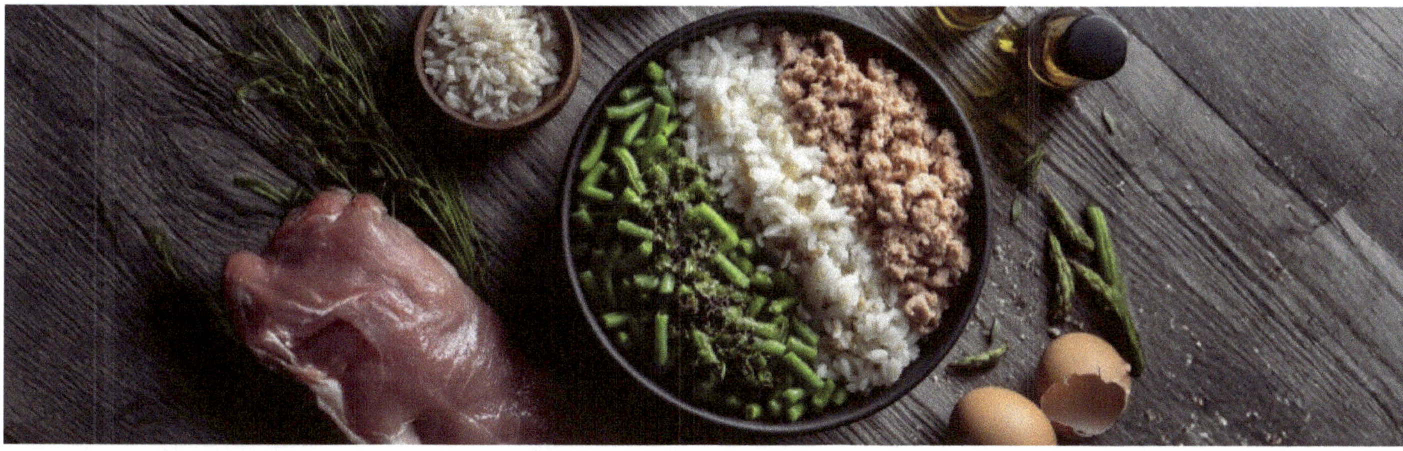

Ingredients:

- 1 lb. (450g) ground lamb (lean, 85%)
- 1 cup (195g) cooked brown rice
- ½ cup (80g) steamed green beans (chopped)
- 1 tsp fish oil (anchovy/salmon oil; source of Omega-3 EPA/DHA + Vitamin D)
- ½ tsp ground eggshell powder (or 500 mg calcium carbonate powder; for calcium balance)

Optional:

- ¼ tsp turmeric powder or green-lipped mussel powder for joint relief
- Add ¼ cup steamed broccoli or spinach for antioxidants

Instructions:

1. Without using any oil, cook ground lamb over medium heat until fully browned. Drain excess fat.
2. Cook brown rice as per package instructions.
3. Steam green beans, then chop finely.
4. Combine lamb, rice, green beans, fish oil, eggshell powder, and optional supplements.
5. Let cool before serving.

Ingredient Substitutions:

- Swap lamb for lean beef or turkey.
- Use quinoa instead of brown rice for higher protein.
- Replace green beans with broccoli for added antioxidants.

Nutrition per 500g serving:

Final Weight	~500g
Calories	~850 kcal
Protein	~40g
Fat	~18g
Carbohydrates	~35g

4. Beef & Oatmeal Bone Support Meal

(A protein-rich, bone-strengthening recipe formulated to support skeletal health, joint function, and anti-inflammatory balance in senior dogs)

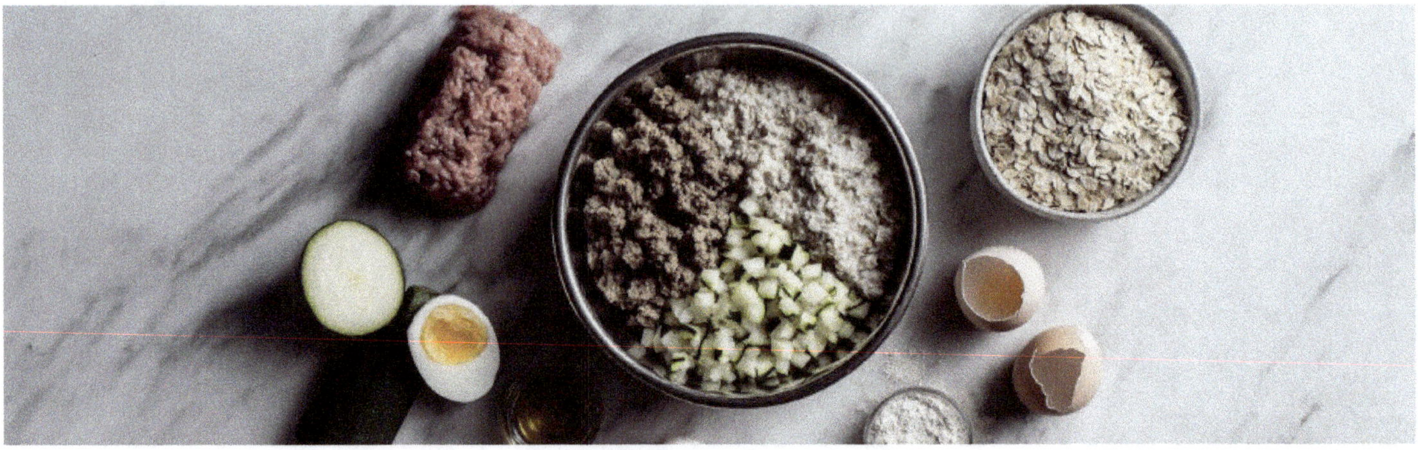

Ingredients:

- 1 lb. (450g) lean ground beef (90% lean)
- 1 cup (80g) cooked oatmeal (plain, unsweetened)
- ½ cup (80g) steamed zucchini (chopped)
- 1 tsp fish oil (anchovy/salmon oil; source of Omega-3 EPA/DHA + Vitamin D)
- ½ tsp ground eggshell powder (or 500 mg calcium carbonate powder; for calcium balance)

Optional:

- ¼ cup steamed carrots, spinach, or green beans for extra antioxidants & fiber

Instructions:

1. Cook ground beef in a pan over medium heat until fully browned (no oil required). Drain excess fat.
2. In another pan, prepare oatmeal using water only (no sugar/milk).
3. Steam zucchini, chop finely.
4. Combine beef, oatmeal, zucchini, fish oil, eggshell powder, and optional veggies.
5. Let cool before serving.

Ingredient Substitutions:

- Use chicken or turkey instead of beef for a leaner option.
- Replace oatmeal with barley for added fiber.
- Swap zucchini with steamed carrots for beta-carotene.

Nutrition per 500g serving:

Final Weight	~500g
Calories	~825 kcal
Protein	~40g
Fat	~18g
Carbohydrates	~30g

5. Mackerel & Barley Inflammation Control Meal

(Omega-3 & antioxidant-rich senior recipe designed to lubricate joints, reduce inflammation, and support mobility)

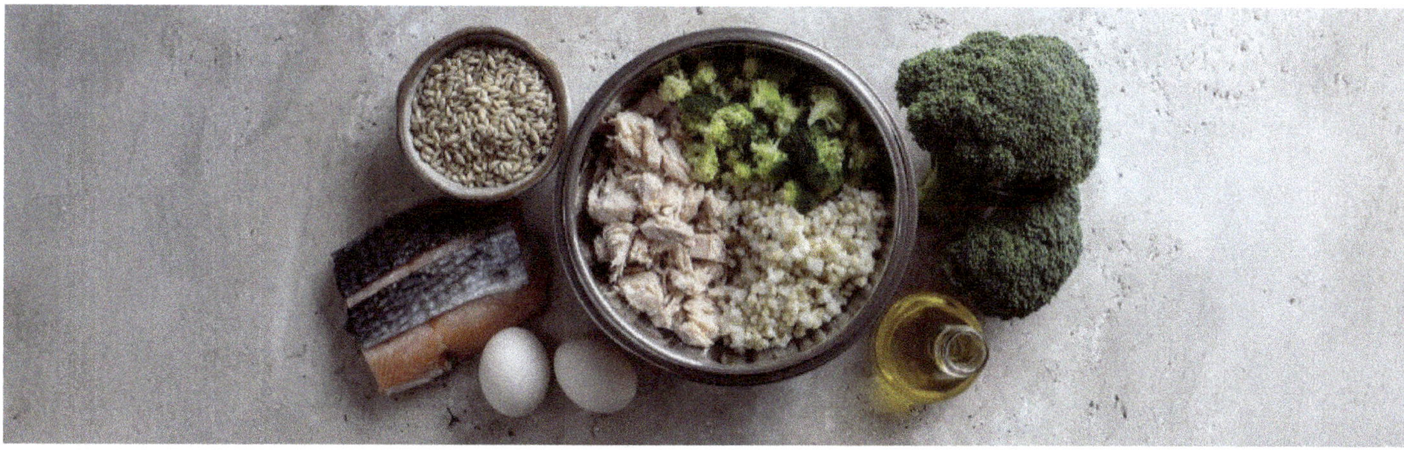

Ingredients:

- 1 lb. (450g) cooked mackerel (or sardines/ salmon; flaked, boneless)
- 1 cup (200g) cooked barley
- ½ cup (90g) steamed broccoli (chopped)
- 1 tsp fish oil (anchovy/salmon oil; extra EPA/DHA + Vitamin D)
- ½ tsp ground eggshell powder (or 500 mg calcium carbonate powder; for calcium balance)

Optional:

- ¼ cup steamed spinach or carrots for extra fiber & antioxidants

Instructions:

1. Bake or steam mackerel until fully cooked, then flake.
2. Cook barley according to package instructions.
3. Steam broccoli, chop finely.
4. Combine all ingredients including fish oil, eggshell powder, and optional veggies.
5. Let cool before serving.

Ingredient Substitutions:

- Swap mackerel for salmon or sardines.
- Use quinoa instead of barley for a grain-free alternative.
- Replace broccoli with zucchini for lower carbs.

Nutrition per 500g serving:

Final Weight	~500g
Calories	~850 kcal
Protein	~42g
Fat	~20g
Carbohydrates	~35g

6. Salmon & Pumpkin Mobility Meal for Seniors

(Omega-3 powerhouse, supports joint lubrication and mobility)

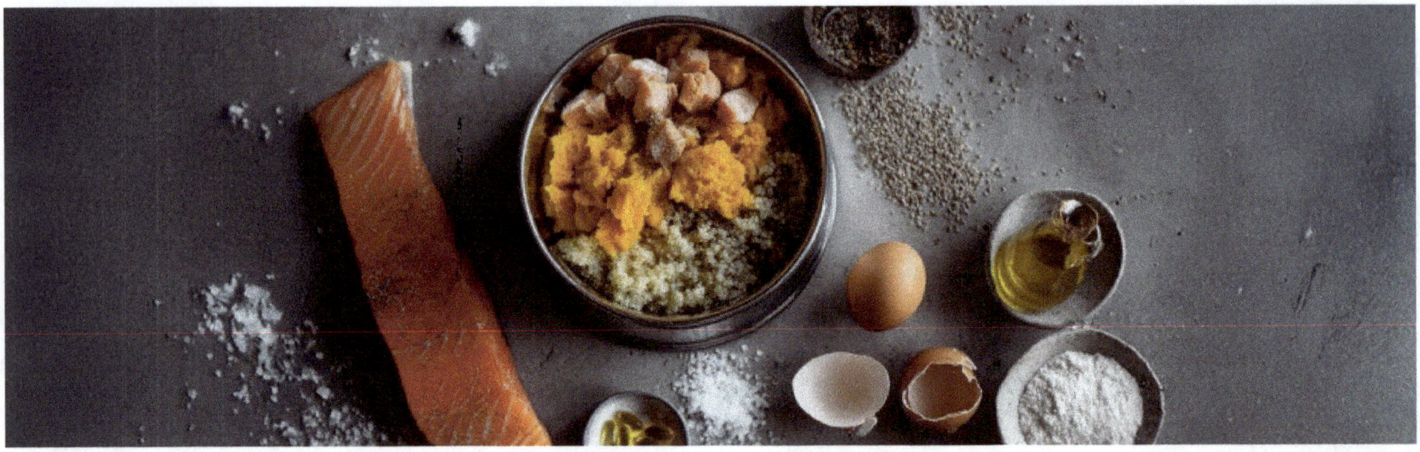

Ingredients:

- 1 lb. cooked boneless salmon (steamed)
- 1 cup cooked pumpkin (mashed)
- ½ cup cooked quinoa
- 2 tsp fish oil (for extra DHA & EPA)
- 1 tsp ground eggshell powder OR 2 crushed calcium tablets
- ½ tsp iodized salt

Optional:

- ¼ tsp turmeric powder (anti-inflammatory)

Instructions:

1. Steam salmon until fully cooked, flake into small pieces.
2. Mix in mashed pumpkin and quinoa.
3. Stir in fish oil, calcium source, salt, and turmeric (optional).
4. Let cool before serving.

Ingredient Substitutions:

- Swap quinoa for brown rice.
- Replace pumpkin with sweet potato.

Nutrition per 500g serving:

Final Weight	~500g
Calories	~600 kcal
Protein	~42g
Fat	~26g
Carbohydrates	~38g

7. Rabbit & Chickpea Joint Support Bowl for Seniors

(Lean protein plus glucosamine boost for cartilage and joints)

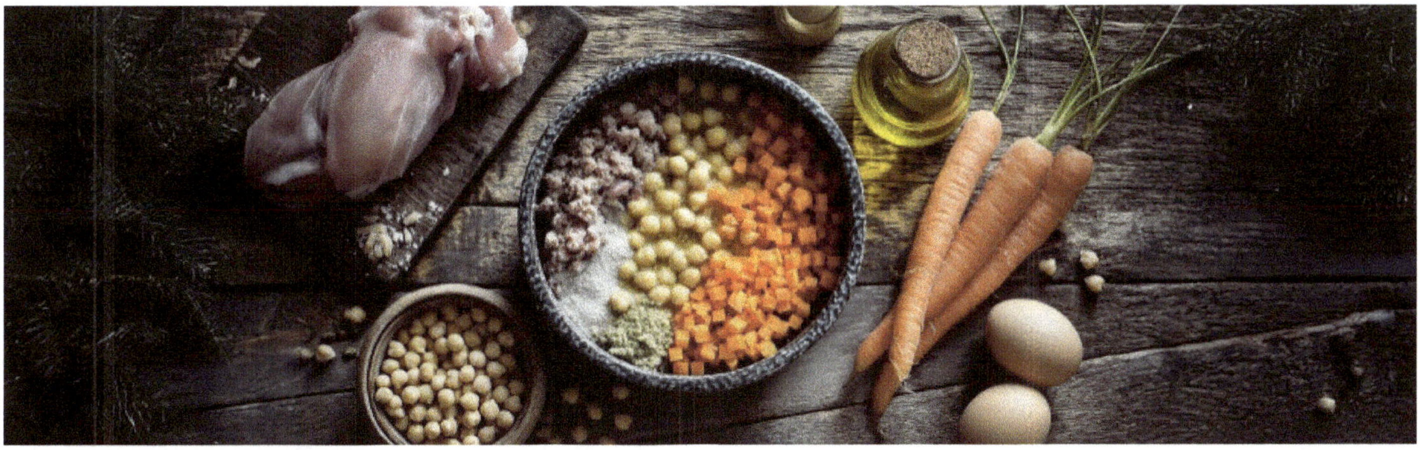

Ingredients:

- 1 lb. (450g) ground rabbit (lean)
- 1 cup (200g) cooked chickpeas (mashed)
- ½ cup (75g) steamed carrots (chopped)
- 1 tsp flaxseed oil
- 1 tsp ground eggshell powder OR 2 crushed calcium tablets

Instructions:

1. Cook rabbit thoroughly and drain excess fat.
2. Stir in cooked chickpeas and steamed carrot
3. Mix in flaxseed oil and your calcium source.
4. Let cool before serving.

Ingredient Substitutions:

- Replace chickpeas with pinto beans.
- Swap rabbit for ground pork loin.

Nutrition per 500g serving:

Final Weight	~500g
Calories	~970 kcal
Protein	~70g
Fat	~20g
Carbohydrates	~45g

8. Lamb & Oats Senior Joint Booster

(Mineral-rich lamb meal for joint support and muscle maintenance)

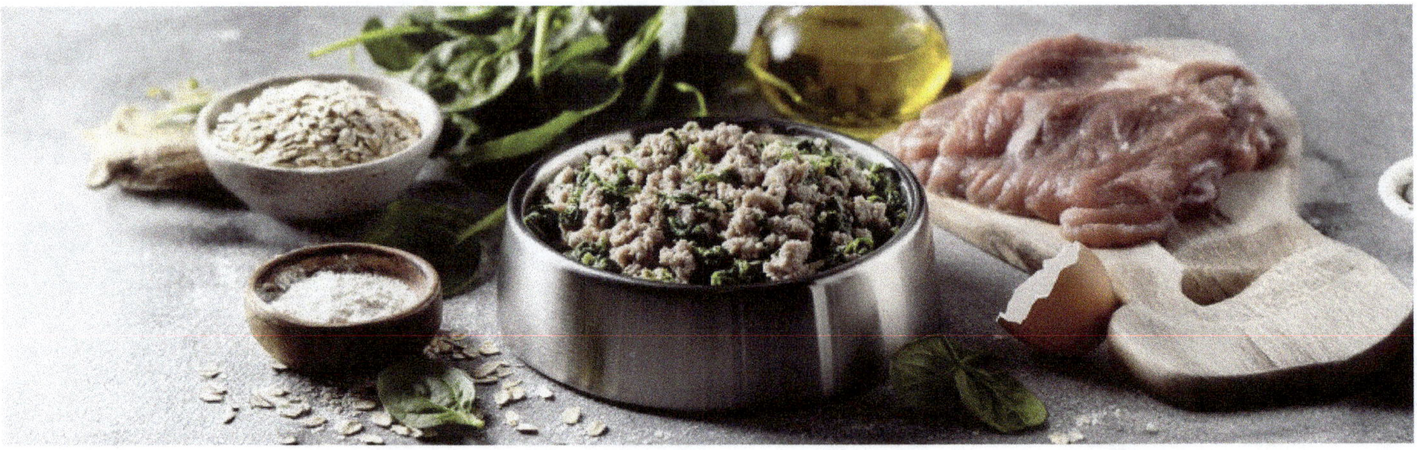

Ingredients:

- 1 lb. ground lamb (85% lean)
- 1 cup cooked oats
- ½ cup steamed spinach (chopped)
- 1 tsp olive oil or 1 tsp fish oil
- 1 tsp ground eggshell powder OR 2 crushed calcium tablets

Optional:

- ¼ tsp turmeric powder

Instructions:

1. Cook lamb in a pan until fully browned.
2. Mix in cooked oats and chopped steamed spinach.
3. Stir in oils, calcium source, and turmeric (optional).
4. Let cool before serving.

Ingredient Substitutions:

- Swap oats for brown rice.
- Replace lamb with lean beef.

Nutrition per 500g serving:

Final Weight	~500g
Calories	~650 kcal
Protein	~40g
Fat	~28g
Carbohydrates	~42g

Easy-To-Chew Options for Aging Dogs

1. Cod & Tapioca Soft Senior Blend

(Easy-to-chew, protein-rich, senior-friendly meal supporting digestion, joint health, and nutrient balance)

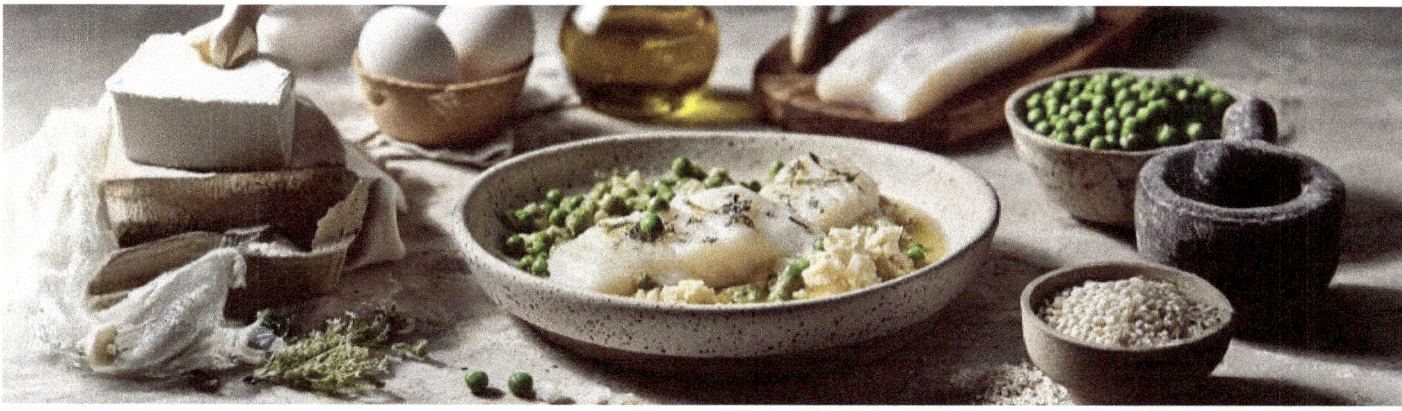

Ingredients:

- 1 lb. (450g) boneless cod
- 1 cup (200g) cooked tapioca
- ½ cup (90g) cooked peas
- 1 tsp fish oil
- ½ tsp ground eggshell powder

Optional:

- ¼ cup steamed carrot or pumpkin for added softness & nutrients

Instructions:

1. In a steamer, cook cod over medium heat until fully cooked, then flake.
2. Boil tapioca pearls (1:3 water ratio) or prepare tapioca starch until soft, mash.
3. Steam peas, mash thoroughly.
4. Combine all ingredients, including fish oil, eggshell powder, and optional veggies.
5. Allow to cool before serving.

Ingredient Substitutions:

- Use tilapia or whitefish instead of cod.
- Replace tapioca with mashed potato for a different texture.
- Swap peas with steamed zucchini or spinach for variety.

Nutrition per 500g serving:

Final Weight	~500g
Calories	~1130g
Protein	~78g
Fat	~20g
Carbohydrates	~60 g

2. Slow-Cooked Chicken & Rice Porridge

(A gentle, soft-textured senior meal tailored for sensitive teeth and digestion, while ensuring nutrient balance and anti-inflammatory support)

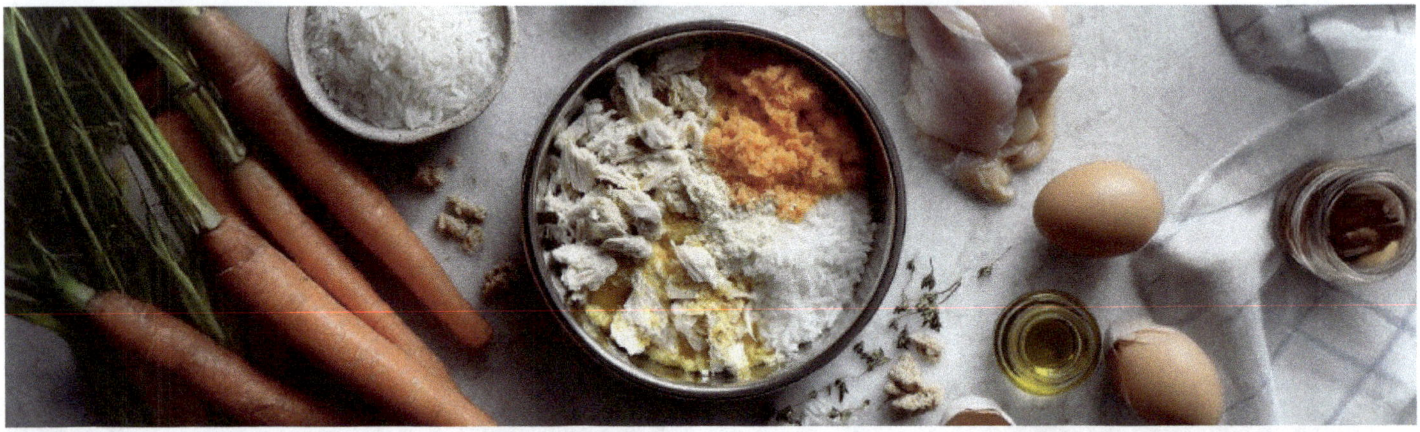

Ingredients:

- 1 lb. (450g) boneless, skinless chicken breast (boiled & shredded)
- 1 cup (195g) cooked white rice (cooked very soft)
- ½ cup (80g) cooked carrots (mashed)
- 1 tsp flaxseed oil (ALA source, skin & coat)
- ½ tsp ground eggshell powder (or 500 mg calcium carbonate powder; for calcium balance)

Optional:

- Add warm water or low-sodium broth for extra hydration
- ¼ cup cooked butternut squash or spinach (mashed) for extra fiber & vitamins

Instructions:

1. Boil chicken breast until fully cooked, shred finely.
2. Cook white rice until very soft and porridge-like.
3. Boil or steam carrots (and optional veggies), mash thoroughly.
4. Mix all ingredients, including flaxseed oil, eggshell powder, and optional broth or water.
5. Serve warm or cooled to desired consistency.

Ingredient Substitutions:

- Replace chicken with turkey or white fish.
- Use quinoa instead of rice for extra protein.
- Swap carrots with butternut squash or pumpkin for more vitamins.

Nutrition per 500g serving:

Final Weight	~500g
Calories	~754g
Protein	~74.1g
Fat	~33.8g
Carbohydrates	~33.8g

3. Beef & Pumpkin Stew

(A moist, soft senior meal designed to promote digestion, joint health, and muscle maintenance while ensuring easy chewing and nutrient balance)

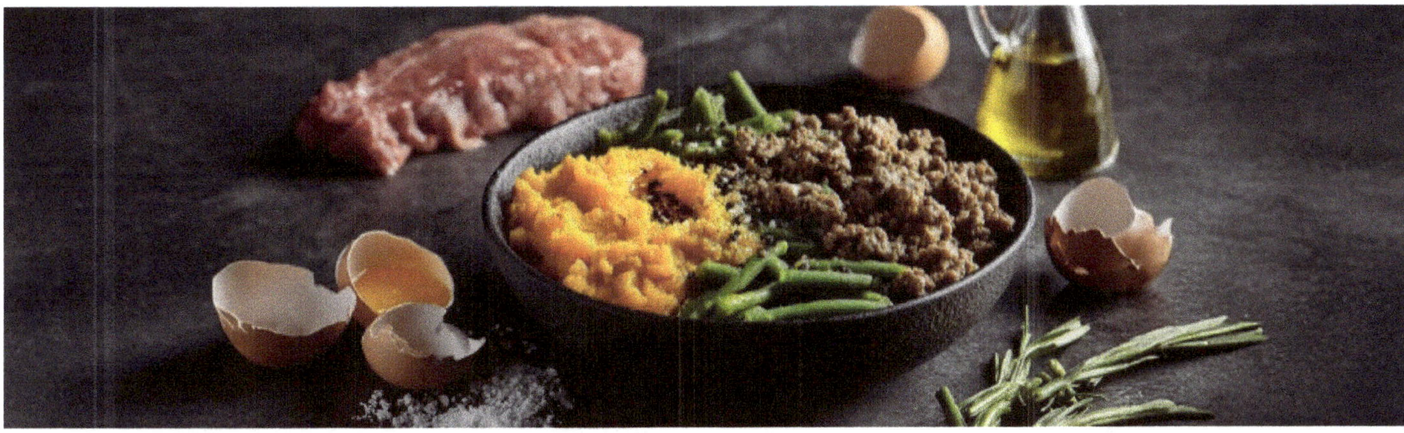

Ingredients:

- 1 lb. (450g) lean ground beef (90% lean)
- 1 cup (245g) cooked pumpkin (mashed)
- ½ cup (90g) cooked green beans (mashed)
- 1 tsp fish oil (anchovy/salmon oil; EPA/DHA + Vitamin D)
- ½ tsp ground eggshell powder (or 500 mg calcium carbonate powder; for calcium balance)

Optional:

- Add warm water or low-sodium broth for stew consistency
- ¼ cup steamed spinach or carrots (mashed) for antioxidants & extra fiber

Instructions:

1. In a non-stick pan, cook ground beef without any oil over medium heat until fully browned. Drain excess fat.
2. Cook pumpkin until soft, mash.
3. Steam green beans (and optional veggies), mash thoroughly.
4. Mix everything together, including fish oil, eggshell powder, and add warm water or broth for desired stew texture.
5. Let cool before serving.

Ingredient Substitutions:

- Use tilapia or whitefish instead of cod.
- Use sweet potatoes instead of pumpkin for added fiber.
- Swap green beans with spinach or carrots for extra antioxidants.

Nutrition per 500g serving:

Final Weight	~500g
Calories	~796 kcal
Protein	~76.1g
Fat	~48.6g
Carbohydrates	~22.5g

4. Fish & Oatmeal Soft Blend

(A brain-boosting, soft-textured senior meal designed to promote cognitive health, joint lubrication, and easy chewing while ensuring balanced nutrition)

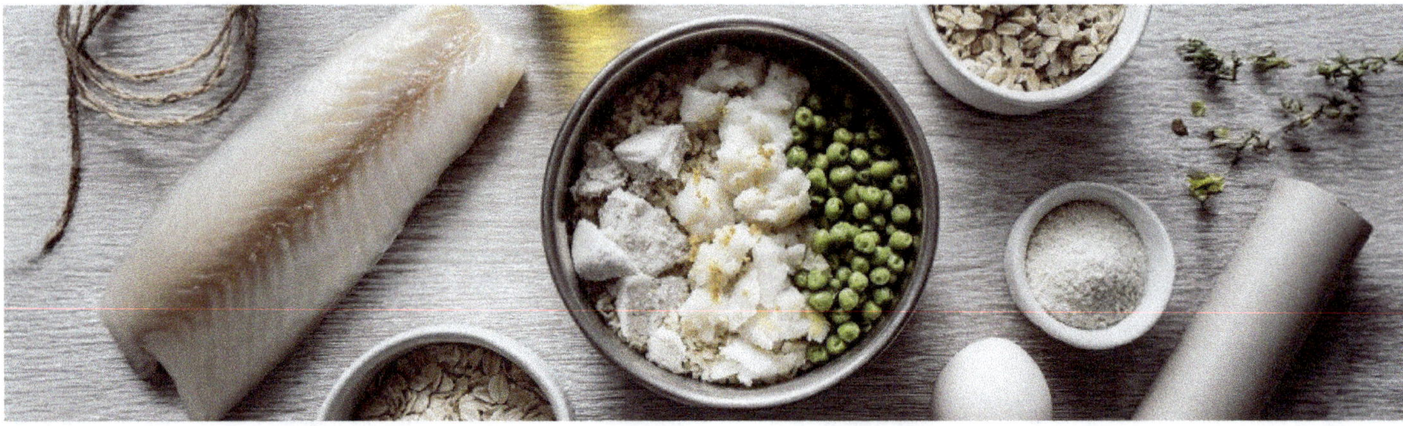

Ingredients:

- 1 lb. (450g) cooked cod (or white fish; flaked, boneless)
- 1 cup (80g) cooked oatmeal (extra water for mushy texture)
- ½ cup (80g) cooked peas (mashed)
- 1 tsp fish oil (anchovy/salmon oil; rich in EPA/ DHA + Vitamin D)
- ½ tsp ground eggshell powder (or 500 mg calcium carbonate powder; for calcium balance)

Optional:

- Add mashed carrots, pumpkin, or spinach for extra vitamins & fiber
- Add warm water or low-sodium broth for smoother texture

Instructions:

1. Bake or steam cod until fully cooked, flake into small pieces.
2. Cook oatmeal with extra water until it becomes soft, porridge-like.
3. Steam peas (and optional veggies), mash thoroughly.
4. Mix everything together, including fish oil, eggshell powder, and warm broth if desired.
5. Let cool slightly before serving.

Ingredient Substitutions:

- Swap cod for salmon for even more omega-3s.
- Replace oatmeal with quinoa for higher protein.
- Use mashed carrots instead of peas for a Vitamin A boost.

Nutrition per 500g serving:

Final Weight	~500g
Calories	~516 kcal
Protein	~89g
Fat	~8g
Carbohydrates	~17g

5. Lamb & Barley Comfort Mash

(A soft, highly digestible senior meal formulated to support joints, immunity, and easy chewing while providing complete nutrient balance)

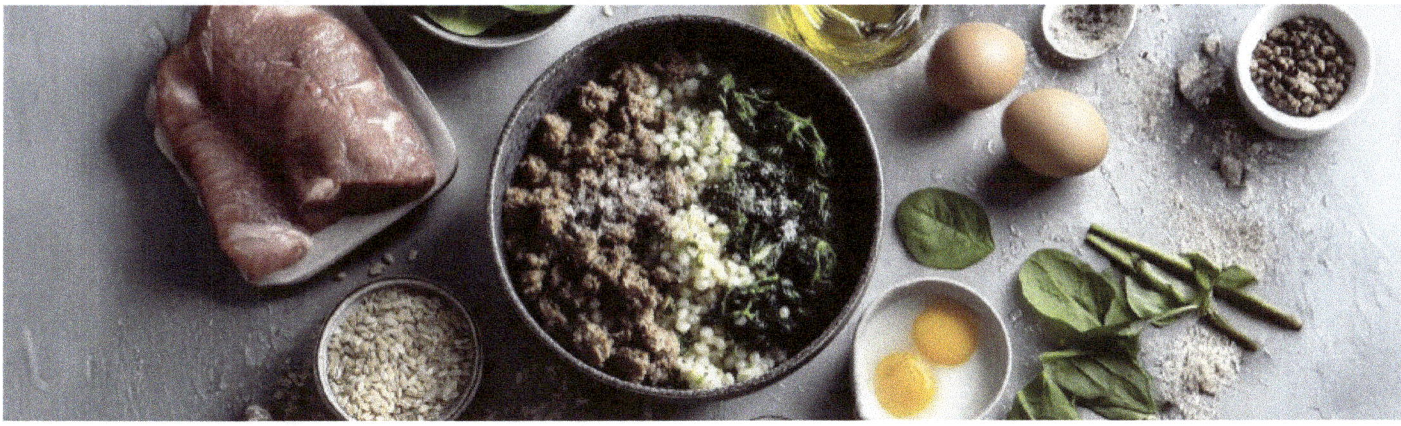

Ingredients:

- 1 lb. (450g) ground lamb (85% lean)
- 1 cup (200g) cooked barley (soft and mushy)
- ½ cup (90g) cooked spinach (mashed)
- 1 tsp coconut oil (MCT source)
- 1 tsp fish oil (anchovy/salmon oil; EPA/DHA + Vitamin D)
- ½ tsp ground eggshell powder (or 500 mg calcium carbonate powder; for calcium balance)

Optional:

- Add warm water or low-sodium broth for soft stew-like texture
- ¼ cup steamed kale, green beans, or pumpkin (mashed) for variety

Instructions:

1. Cook ground lamb in a pan over medium heat until fully browned (no oil). Drain excess fat.
2. Cook barley until very soft and mushy.
3. Steam spinach (and optional veggies), mash thoroughly.
4. Mix all ingredients together, adding coconut oil, fish oil, eggshell powder, and warm water/broth to desired softness.
5. Let cool before serving.

Ingredient Substitutions:

- Swap lamb for turkey or chicken.
- Replace barley with white rice for easier digestion.
- Use kale instead of spinach for more Vitamin C.

Nutrition per 500g serving:

Final Weight	~500g
Calories	~1114 kcal
Protein	~80g
Fat	~70g
Carbohydrates	~40g

6. Chicken & Pumpkin Senior Porridge

(Soft-textured, easy-to-digest, and nutrient-rich)

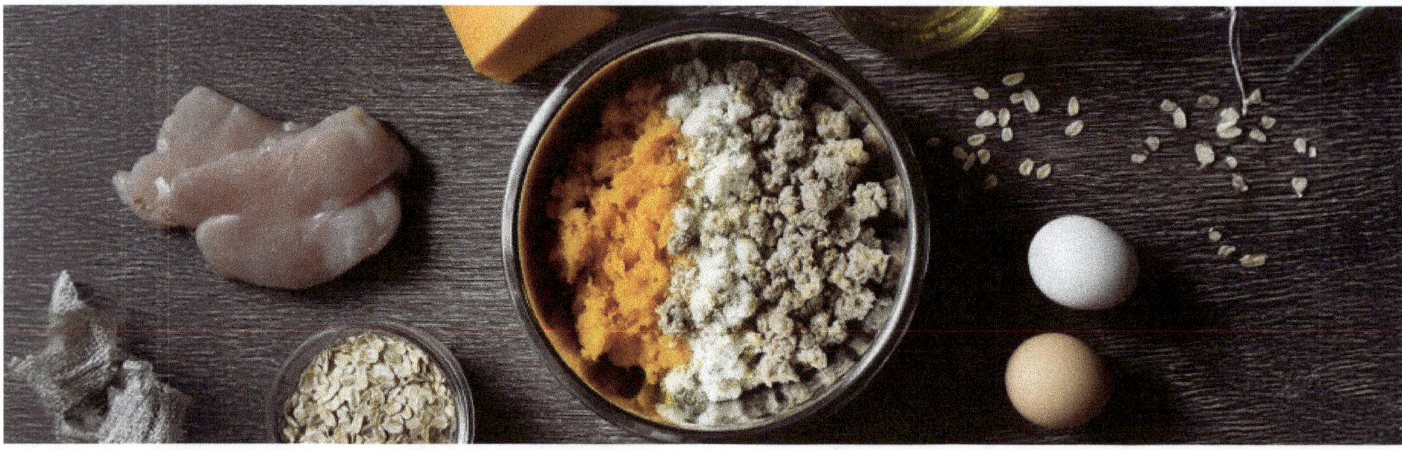

Ingredients:

- 1 lb. ground chicken (or finely minced)
- 1 cup cooked pumpkin (mashed)
- ½ cup cooked oats (soft)
- 1 tsp fish oil (for EPA/DHA)
- 1 tsp ground eggshell powder OR 2 crushed calcium tablets

Instructions:

1. Cook chicken until soft, no browning needed.
2. Stir in mashed pumpkin and soft-cooked oats.
3. Add fish oil and eggshell powder/calcium tablets.
4. Let cool before serving.

Ingredient Substitutions:

- Swap oats for rice.
- Replace pumpkin with mashed carrots.

Nutrition per 500g serving:

Final Weight	~500g
Calories	~590 kcal
Protein	~38g
Fat	~20g
Carbohydrates	~42g

7. Whitefish & Sweet Potato Soft Mash for Seniors

(Low-fat, soft meal ideal for sensitive stomachs and dental issues)

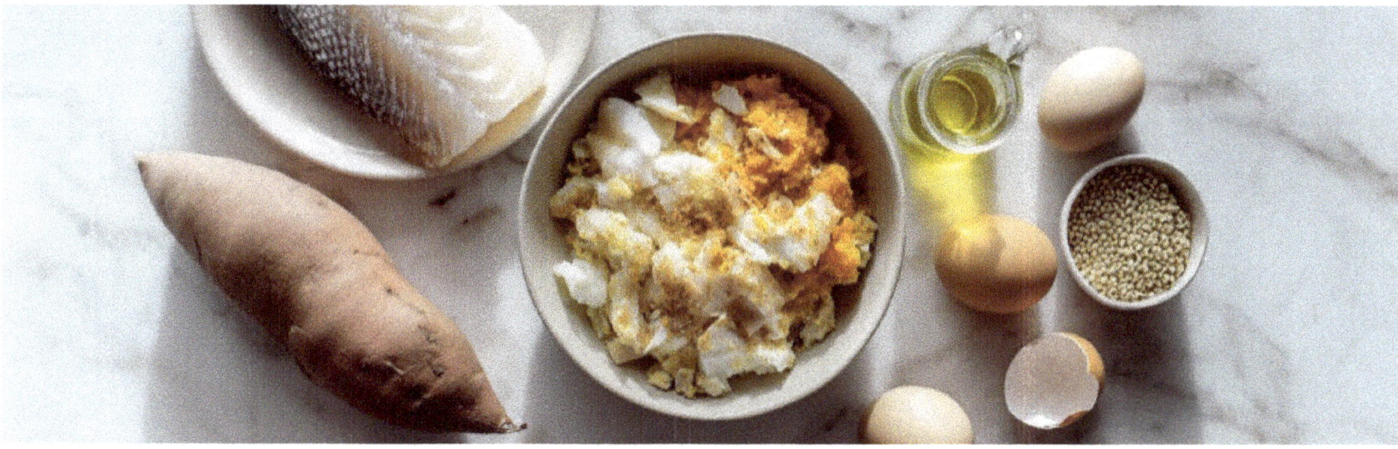

Ingredients:

- 1 lb. boneless whitefish (cod or tilapia, steamed)
- 1 cup cooked sweet potato (mashed)
- ½ cup cooked millet (soft)
- 1 tsp fish oil (for EPA/DHA)
- 1 tsp ground eggshell powder OR 2 crushed calcium tablets

Instructions:

1. Steam fish until fully done, flake into small pieces.
2. Mix mashed sweet potato and soft-cooked millet.
3. Add fish oil and eggshell powder/calcium tablets.
4. Let cool before serving.

Ingredient Substitutions:

- Replace millet with oats.
- Swap sweet potato for pumpkin.

Nutrition per 500g serving:

Final Weight	~500g
Calories	~580 kcal
Protein	~40g
Fat	~20g
Carbohydrates	~46g

8. Egg & Yogurt Soft Senior Meal

(High-calcium, protein-packed, extra soft for easy chewing)

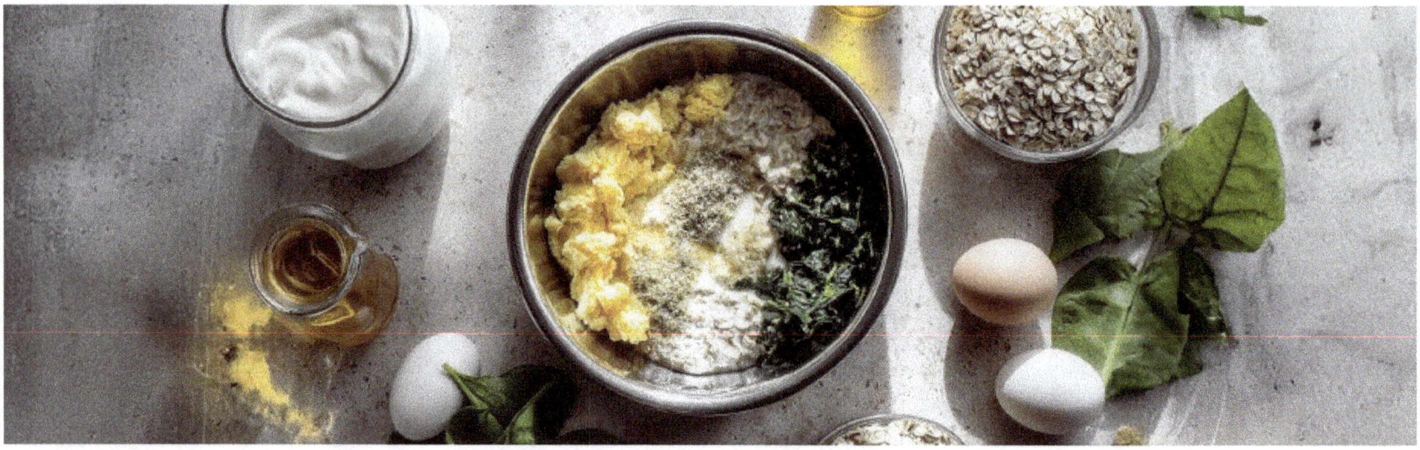

Ingredients:

- 3 large scrambled eggs
- ½ cup plain Greek yogurt (calcium-rich)
- ½ cup cooked oatmeal (soft)
- ½ cup steamed spinach (chopped finely)
- 1 tsp fish oil (EPA/DHA)
- 1 tsp ground eggshell powder OR 2 crushed calcium tablets

Instructions:

1. Scramble eggs gently.
2. Stir in soft-cooked oats, Greek yogurt, and steamed spinach.
3. Add fish oil and eggshell powder/calcium tablets.
4. Mix thoroughly and let cool.

Ingredient Substitutions:

- Replace oatmeal with rice.
- Use kefir instead of yogurt.

Nutrition per 500g serving:

Final Weight	~500g
Calories	~600 kcal
Protein	~36g
Fat	~24g
Carbohydrates	~30g

Anti-Inflammatory Recipes for Arthritis

1. Omega-3 Salmon & Pumpkin Comfort Meal

(Anti-inflammatory, arthritis-supportive meal packed with Omega-3s, antioxidants, and balanced nutrients to promote mobility and reduce joint pain)

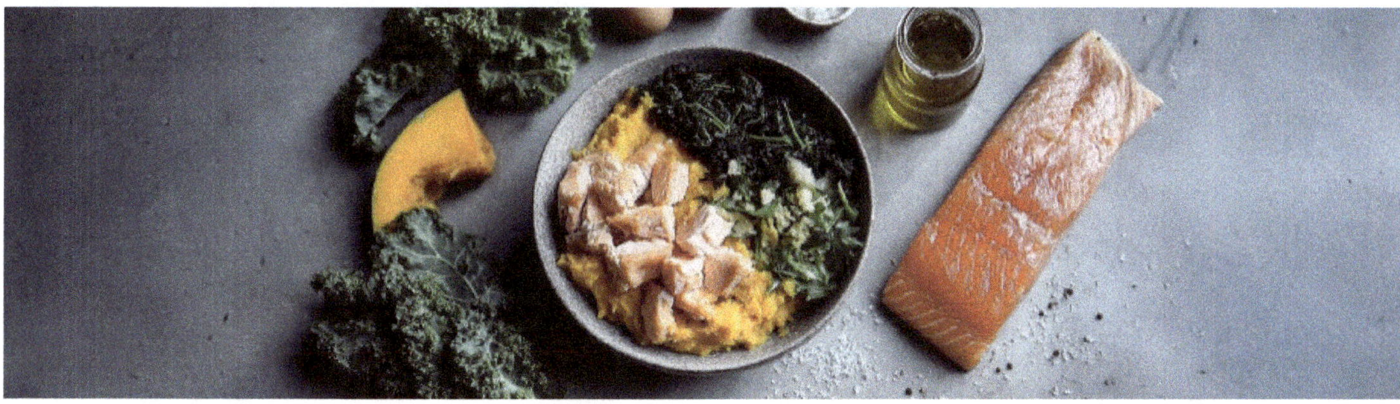

Ingredients:

- 1 lb. (450g) cooked salmon (or sardines/mackerel; flaked, boneless)
- 1 cup (245g) cooked pumpkin (plain, unsweetened, mashed)
- ½ cup (90g) steamed kale (chopped finely)
- 1 tsp fish oil (anchovy/salmon oil; extra EPA/DHA + Vitamin D)
- ½ tsp ground eggshell powder (or 500 mg calcium carbonate powder; for calcium balance)

Optional:

- ¼ tsp turmeric powder or green-lipped mussel powder for additional joint support
- Add warm water or low-sodium broth for extra hydration

Instructions:

1. Bake or steam salmon until fully cooked, flake finely.
2. Cook pumpkin until soft, mash thoroughly.
3. Steam kale, chop finely.
4. Mix all ingredients together, including fish oil, eggshell powder, and optional joint supplements.
5. Let cool before serving.

Ingredient Substitutions:

- Swap salmon for mackerel or sardines for even more DHA.
- Replace pumpkin with sweet potatoes for added fiber.
- Use spinach instead of kale for a milder, gentler option.

Nutrition per 500g serving:

Calories	~709 kcal
Protein	~68g
Fat	~41g
Carbohydrates	~23g
Carbohydrates	~46g

2. Turkey & Turmeric Anti-Inflammatory Meal

(Joint-soothing, anti-inflammatory senior meal with turmeric, glucosamine-rich protein, and balanced nutrients to reduce arthritis discomfort)

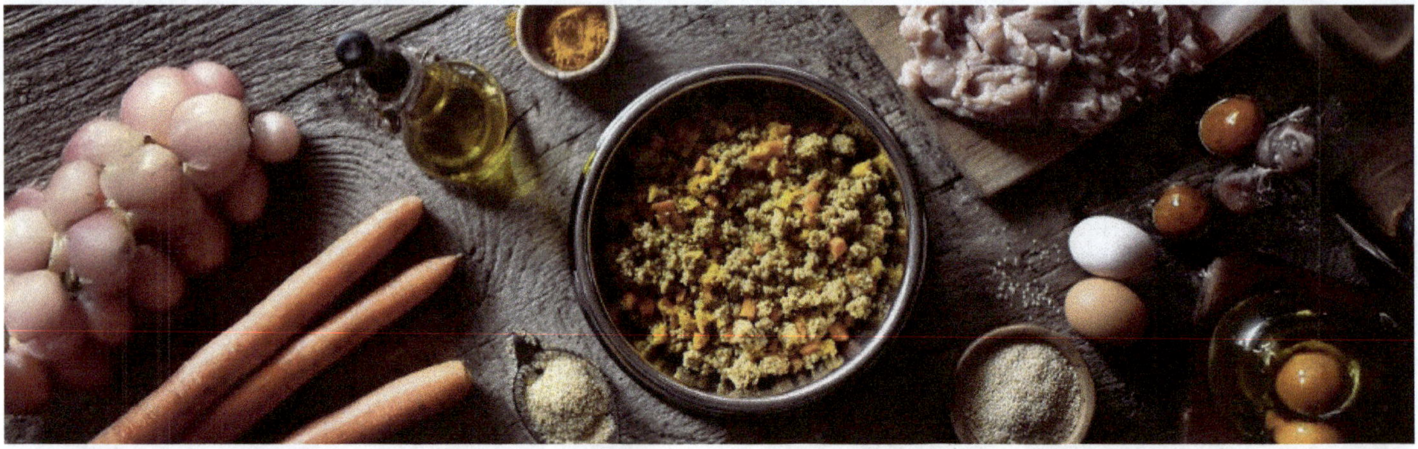

Ingredients:

- 1 lb. (450g) ground turkey (lean, 93%)
- 1 cup (185g) cooked quinoa
- ½ cup (80g) steamed carrots (mashed)
- ½ tsp turmeric powder
- 1 tsp fish oil (anchovy/salmon oil; Omega-3 EPA/DHA + Vitamin D)
- ½ tsp ground eggshell powder (or 500 mg calcium carbonate powder; for calcium balance)

Optional

- Add steamed spinach, pumpkin, or green beans for fiber & vitamins

Instructions:

1. Cook ground turkey in a pan over medium heat until fully browned (no oil required). Drain excess fat.
2. Cook quinoa as per package instructions.
3. Steam carrots and optional veggies, mash well.
4. Mix in turmeric powder, fish oil, eggshell powder, and all ingredients together.
5. Let cool before serving.

Ingredient Substitutions:

- Use chicken or lean beef instead of turkey.
- Swap quinoa for brown rice if needed.
- Replace carrots with pumpkin for digestion support.

Nutrition per 500g serving:

Final Weight	~500g
Calories	~739 kcal
Protein	~75g
Fat	~34g
Carbohydrates	~32g

3. Lamb & Blueberry Joint Protection Meal

(Antioxidant-packed, joint-protective recipe for dogs prone to inflammation and arthritis, ensuring balanced nutrients and joint support)

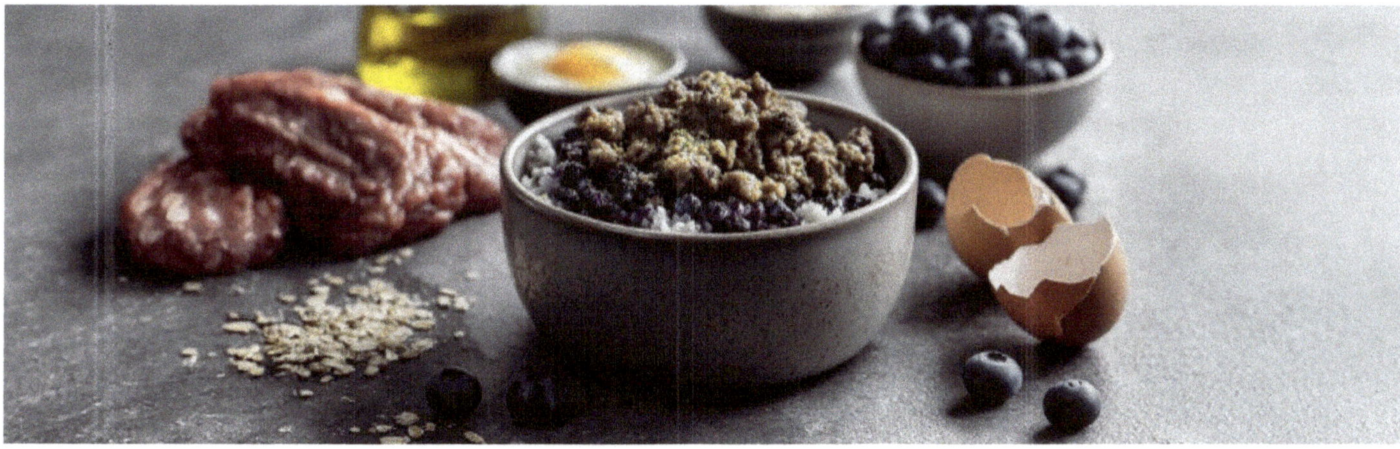

Ingredients:

- 1 lb. (450g) ground lamb (85% lean)
- 1 cup (195g) cooked brown rice
- ½ cup (75g) mashed blueberries
- 1 tsp fish oil (anchovy/salmon oil; EPA/DHA + Vitamin D)
- ½ tsp ground eggshell powder (or 500 mg calcium carbonate powder; for calcium balance)

Optional:

- ¼ tsp turmeric powder for additional anti-inflammatory effect
- Add steamed spinach, green beans, or pumpkin for extra fiber & vitamins

Instructions:

1. Cook ground lamb in a pan over medium heat until fully browned (no oil). Drain excess fat.
2. Cook brown rice until soft.
3. Mash blueberries into a puree.
4. Mix all ingredients together, including fish oil, eggshell powder, and optional turmeric/veggies.
5. Let cool before serving.

Ingredient Substitutions:

- Use lean beef instead of lamb.
- Replace brown rice with quinoa for more protein.
- Swap blueberries with strawberries or blackberries for different antioxidants.

Nutrition per 500g serving:

Final Weight	~500g
Calories	~1156 kcal
Protein	~81g
Fat	~72g
Carbohydrates	~42g

4. Sardine & Chia Seed Pain Relief Mix

(An Omega-3-packed, antioxidant-rich meal designed to lubricate joints, reduce pain, and support digestion in arthritic dogs)

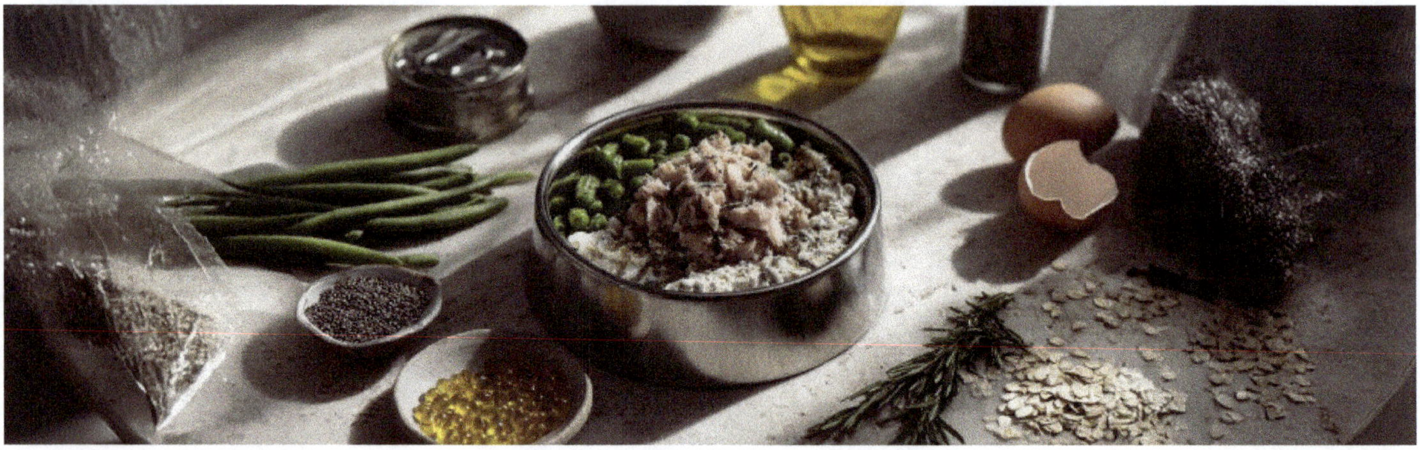

Ingredients:

- 1 lb. (450g) canned sardines in water (no salt, with soft bones)
- 1 cup (80g) cooked oatmeal (soft texture, extra water)
- ½ cup (80g) steamed green beans (chopped finely)
- 1 tsp chia seeds (soaked in water for 10 minutes)
- 1 tsp fish oil (anchovy/salmon oil; EPA/DHA + Vitamin D)
- ½ tsp ground eggshell powder (or 500 mg calcium carbonate powder; for calcium balance)

Optional:

- ¼ tsp turmeric powder or green-lipped mussel powder for additional joint relief

Instructions:

1. Mash sardines in a bowl, ensuring soft bones are evenly mixed.
2. Cook oatmeal using extra water for a soft, porridge-like texture.
3. Steam green beans (and optional veggies if desired), chop finely.
4. Soak chia seeds in water for 10 minutes.
5. Mix all ingredients together, including fish oil, eggshell powder, and optional joint supplements.
6. Let cool before serving.

Ingredient Substitutions:

- Swap sardines for salmon or mackerel.
- Use quinoa instead of oatmeal for higher protein.
- Replace green beans with zucchini for a softer texture.

Nutrition per 500g serving:

Final Weight	~500g
Calories	~891 kcal
Protein	~93g
Fat	~49g
Carbohydrates	~16g

5. Beef & Flaxseed Arthritis Support Meal

(Collagen-rich, anti-inflammatory senior meal designed to reduce arthritis symptoms, support joint cartilage, and maintain muscle mass)

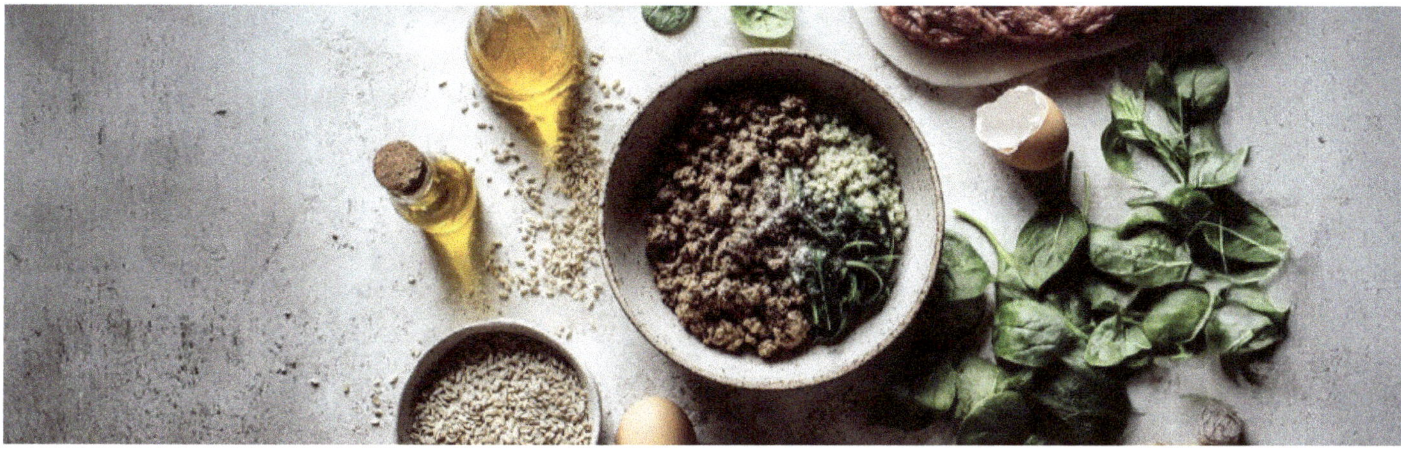

Ingredients:

- 1 lb. (450g) lean ground beef (90% lean)
- 1 cup (200g) cooked barley (very soft)
- ½ cup (90g) steamed spinach (mashed)
- 1 tsp flaxseed oil (ALA Omega-3 source)
- ½ tsp ground eggshell powder (or 500 mg calcium carbonate powder; for calcium balance)

Optional:

- ¼ tsp turmeric powder or green-lipped mussel powder for added joint support
- Add warm water or low-sodium broth for a softer stew-like texture

Instructions:

1. Cook ground beef in a non-stick pan over medium heat until fully browned (no oil). Drain excess fat.
2. Cook barley until very soft.
3. Steam spinach (and optional veggies), mash thoroughly.
4. Mix all ingredients together, adding flaxseed oil, eggshell powder, and optional turmeric.
5. Add broth or water as needed. Let cool before serving.

Ingredient Substitutions:

- Swap beef for chicken or turkey for a leaner option.
- Replace barley with oatmeal for a softer texture.
- Use steamed kale instead of spinach for more Vitamin C.

Nutrition per 500g serving:

Final Weight	~500g
Calories	~947 kcal
Protein	~83g
Fat	~58g
Carbohydrates	~40g

6. Beef & Turmeric Anti-Inflammatory Bowl for Seniors

(Anti-inflammatory, rich in iron, designed to support mobility & digestion)

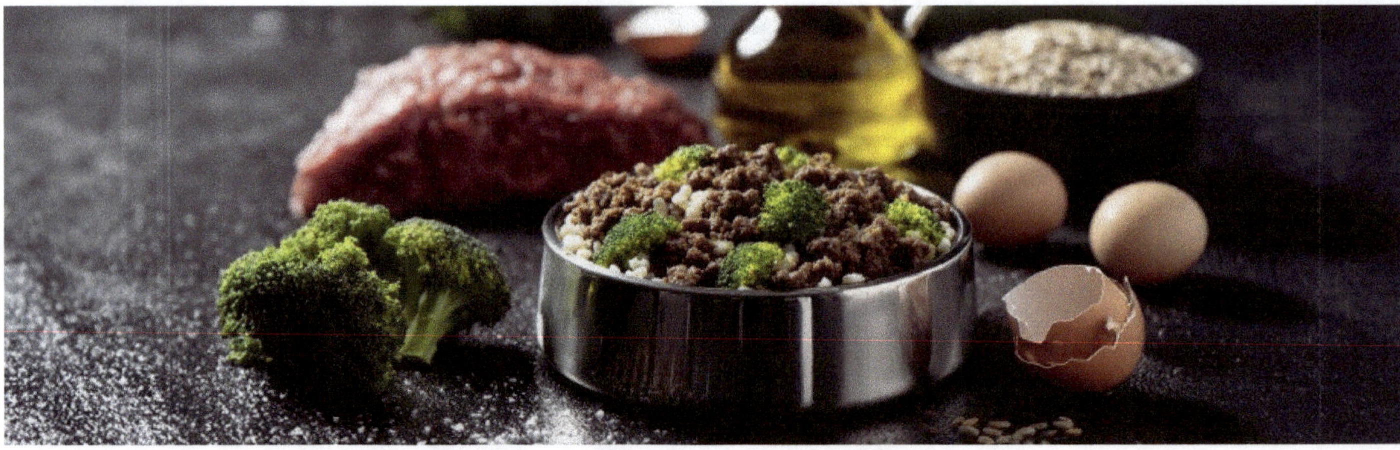

Ingredients:

- 1 lb. lean ground beef (90%)
- 1 cup cooked barley
- ½ cup steamed broccoli (chopped)
- 1 tsp olive oil or 1 tsp fish oil
- 1 tsp ground eggshell powder OR 2 crushed calcium tablets

Optional:

- ¼ tsp turmeric powder

Instructions:

1. Cook beef until fully browned.
2. Mix in cooked barley and steamed broccoli.
3. Stir in oils, calcium, and turmeric if using.
4. Let cool before serving.

Ingredient Substitutions:

- Replace barley with brown rice.
- Swap broccoli for spinach.

Nutrition per 500g serving:

Final Weight	~500g
Calories	~650 kcal
Protein	~42g
Fat	~24g
Carbohydrates	~40g

7. Elk & Millet Anti-Inflammatory Stew for Seniors

(Rich in omega-6 & antioxidants, joint-friendly, immune-supporting)

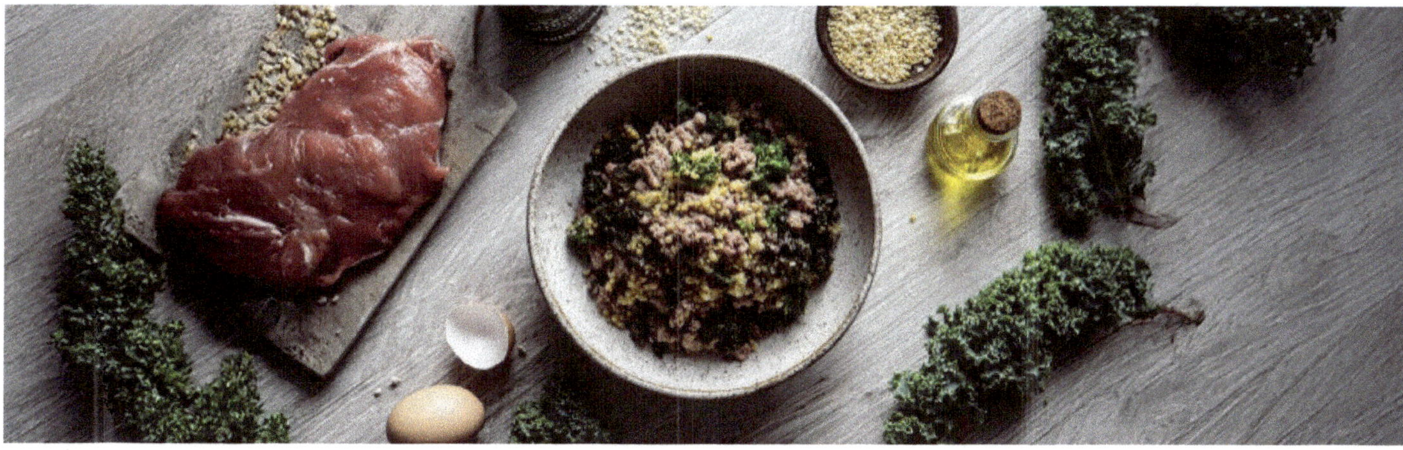

Ingredients:

- 1 lb. (450g) ground elk (lean)
- 1 cup (200g) cooked millet
- ½ cup (75g) steamed kale (chopped)
- 1 tsp flaxseed oil OR 1 tsp fish oil
- 1 tsp ground eggshell powder OR 2 crushed calcium tablets

Instructions:

1. Brown elk, drain excess fat.
2. Mix in cooked millet and steamed kale
3. Stir in oils and calcium source.
4. Let cool before serving.

Ingredient Substitutions:

- Replace kale with steamed spinach.
- Swap millet for couscous

Nutrition per 500g serving:

Final Weight	~500g
Calories	~860 kcal
Protein	~60g
Fat	~20g
Carbohydrates	~50g

8. Whitefish & Zucchini Inflammation Soother for Seniors

(Low-fat, light, packed with omega-3s and antioxidants)

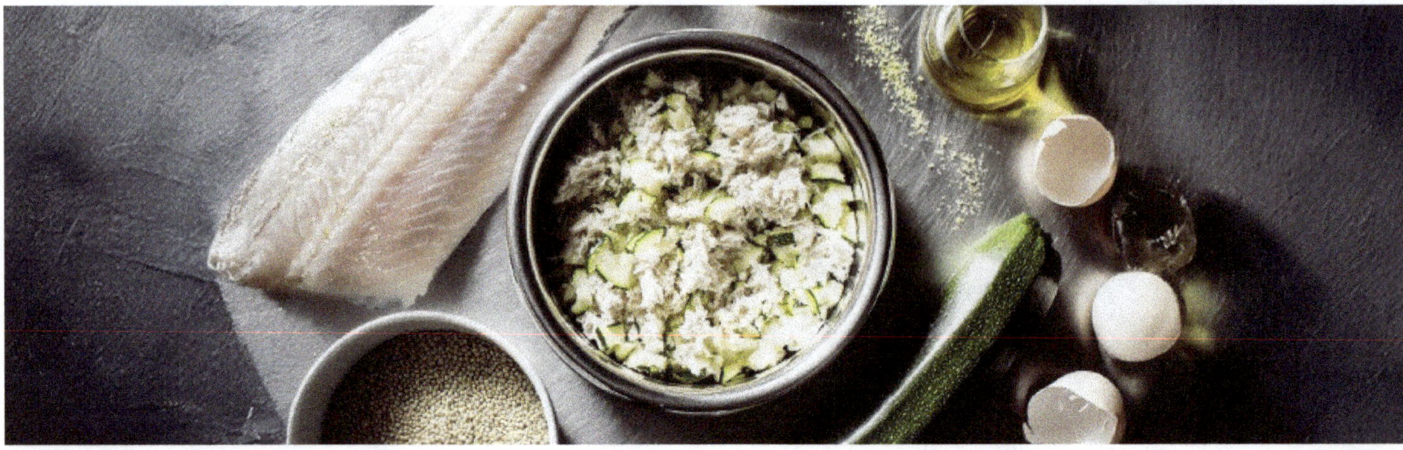

Ingredients:

- 1 lb. boneless whitefish (steamed)
- 1 cup cooked millet
- ½ cup steamed zucchini (chopped)
- 1 tsp fish oil (for EPA/DHA) or 1 tsp olive oil
- 1 tsp ground eggshell powder OR 2 crushed calcium tablets

Optional:

- ¼ tsp turmeric powder

Instructions:

1. Steam fish until fully cooked, flake.
2. Mix in cooked millet and steamed zucchini.
3. Stir in oils, calcium source, and turmeric if using.
4. Let cool before serving.

Ingredient Substitutions:

- Replace millet with oats.
- Swap zucchini for green beans.

Nutrition per 500g serving:

Final Weight	~500g
Calories	~580 kcal
Protein	~38g
Fat	~22g
Carbohydrates	~40g

Key Takeaways:

- Every dog needs food that matches their life stage, whether it's a puppy, adult, or senior.
- Sticking to portion sizes and cooking methods is extremely important to keep meals nutritious.
- Puppies should be fed meals that help them grow, build strong bones, and digest easily.
- Adult dogs should be fed food that keeps their coat shiny and helps with weight control.
- Soft, joint-friendly meals are good for senior dogs to keep them active and healthy.

Get the most of what you have just learned:

- Offer a mix of proteins like beef, chicken, fish, and veggies for variety.
- Follow the recipe as is; don't change cooking methods as it can affect nutrition. If the recipe says, boil, then boil the ingredients (do not steam or roast).
- Don't swap ingredients unless the recipe allows—it can change the nutrition.

Now that you've learned how to create balanced meals, let's explore something just as important—your dog's unique dietary needs. If your pup has allergies or sensitivities, choosing the right ingredients is crucial. In the next chapter, we'll discuss common allergens, how to spot them, and recipes designed for dogs with special dietary requirements. With this knowledge, you'll be able to give your dog the safest, healthiest, and tastiest meals possible.

So, are you ready?

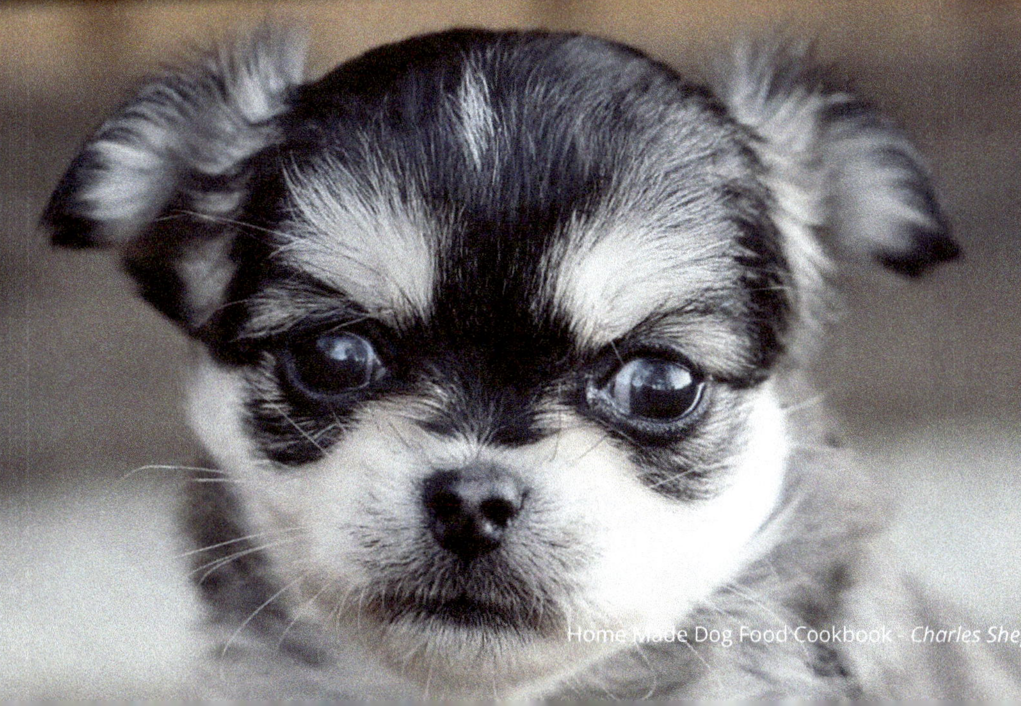

CHAPTER 4:

Allergy-Friendly and Special Diet Recipes

"Did you know that up to 20% of dogs suffer from food allergies? The right diet can eliminate symptoms and improve quality of life."

Dog owners sometimes don't realize their furry friend has a food allergy until it's too late. By the time symptoms appear, your dog may already be suffering from itchy skin, digestive issues, or chronic infections. Surprisingly, even basic ingredients in pup food—like beef, chicken, and grains—make up the most common allergens. Studies indicate that beef is the leading cause of canine adverse food reactions (CAFRs), affecting approximately 34% of reported cases. Chicken follows closely, triggering allergic responses in about 15% of dogs. Grains, particularly wheat, is a notorious culprit, with 13% of affected dogs experiencing reactions (Mueller, Olivry, & Prélaud, 2016). Feeding your dog these allergens can cause a lot of health problems:

- Chicken can cause itchy skin, ear infections, and digestive upset.
- Beef leads to skin rashes, excessive licking, and diarrhea.
- Grains can trigger bloating, stomach pain, and chronic itching.

This is why identifying these allergens is the first step in managing food allergies. Knowing what your dog is allergic to makes it easier to prepare healthy and safe homemade meals.

Food Allergies Vs Intolerances

Food allergies are not the same as food intolerances. Your dog could be allergic to an ingredient but not necessarily intolerant to it. Both require specific meal management and precautions to ensure a healthy life.

A food allergy is an immune system response where the body mistakenly identifies a food source as a threat. Allergens can trigger symptoms like itching, skin rashes, ear infections, and gastrointestinal issues. On the other hand, food intolerance does not involve the immune system and usually stems from the digestive system's inability to process certain ingredients. Hence, food intolerances are not as severe and may include bloating, diarrhea, or gas (which can be managed unlike reactions caused by allergens). Also, while allergies require complete avoidance of the offending food source, intolerances can sometimes be managed by adjusting portion sizes or opting for alternative cooking methods.

Always choose your pet's diet based on whether they have an allergy or an intolerance. The best way to know your pup's allergies or intolerances is by using the elimination diet method. It's a comprehensive way to ensure your furry friend gets all the nutrients they need without sudden health reactions.

Identifying Allergens: The Elimination Diet Method

It may be challenging, but not impossible, to find the exact ingredient causing a reaction in your pup. With the Elimination Diet Method, you can pinpoint problem foods by removing potential allergens and gradually reintroducing them while monitoring symptoms. This process makes it easier to determine whether a dog has a food allergy (immune response) or a food intolerance (digestive issue).

I have classified this into two:

- For dogs that have been eating certain ingredients without issues but need to identify any potential allergens.
- For dogs that had allergic reactions or intolerances in their previous diet and need to pinpoint the problem ingredient.

If you're switching your dog's diet for a healthier option and they haven't had any issues with their previous diet, choose the first option. However, if transitioning to homemade meals is a necessity due to any adverse food reactions in the past, you should follow the second approach to carefully identify the offending ingredient. The elimination diet method will give you a clear understanding of what ingredients your dog can safely eat without triggering allergies or intolerances.

Approach 1: Identifying New Allergens While Keeping a Familiar Diet

Ideal for dogs that have been safely eating certain ingredients in their previous diet without any issues but need to identify potential allergens in home-cooked meals.

Step-by-Step Process:

1. At the start, stick to ingredients your dog has been eating without reactions: For example, if they have been eating chicken in kibble or wet food and showed no symptoms, you can safely use chicken in homemade meals.
2. Introduce one new ingredient at a time: Add a single new protein (such as beef, turkey, or fish) or a new grain (like wheat, rice quinoa, or oats) to the familiar diet.
3. Keep the diet the same except for that one new ingredient for the next 7–14 days and monitor symptoms (like itching, vomiting, diarrhea, etc.).
4. If a reaction occurs, remove the newly introduced ingredient and allow symptoms to clear up before trying another. However, if no reaction happens, that ingredient is safe to keep in their diet.
5. Continue testing one ingredient at a time: Repeat this process with different proteins, grains, and vegetables until you have a safe, allergen-free homemade diet.

Approach 2: Finding the Problem Ingredient for Dogs with Allergies/Intolerances

For dogs that had allergic reactions or intolerances to their previous diet and need a safer home-cooked diet without the problem ingredients.

Step-by-Step Process:

1. Start with a basic elimination diet. Remove all ingredients from the previous diet and start fresh with a single-protein and single-carb meal. For example, choose a mild, easily digestible protein (e.g., turkey, rabbit, or whitefish) and a simple carbohydrate (e.g., pumpkin, sweet potato, or quinoa).
2. Feed This Diet for 2–4 Weeks. No treats, table scraps, or flavored supplements during this time. If symptoms improve, it means something in the old diet was causing a reaction.
3. Slowly reintroduce ingredients from the old diet. Add one previous ingredient back at a time (like chicken or beef). Watch for any signs of allergies/intolerances for 7–14 days. If symptoms return, it means that the new ingredient is likely the problem. Remove it from the diet permanently and let the symptoms heal while feeding the previous basic elimination diet.
4. Continue testing until you identify all the allergens to build a safe homemade diet.

To make things easier, here is an Elimination Diet Tracking Template! You can use this chart to monitor your dog's reaction to different ingredients and identify any potential allergies or intolerances. This will help you keep track of symptoms, severity, and whether to continue or remove an ingredient from their diet.

Here is example template to help you understand how to use the Elimination Diet Tracking Chart:

Date	Ingredient Introduced	Symptoms (Yes/No)	Reaction Noticed (If Any)	Severity (Mild/ Moderate/ Severe)	Notes (Changes, Improvements, Reactions)	Continue or Remove?
07/01	Chicken	No	—	—	No reaction, well tolerated	Continue
07/03	Beef	Yes	Itching, diarrhea	Moderate	Symptoms appeared within hours	Remove
07/05	Wheat	No	—	—	No issues, digestion normal	Continue

Each time you introduce a new ingredient, add it to the chart under the correct day. Monitor your dog for any signs of allergic reactions or intolerances like itching, diarrhea, vomiting, or ear infections. If no reaction occurs after 48 hours, mark the ingredient as safe in the chart and proceed to introduce the next one. If a reaction happens, highlight that ingredient and remove it immediately. Then, allow your dog's symptoms to heal before testing another new ingredient. Keep notes on any symptoms, their severity, and how long they lasted to identify problem foods accurately.

Follow this step-by-step introduction order for testing allergens and intolerances:

- Proteins – Start with a single protein source (e.g., chicken, beef, fish, pork, lamb).
- Carbohydrates – Add one grain or starch (e.g., rice, wheat, corn).
- Dairy – Introduce small amounts of dairy (e.g., milk, cheese, yogurt).

- Eggs – Test with a small portion of an egg.
- Legumes & Soy – Add peas, lentils, or soy-based ingredients.
- Fats – Try small amounts of animal fats or plant oils like fish or olive oil.
- Vegetables – Introduce non-toxic veggies (e.g., carrots, spinach) while avoiding onions/garlic.

Elimination Diet Tracking Chart

Keep this chart handy when introducing new foods to your dog and update it regularly to track any reactions. Track changes for these ingredients: chicken, beef, dairy, wheat, lamb, soy, egg, corn, pork, fish, rice, gluten, oils, legumes, and vegetables.

Date	Ingredient Introduced	Symptoms (Yes/No)	Reaction Noticed (If Any)	Severity (Mild/ Moderate/ Severe)	Notes (Changes, Improvements, Reactions)	Continue or Remove?

Allergen-Friendly and Special Diet Recipes

In this section, we will cover allergen-friendly and special diet recipes, so your pup can enjoy their meal times without adverse health reactions. These recipes are particularly designed to give your furry friend the best of home-cooked meals while meeting their nutritional levels.

Single-Protein Recipes

1. Duck & Quinoa Gentle Meal

(Novel protein, grain-free, ideal for sensitive stomachs and allergies)

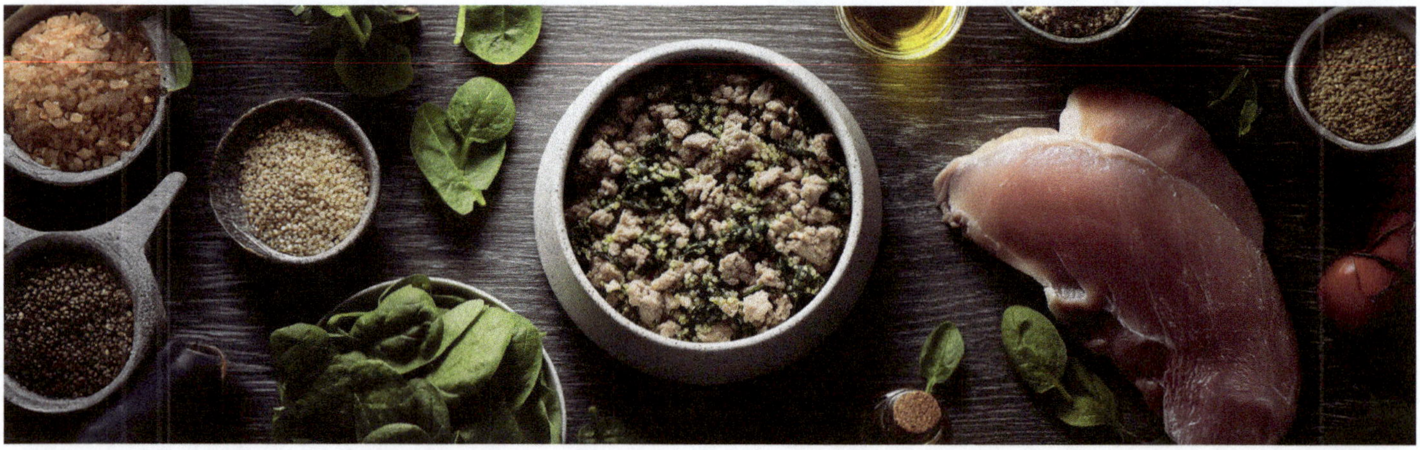

Ingredients:

- 1 lb. ground duck (skin removed)
- 1 cup cooked quinoa
- ½ cup steamed spinach (chopped)
- 1 tsp flaxseed oil
- 1 tsp olive oil

Instructions:

1. Cook duck thoroughly.
2. Mix in cooked quinoa and steamed spinach.
3. Stir in oils.
4. Let cool before serving.

Ingredient Substitutions:

- Replace quinoa with millet.
- Swap spinach with green beans.

Nutrition per 500g serving:

Final Weight	~500g
Calories	~600 kcal
Protein	~40g
Fat	~26g
Carbohydrates	~40g

2. Rabbit & Sweet Potato Sensitive Meal

(Rich in omega-6 & antioxidants, joint-friendly, immune-supporting)

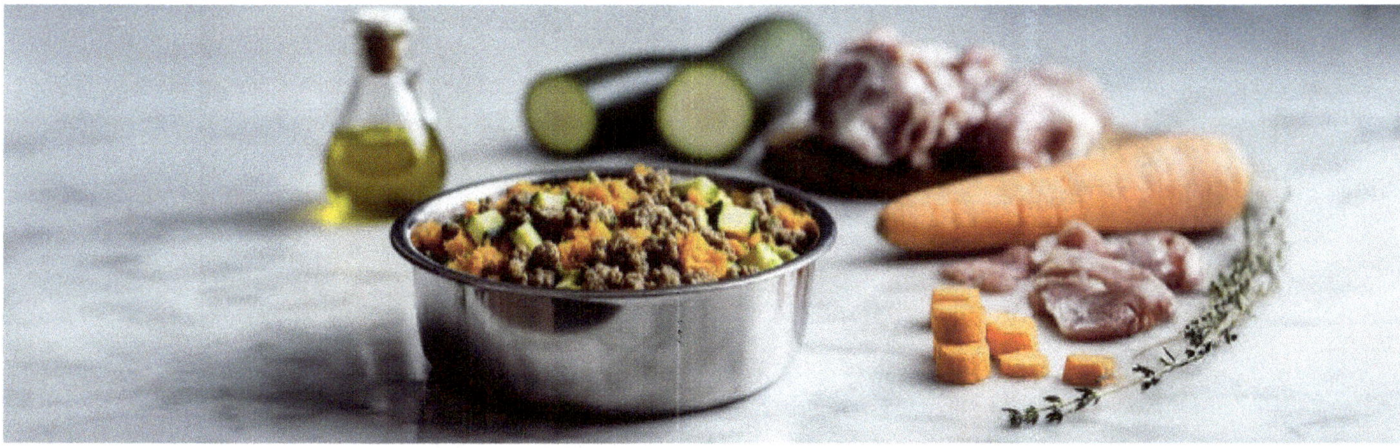

Ingredients:

- 1 lb. ground rabbit
- 1 cup mashed sweet potato
- ½ cup steamed zucchini (chopped)
- 1 tsp flaxseed oil
- 1 tsp olive oil

Instructions:

1. Cook rabbit thoroughly.
2. Stir in mashed sweet potato and zucchini.
3. Mix in oils.
4. Let cool before serving.

Ingredient Substitutions:

- Replace sweet potato with pumpkin.
- Swap zucchini with spinach.

Nutrition per 500g serving:

Final Weight	~500g
Calories	~580 kcal
Protein	~40g
Fat	~22g
Carbohydrates	~38g

3. Venison & Millet Allergy-Friendly Bowl

(Rich, lean novel protein with fiber-rich millet, no grains or dairy)

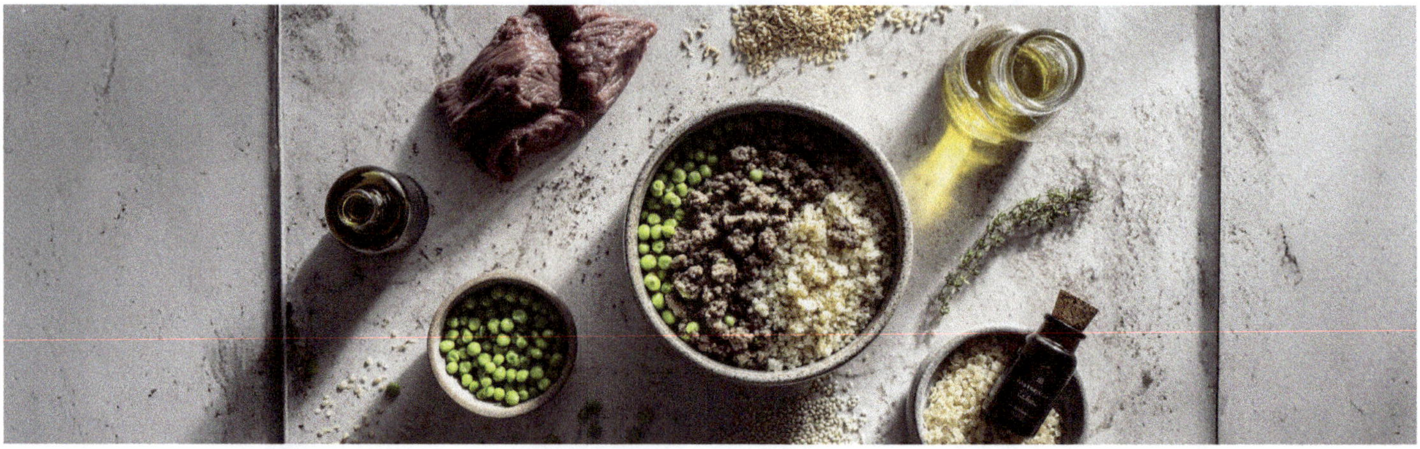

Ingredients:

- 1 lb. ground venison
- 1 cup cooked millet
- ½ cup steamed peas
- 1 tsp flaxseed oil
- 1 tsp olive oil

Instructions:

1. Cook venison thoroughly.
2. Stir in cooked millet and peas.
3. Mix in oils.
4. Let cool before serving.

Ingredient Substitutions:

- Replace millet with quinoa.
- Swap peas with green beans.

Nutrition per 500g serving:

Final Weight	~500g
Calories	~610 kcal
Protein	~42g
Fat	~24g
Carbohydrates	~40g

4. Whitefish & Pumpkin Hypoallergenic Meal

(Light, low-fat, ideal for skin sensitivities and digestive comfort)

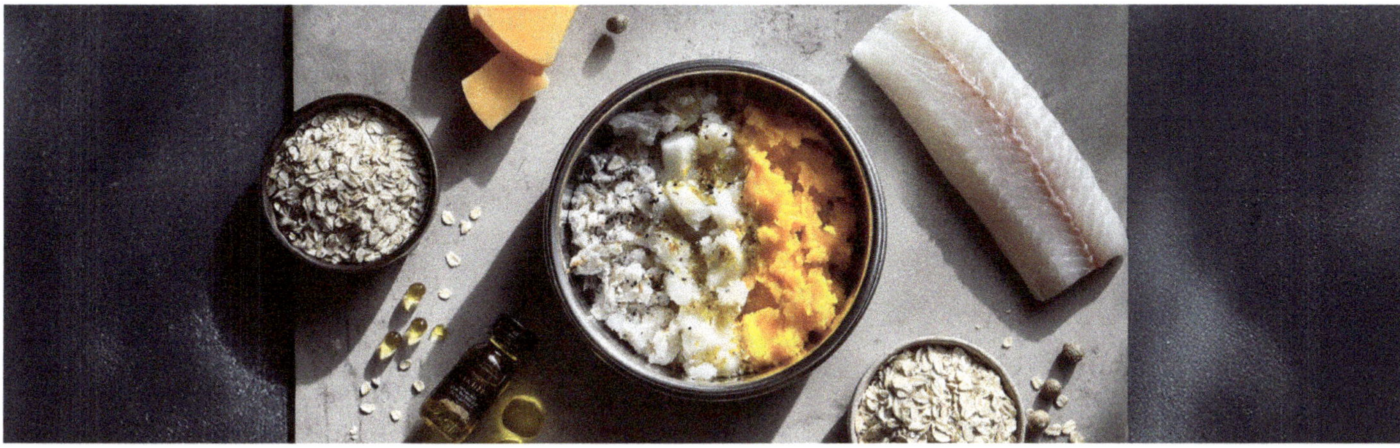

Ingredients:

- 1 lb. boneless whitefish (cod or tilapia, steamed)
- 1 cup mashed pumpkin
- ½ cup cooked oats
- 1 tsp fish oil
- 1 tsp olive oil

Instructions:

1. Steam fish until cooked, flake.
2. Stir in pumpkin and oats.
3. Mix in oils.
4. Let cool before serving.

Ingredient Substitutions:

- Replace oats with quinoa.
- Swap pumpkin with sweet potato.

Nutrition per 500g serving:

Final Weight	~500g
Calories	~560 kcal
Protein	~38g
Fat	~20g
Carbohydrates	~36g

5. Kangaroo & Tapioca Allergy Relief Meal

(Novel red meat option, gluten-free, and balanced for sensitivities)

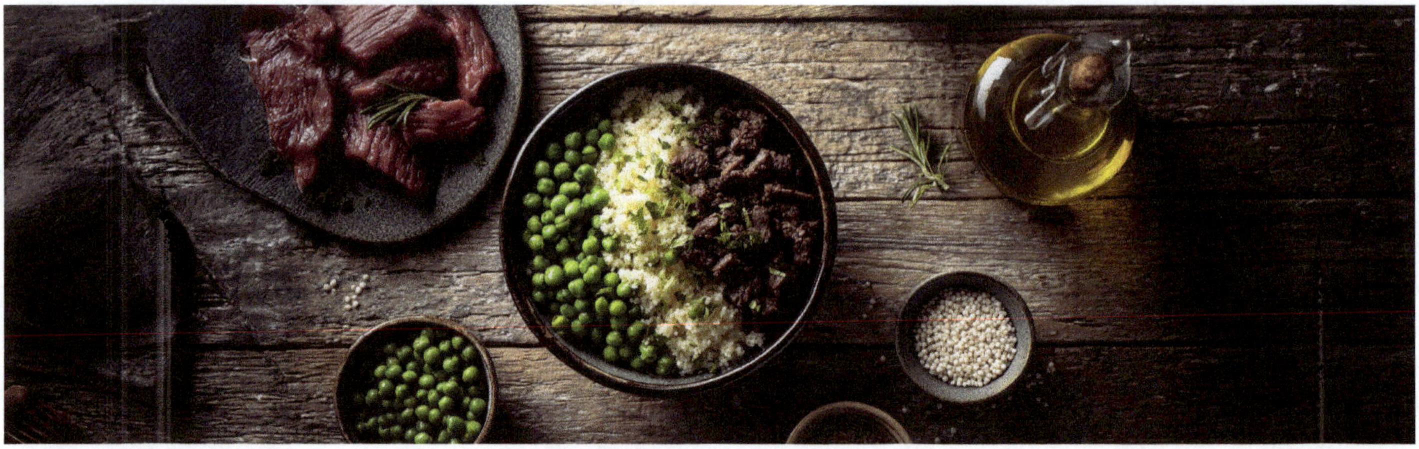

Ingredients:

- 1 lb. (450g) ground kangaroo (lean)
- 1 cup (200g) cooked tapioca (mashed, from pearls or starch)
- ½ cup (75g) steamed peas (chopped)
- 1 tsp flaxseed oil
- 1 tsp olive oil

Instructions:

1. Brown kangaroo thoroughly.
2. Mix in tapioca and steamed peas
3. Stir in oils.
4. Let cool before serving.

Ingredient Substitutions:

- Replace tapioca with mashed potato
- Swap peas with steamed spinach

Nutrition per 500g serving:

Final Weight	~500g
Calories	~740 kcal
Protein	~70g
Fat	~25g
Carbohydrates	~55g

6. Pork & Pumpkin Digestive Ease Meal

(Gentle novel protein, grain-free, supports sensitive stomachs)

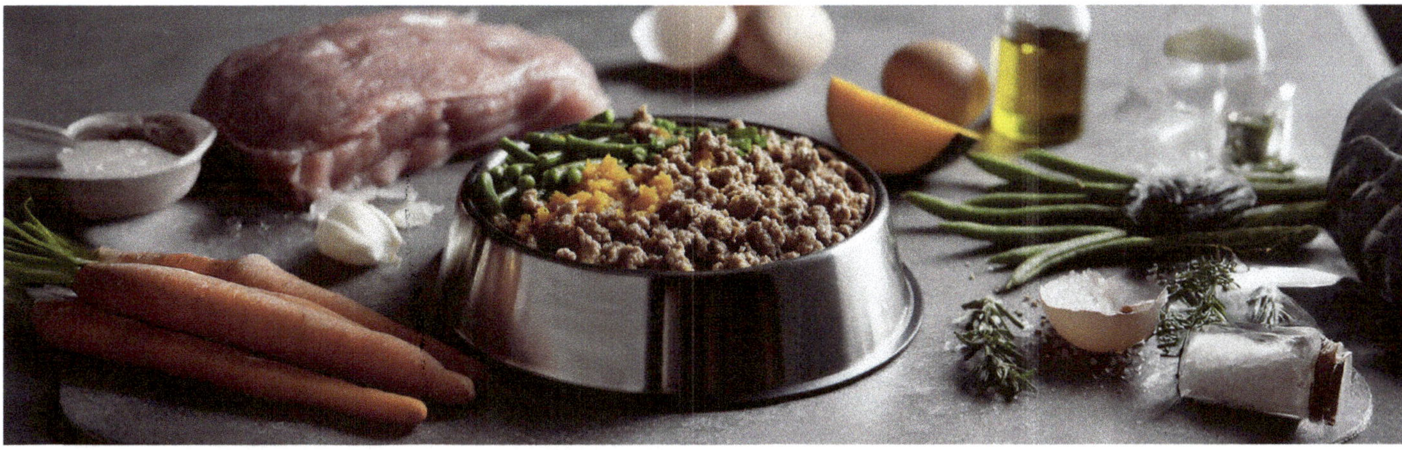

Ingredients:

- 1 lb. ground pork (90% lean)
- 1 cup cooked pumpkin (mashed)
- ½ cup steamed green beans (chopped)
- 2 tsp flaxseed oil
- 1 tsp ground eggshells OR 2 crushed calcium tablets
- ½ tsp iodized salt

Instructions:

1. In a pan, cook the ground pork until fully browned (no added oil).
2. Add the mashed pumpkin and chopped green beans. Mix well.
3. Stir in flaxseed oil, ground eggshells (or calcium tablets), and iodized salt.
4. Cool before serving.

Ingredient Substitutions:

- Replace pumpkin with sweet potato.
- Use ground turkey instead of pork.

Nutrition per 500g serving:

Final Weight	~500g
Calories	~650 kcal
Protein	~45g
Fat	~35g
Carbohydrates	~25g

7. Bison & Millet Allergy Relief Bowl

(Lean novel protein, gluten-free, ideal for dogs with beef or chicken allergies)

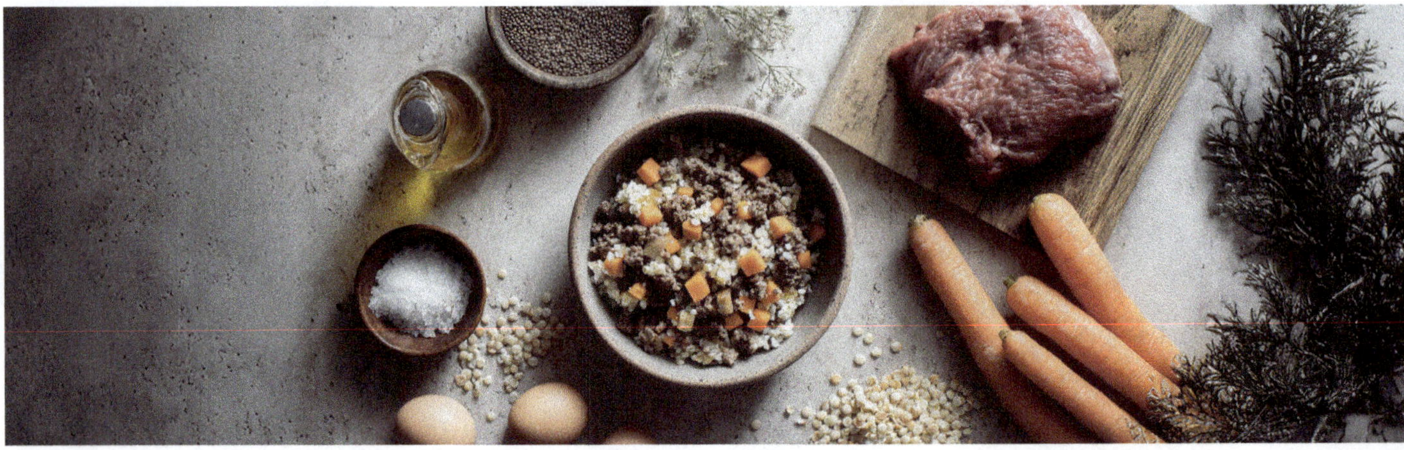

Ingredients:

- 1 lb. ground bison (90% lean)
- 1 cup cooked millet
- ½ cup steamed carrots (chopped)
- 2 tsp fish oil
- 1 tsp ground eggshells OR 2 crushed calcium tablets
- ½ tsp iodized salt

Instructions:

1. In a pan, cook the ground bison until browned (no added oil).
2. Add the cooked millet and chopped carrots. Mix thoroughly.
3. Stir in fish oil, ground eggshells (or calcium tablets), and iodized salt.
4. Cool before serving.

Ingredient Substitutions:

- Replace millet with quinoa.
- Use ground venison instead of bison.

Nutrition per 500g serving:

Final Weight	~500g
Calories	~700 kcal
Protein	~50g
Fat	~30g
Carbohydrates	~35g

8. Rabbit & Zucchini Sensitive Skin Meal

(Novel protein, grain-free, gentle on digestion and skin)

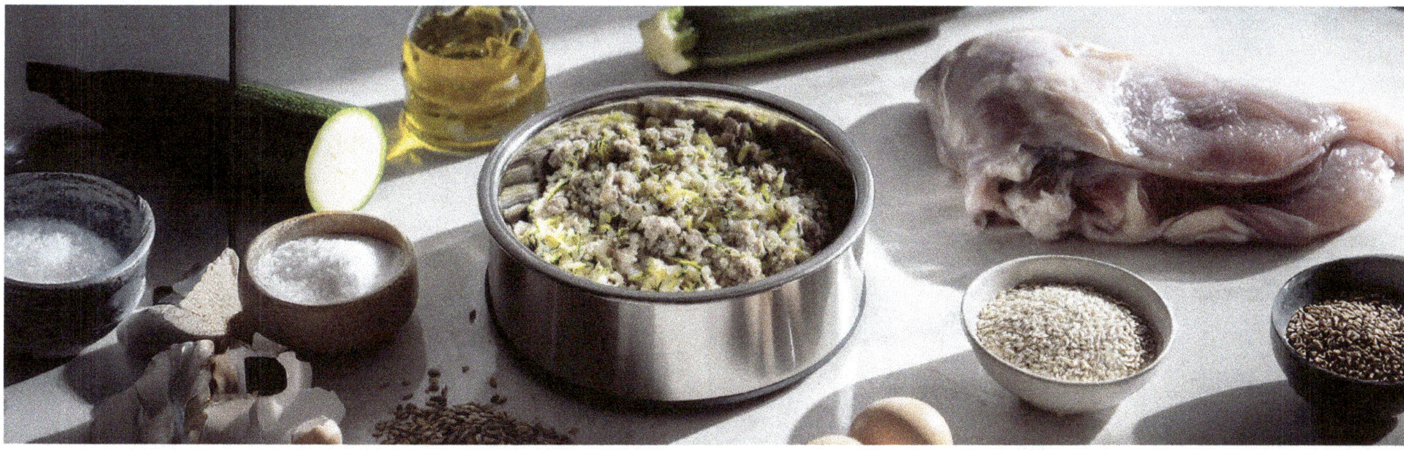

Ingredients:

- 1 lb. ground rabbit
- 1 cup steamed zucchini (mashed)
- ½ cup cooked millet
- 2 tsp flaxseed oil
- 1 tsp ground eggshells OR 2 crushed calcium tablets
- ½ tsp iodized salt

Instructions:

1. In a pan, cook the ground rabbit until fully browned (no added oil).
2. Add the mashed zucchini and cooked millet. Mix well.
3. Stir in flaxseed oil, ground eggshells (or calcium tablets), and iodized salt.
4. Cool before serving.

Ingredient Substitutions:

- Replace zucchini with pumpkin.
- Use ground turkey instead of rabbit.

Nutrition per 500g serving:

Final Weight	~500g
Calories	~600 kcal
Protein	~50g
Fat	~25g
Carbohydrates	~20g

Grain-Free and Gluten-Free Meals

1. Turkey & Pumpkin Grain-Free Meal

(Lean, easy-to-digest, no grains, perfect for sensitive dogs)

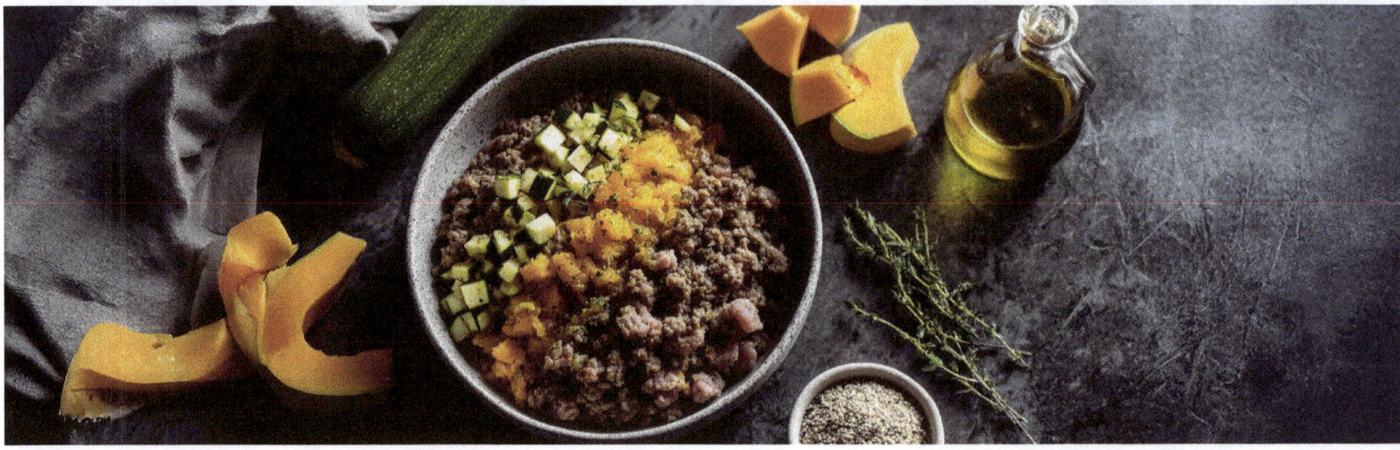

Ingredients:

- 1 lb. ground turkey (93% lean)
- 1 cup mashed pumpkin
- ½ cup steamed zucchini (chopped)
- 1 tsp flaxseed oil
- 1 tsp olive oil

Instructions:

1. Cook turkey thoroughly.
2. Mix in mashed pumpkin and zucchini.
3. Stir in oils.
4. Let cool before serving.

Ingredient Substitutions:

- Replace zucchini with spinach.
- Swap turkey with rabbit or duck.

Nutrition per 500g serving:

Final Weight	~500g
Calories	~580 kcal
Protein	~40g
Fat	~22g
Carbohydrates	~36g

2. Beef & Sweet Potato Grain-Free Bowl

(Rich in iron, high in fiber, gluten-free, and balanced)

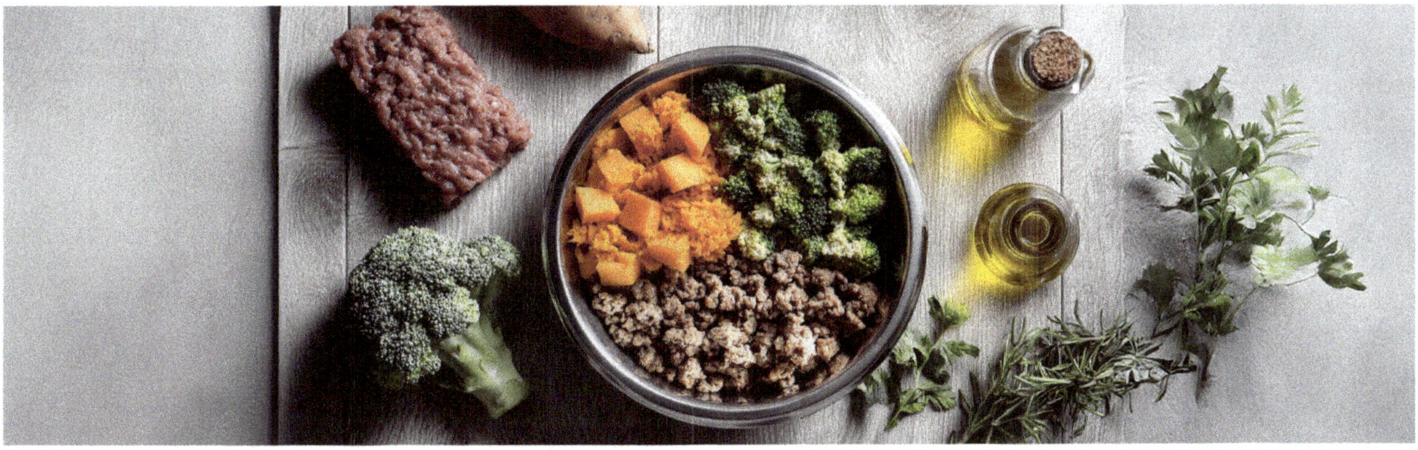

Ingredients:

- 1 lb. lean ground beef (90% lean)
- 1 cup mashed sweet potato
- ½ cup steamed broccoli (chopped)
- 1 tsp flaxseed oil
- 1 tsp olive oil

Instructions:

1. Brown beef thoroughly.
2. Mix in mashed sweet potato and broccoli.
3. Stir in oils.
4. Let cool before serving.

Ingredient Substitutions:

- Replace sweet potato with pumpkin.
- Swap broccoli with green beans.

Nutrition per 500g serving:

Final Weight	~500g
Calories	~620 kcal
Protein	~40g
Fat	~26g
Carbohydrates	~38g

3. Salmon & Quinoa Allergy-Free Meal

(Gluten-free, omega-3 rich, promotes healthy skin & digestion)

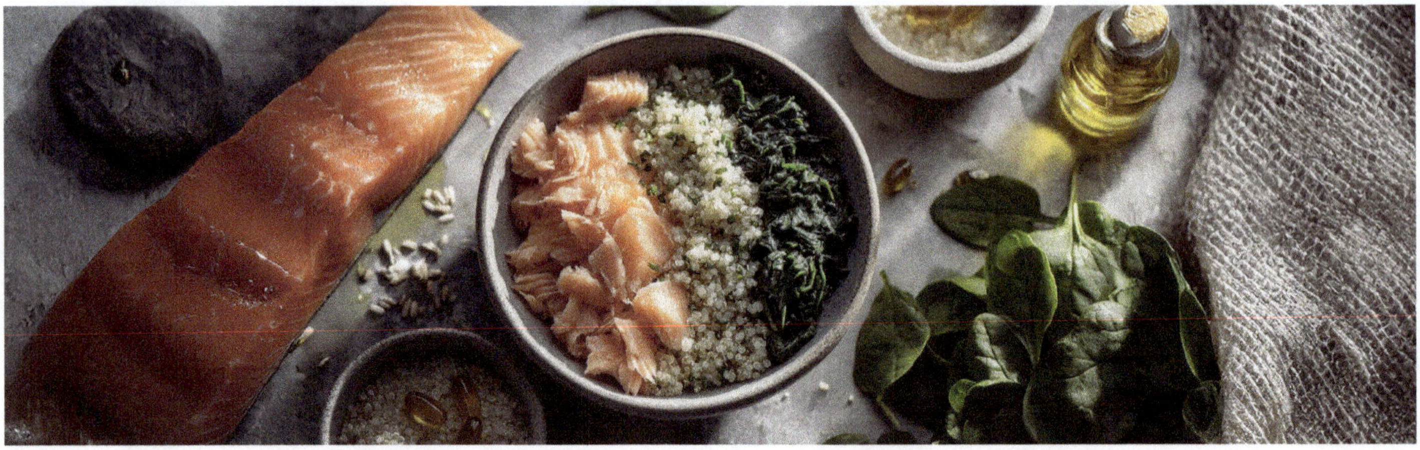

Ingredients:

- 1 lb. boneless salmon (steamed)
- 1 cup cooked quinoa
- ½ cup steamed spinach (chopped)
- 1 tsp fish oil
- 1 tsp olive oil

Instructions:

1. Steam salmon until fully cooked, flake.
2. Stir in quinoa and spinach.
3. Mix in oils.
4. Let cool before serving.

Ingredient Substitutions:

- Replace quinoa with millet.
- Swap spinach with broccoli.

Nutrition per 500g serving:

Final Weight	~500g
Calories	~610 kcal
Protein	~42g
Fat	~26g
Carbohydrates	~38g

4. Rabbit & Green Bean Grain-Free Stew

(Novel protein, no grains, gentle for digestive sensitivities)

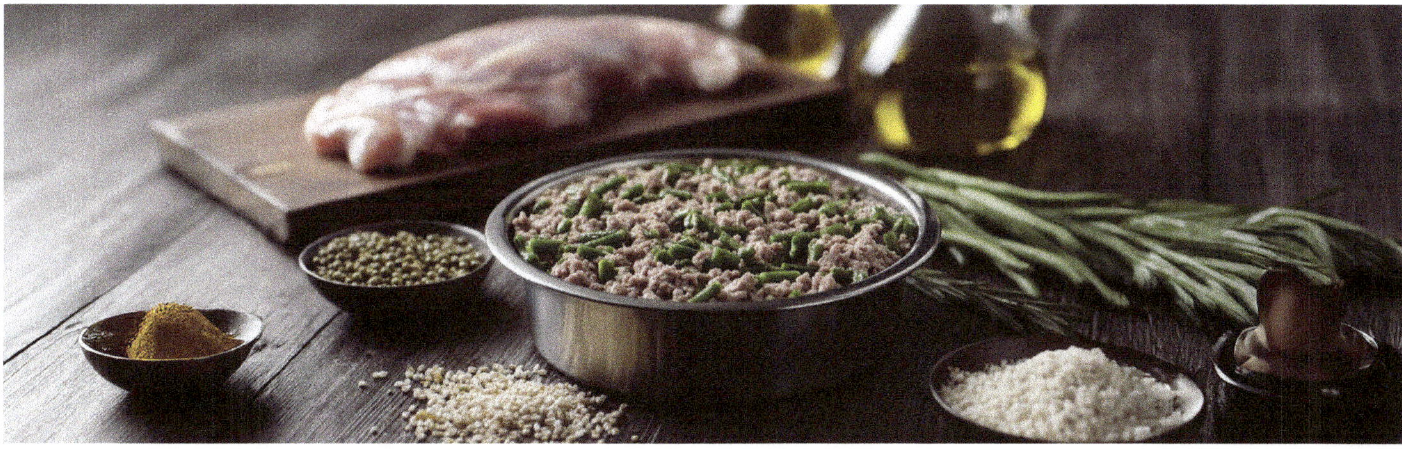

Ingredients:

- 1 lb. ground rabbit
- 1 cup steamed green beans (chopped)
- ½ cup cooked millet
- 1 tsp flaxseed oil
- 1 tsp olive oil

Instructions:

1. Cook rabbit thoroughly.
2. Mix in green beans and millet.
3. Stir in oils.
4. Let cool before serving.

Ingredient Substitutions:

- Replace millet with quinoa.
- Swap green beans with peas.

Nutrition per 500g serving:

Final Weight	~500g
Calories	~590 kcal
Protein	~40g
Fat	~22g
Carbohydrates	~36g

5. Chicken & Carrot Grain-Free Energy Bowl

(Lean, fiber-rich, no grains, supports energy and gut health)

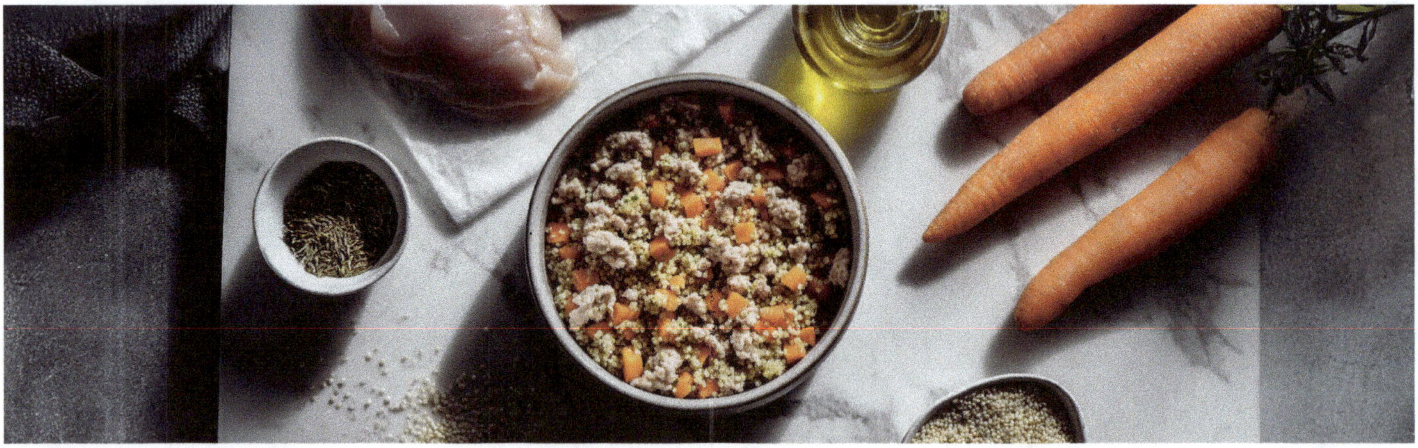

Ingredients:

- 1 lb. ground chicken (93% lean)
- 1 cup steamed carrots (chopped)
- ½ cup cooked quinoa
- 1 tsp flaxseed oil
- 1 tsp olive oil

Instructions:

1. Cook chicken thoroughly.
2. Stir in carrots and quinoa.
3. Mix in oils.
4. Let cool before serving.

Ingredient Substitutions:

- Replace quinoa with millet.
- Swap carrots with zucchini.

Nutrition per 500g serving:

Final Weight	~500g
Calories	~560 kcal
Protein	~38g
Fat	~20g
Carbohydrates	~36g

6. Trout & Sweet Potato Skin Soother Meal

(Low-fat, omega-3 rich, grain-free, promotes skin healing)

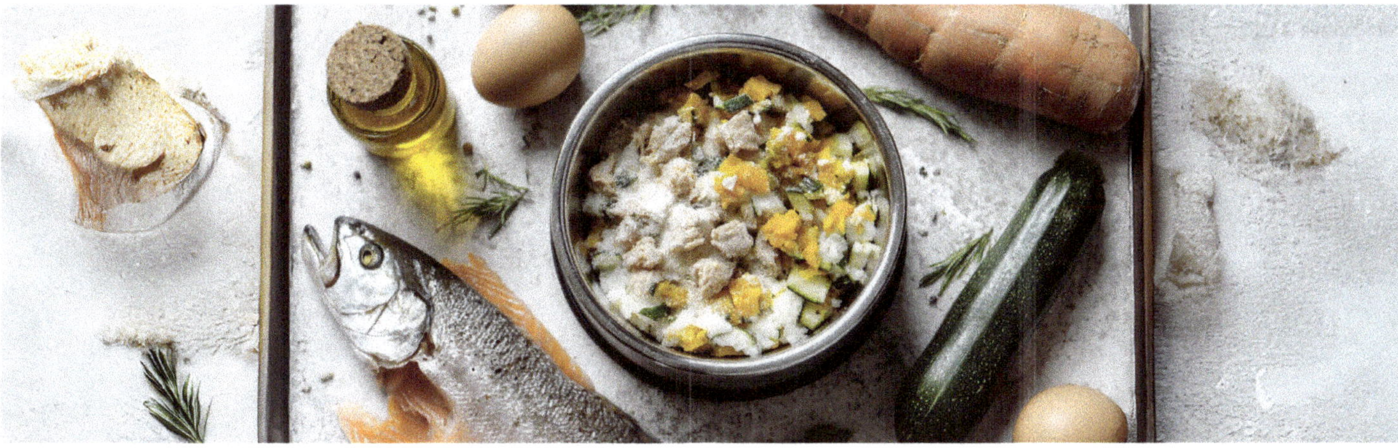

Ingredients:

- 1 lb. boneless trout (steamed and flaked)
- 1 cup cooked sweet potato (mashed)
- ½ cup steamed zucchini (chopped)
- 2 tsp fish oil
- 1 tsp ground eggshells OR 2 crushed calcium tablets
- ½ tsp iodized salt

Instructions:

1. Steam the trout until fully cooked, then flake into small pieces.
2. Mix in the mashed sweet potato and chopped zucchini.
3. Stir in fish oil, ground eggshells (or calcium tablets), and iodized salt.
4. Cool before serving.

Ingredient Substitutions:

- Replace sweet potato with pumpkin.
- Use whitefish instead of trout.

Nutrition per 500g serving:

Final Weight	~500g
Calories	~600 kcal
Protein	~40g
Fat	~25g
Carbohydrates	~30g

7. Salmon & Carrot Grain-Free Glow Meal

(Omega-3 rich, grain-free, supports skin and digestion)

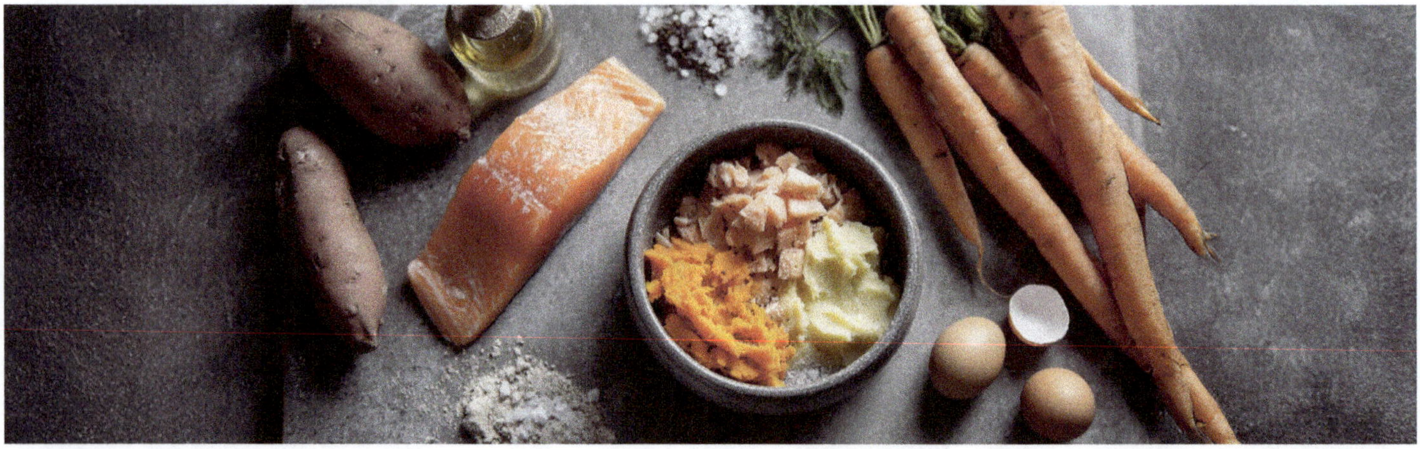

Ingredients:

- 1 lb. boneless salmon (steamed and flaked)
- 1 cup steamed carrots (mashed)
- ½ cup cooked sweet potato (mashed)
- 2 tsp fish oil
- 1 tsp ground eggshells OR 2 crushed calcium tablets
- ½ tsp iodized salt

Instructions:

1. Steam the salmon until fully cooked, then flake into small pieces.
2. Mix in the mashed carrots and sweet potato.
3. Stir in fish oil, ground eggshells (or calcium tablets), and iodized salt.
4. Cool before serving.

Ingredient Substitutions:

- Replace carrots with green beans.
- Use trout instead of salmon.

Nutrition per 500g serving:

Final Weight	~500g
Calories	~650 kcal
Protein	~40g
Fat	~30g
Carbohydrates	~25g

Low-Fat Recipes for Pancreatitis

1. Whitefish & Green Bean Lean Meal

(Low-fat, light, packed with omega-3s, easy on the stomach)

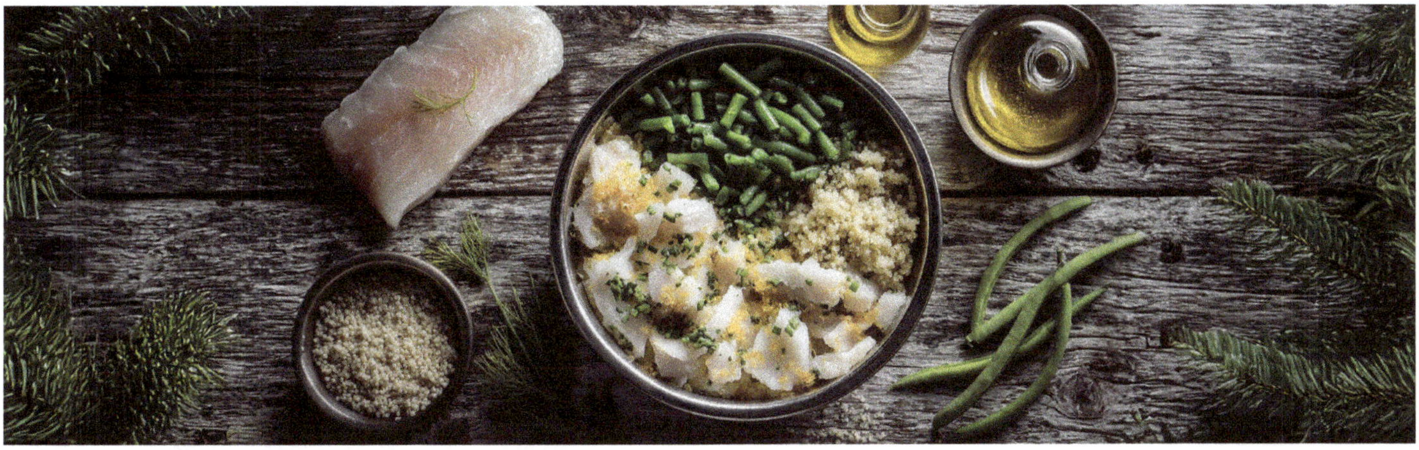

Ingredients:

- 1 lb. boneless whitefish (cod or tilapia, steamed)
- 1 cup steamed green beans (chopped)
- ½ cup cooked quinoa
- 1 tsp fish oil
- 1 tsp olive oil

Instructions:

1. Steam fish until fully cooked, flake.
2. Stir in green beans and quinoa.
3. Mix in oils.
4. Let cool before serving.

Ingredient Substitutions:

- Replace quinoa with millet.
- Swap green beans with spinach.

Nutrition per 500g serving:

Final Weight	~500g
Calories	~510 kcal
Protein	~38g
Fat	~16g
Carbohydrates	~32g

2. Turkey & Zucchini Light Meal

(Lean, low-fat protein source, rich in fiber and nutrients)

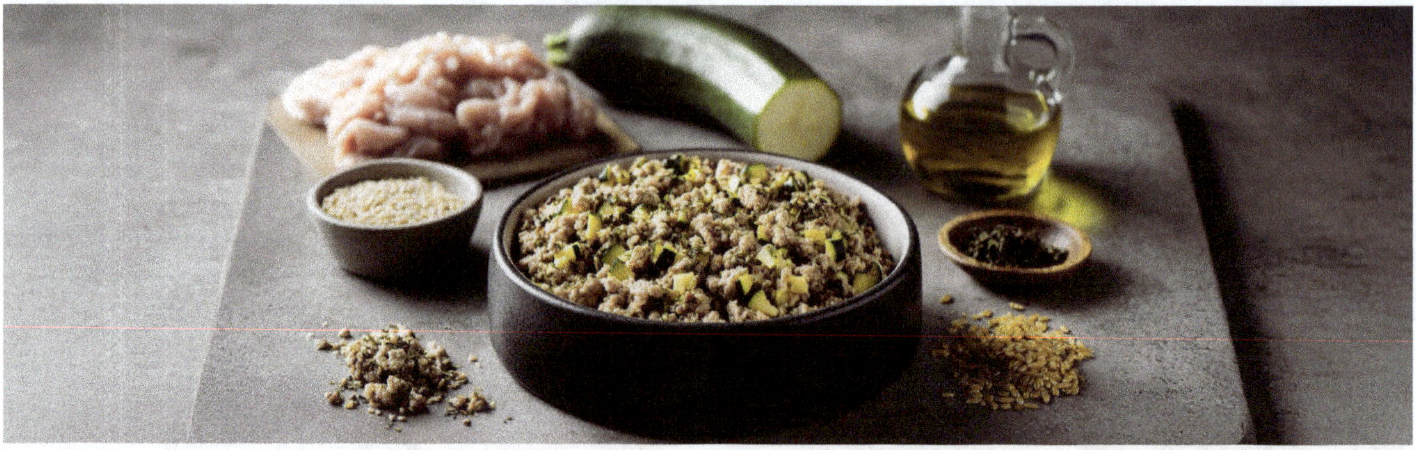

Ingredients:

- 1 lb. ground turkey (93% lean)
- 1 cup steamed zucchini (chopped)
- ½ cup cooked millet
- 1 tsp flaxseed oil
- 1 tsp olive oil

Instructions:

1. Cook turkey thoroughly.
2. Stir in zucchini and millet.
3. Mix in oils.
4. Let cool before serving.

Ingredient Substitutions:

- Replace millet with quinoa.
- Swap zucchini with green beans.

Nutrition per 500g serving:

Final Weight	~500g
Calories	~520 kcal
Protein	~40g
Fat	~18g
Carbohydrates	~30g

3. Chicken & Broccoli Low-Fat Bowl

(Low-fat, fiber-packed, easily digestible)

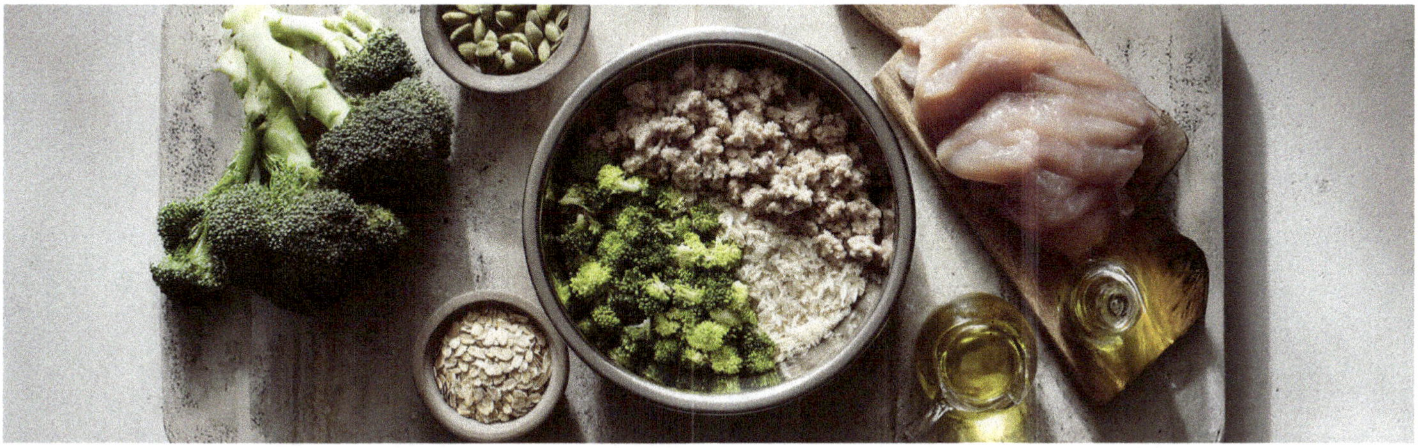

Ingredients:

- 1 lb. ground chicken (93% lean)
- 1 cup steamed broccoli (chopped)
- ½ cup cooked oats
- 1 tsp flaxseed oil
- 1 tsp olive oil

Instructions:

1. Cook chicken thoroughly.
2. Stir in broccoli and oats.
3. Mix in oils.
4. Let cool before serving.

Ingredient Substitutions:

- Replace oats with brown rice.
- Swap broccoli with green beans.

Nutrition per 500g serving:

Final Weight	~500g
Calories	~530 kcal
Protein	~38g
Fat	~18g
Carbohydrates	~32g

4. Egg & Spinach Lean Meal

(Soft-textured, lower fat, nutrient-dense, gentle on digestion)

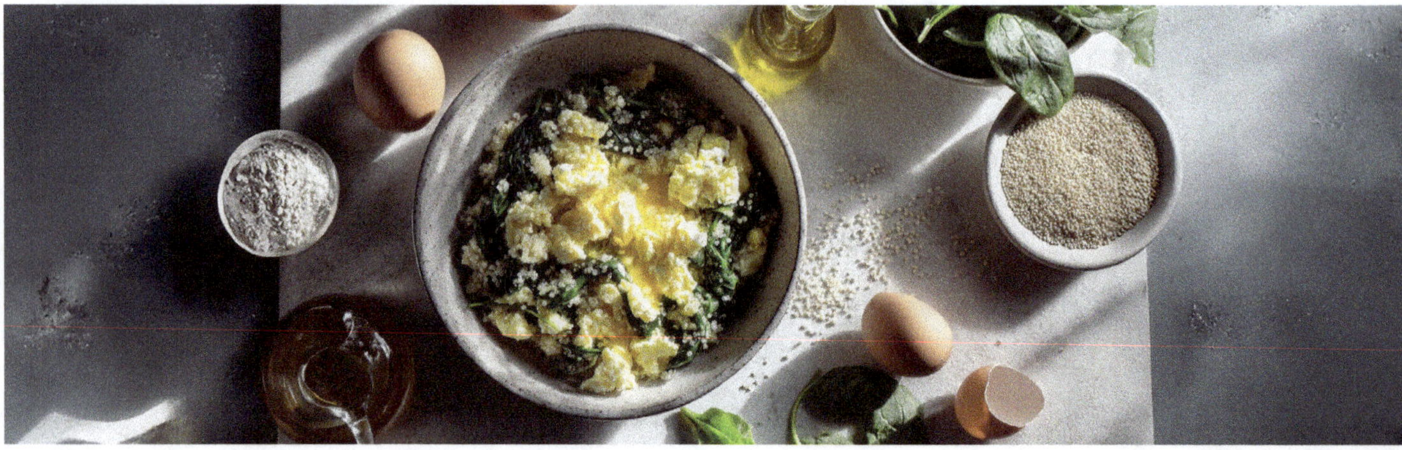

Ingredients:

- 3 large scrambled eggs
- 1 cup steamed spinach (chopped)
- ½ cup cooked quinoa
- 1 tsp flaxseed oil
- 1 tsp olive oil

Instructions:

1. Scramble eggs gently.
2. Stir in spinach and quinoa.
3. Mix in oils.
4. Let cool before serving.

Ingredient Substitutions:

- Replace quinoa with millet.
- Swap spinach with broccoli.

Nutrition per 500g serving:

Final Weight	~500g
Calories	~520 kcal
Protein	~36g
Fat	~18g
Carbohydrates	~30g

5. Rabbit & Carrot Low-Fat Meal

(Novel protein, low in fat, easy on sensitive digestion)

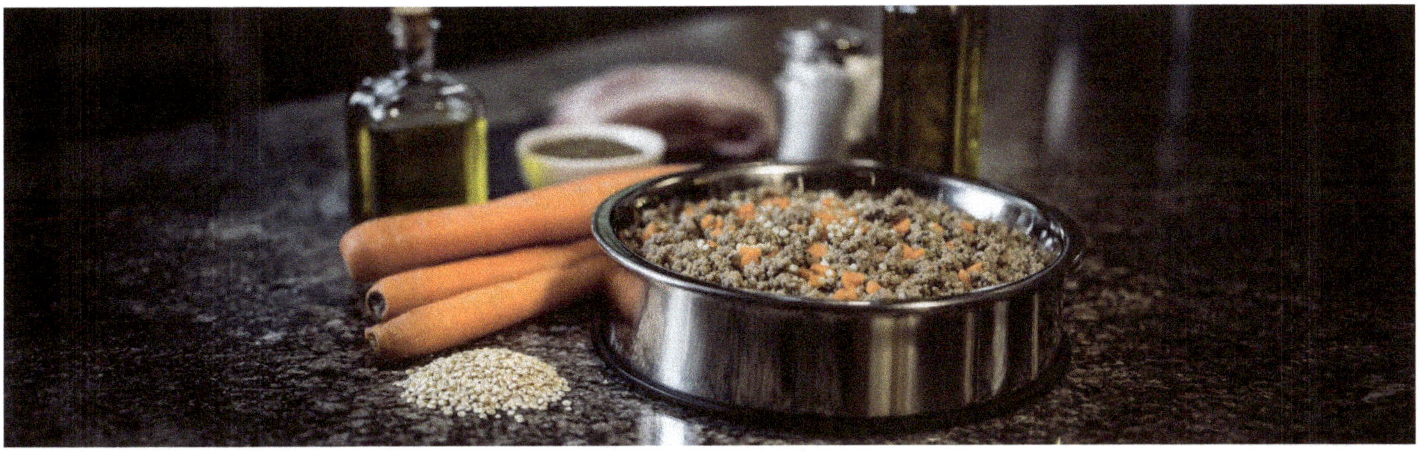

Ingredients:

- 1 lb. ground rabbit
- 1 cup steamed carrots (chopped)
- ½ cup cooked millet
- 1 tsp flaxseed oil
- 1 tsp olive oil

Instructions:

1. Cook rabbit thoroughly.
2. Stir in carrots and millet.
3. Mix in oils.
4. Let cool before serving.

Ingredient Substitutions:

- Replace millet with quinoa.
- Swap carrots with green beans.

Nutrition per 500g serving:

Final Weight	~500g
Calories	~520 kcal
Protein	~40g
Fat	~18g
Carbohydrates	~28g

6. Turkey & Pea Low-Fat Energy Meal

(Lean protein, low-fat, fiber-rich, suitable for pancreatitis management)

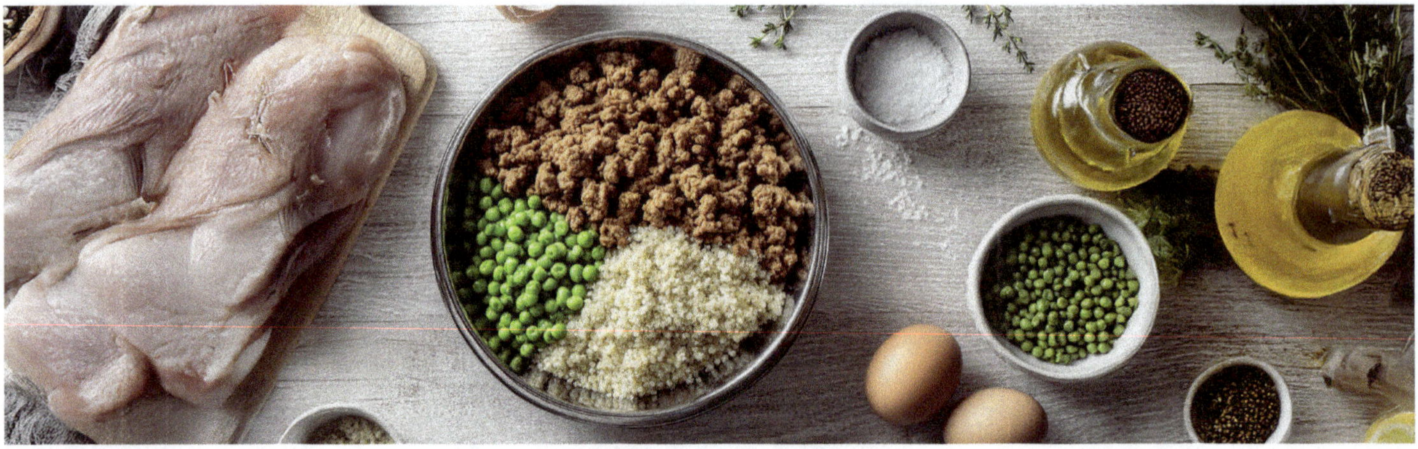

Ingredients:

- 1 lb. ground turkey (93% lean)
- 1 cup steamed peas (mashed)
- ½ cup cooked quinoa
- 2 tsp flaxseed oil
- 1 tsp ground eggshells OR 2 crushed calcium tablets
- ½ tsp iodized salt

Instructions:

1. In a pan, cook the ground turkey until fully browned (no added oil).
2. Add the mashed peas and cooked quinoa. Mix well.
3. Stir in flaxseed oil, ground eggshells (or calcium tablets), and iodized salt.
4. Cool before serving.

Ingredient Substitutions:

- Replace peas with green beans.
- Use millet instead of quinoa.

Nutrition per 500g serving:

Final Weight	~500g
Calories	~550 kcal
Protein	~45g
Fat	~20g
Carbohydrates	~30g

7. Chicken & Pumpkin Low-Fat Comfort Meal

(Lean protein, low-fat, easy on the pancreas and digestion)

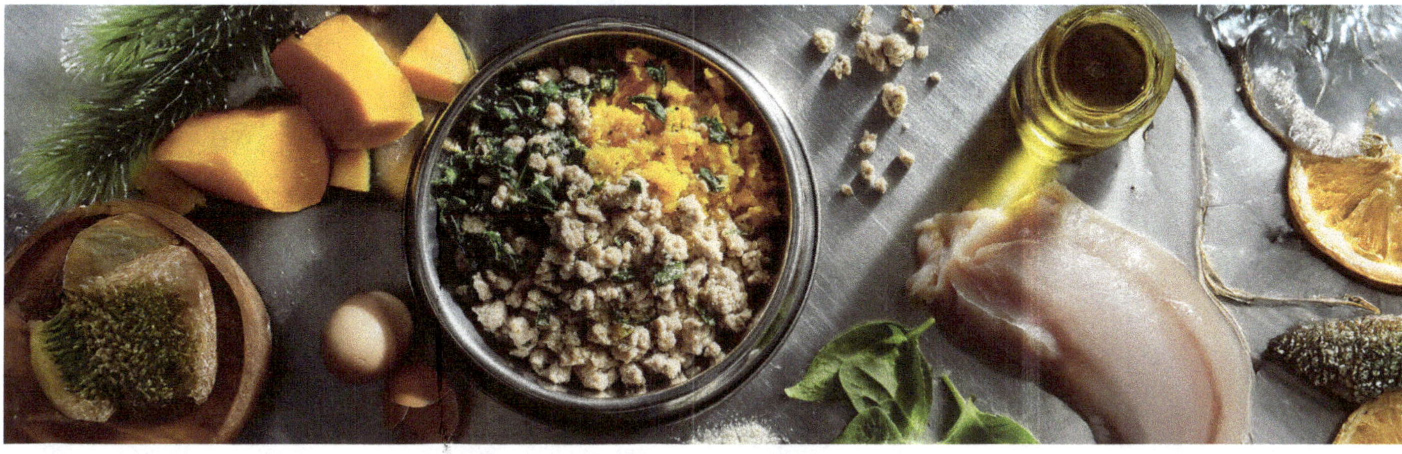

Ingredients:

- 1 lb. ground chicken (93% lean)
- 1 cup cooked pumpkin (mashed)
- ½ cup steamed spinach (chopped)
- 2 tsp flaxseed oil
- 1 tsp ground eggshells OR 2 crushed calcium tablets
- ½ tsp iodized salt

Instructions:

1. In a pan, cook the ground chicken until fully browned (no added oil).
2. Add the mashed pumpkin and chopped spinach. Mix well.
3. Stir in flaxseed oil, ground eggshells (or calcium tablets), and iodized salt.
4. Cool before serving.

Ingredient Substitutions:

- Replace pumpkin with sweet potato.
- Use turkey instead of chicken.

Nutrition per 500g serving:

Final Weight	~500g
Calories	~500 kcal
Protein	~45g
Fat	~15g
Carbohydrates	~25g

Kidney-Friendly Meals

1. Whitefish & Pumpkin Kidney Support Meal

(Low-phosphorus, light, gentle on kidneys and digestion)

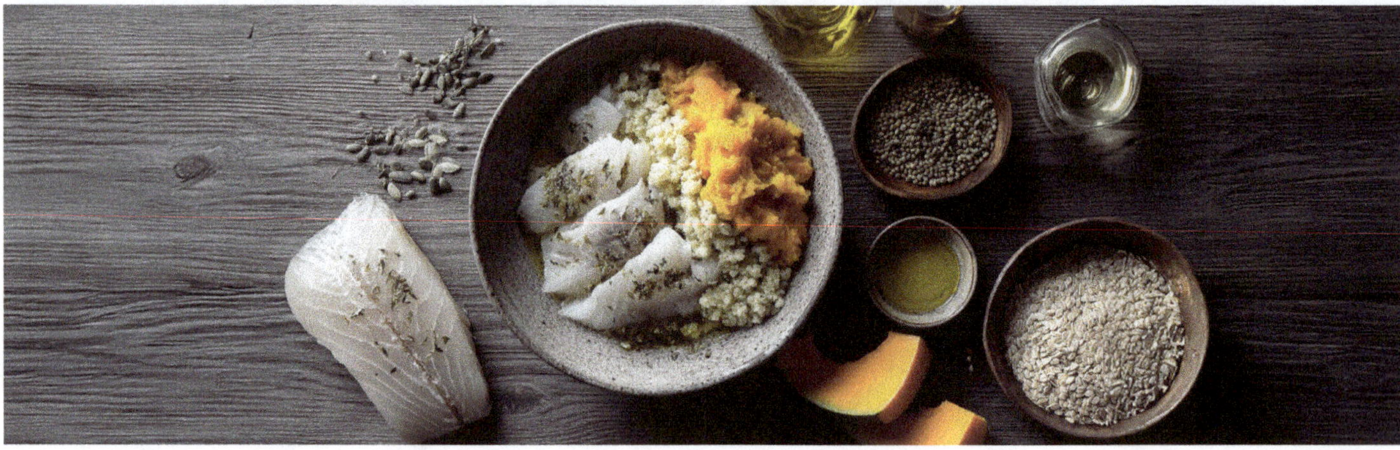

Ingredients:

- 1 lb. boneless whitefish (cod or tilapia, steamed)
- 1 cup mashed pumpkin
- ½ cup cooked millet
- 1 tsp fish oil
- 1 tsp olive oil

Instructions:

1. Steam fish until fully cooked, flake.
2. Stir in mashed pumpkin and millet.
3. Mix in oils.
4. Let cool before serving.

Ingredient Substitutions:

- Replace millet with white rice.
- Swap pumpkin with sweet potato.

Nutrition per 500g serving:

Final Weight	~500g
Calories	~540 kcal
Protein	~36g
Fat	~22g
Carbohydrates	~34g

2. Turkey & Sweet Potato Kidney Care Meal

(Moderate protein, easily digestible carbs, low phosphorus)

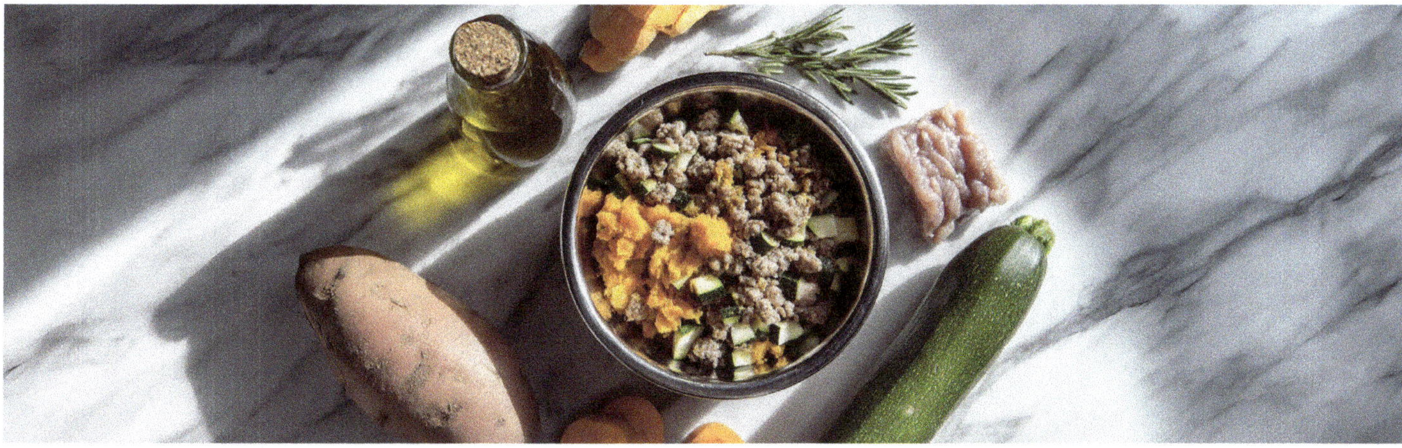

Ingredients:

- 1 lb. ground turkey (93% lean)
- 1 cup mashed sweet potato
- ½ cup steamed zucchini (chopped)
- 1 tsp flaxseed oil
- 1 tsp olive oil

Instructions:

1. Cook turkey thoroughly.
2. Stir in sweet potato and zucchini.
3. Mix in oils.
4. Let cool before serving.

Ingredient Substitutions:

- Replace zucchini with carrots.
- Swap turkey with chicken breast.

Nutrition per 500g serving:

Final Weight	~500g
Calories	~550 kcal
Protein	~38g
Fat	~22g
Carbohydrates	~32g

3. Egg & Rice Kidney-Friendly Bowl

(Lower phosphorus, soft texture, gentle on kidneys)

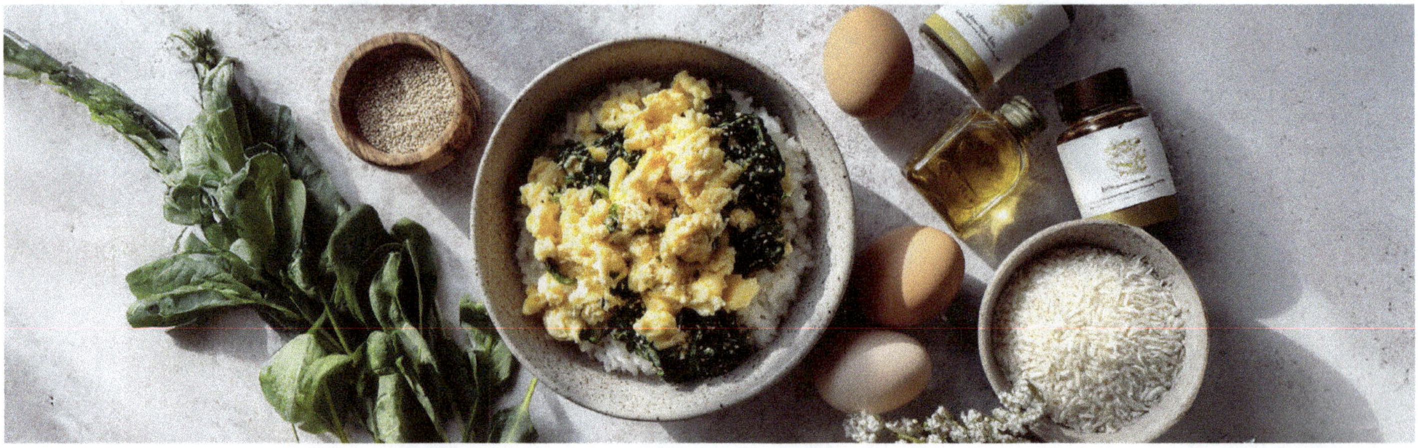

Ingredients:

- 3 large scrambled eggs
- 1 cup cooked white rice
- ½ cup steamed spinach (chopped)
- 1 tsp flaxseed oil
- 1 tsp olive oil

Instructions:

1. Scramble eggs gently.
2. Stir in cooked rice and spinach.
3. Mix in oils.
4. Let cool before serving.

Ingredient Substitutions:

- Replace spinach with green beans.
- Swap rice with millet.

Nutrition per 500g serving:

Final Weight	~500g
Calories	~520 kcal
Protein	~34g
Fat	~20g
Carbohydrates	~34g

4. Lamb & Green Bean Kidney Support Stew

(Moderate protein, nutrient-rich, with lower phosphorus content)

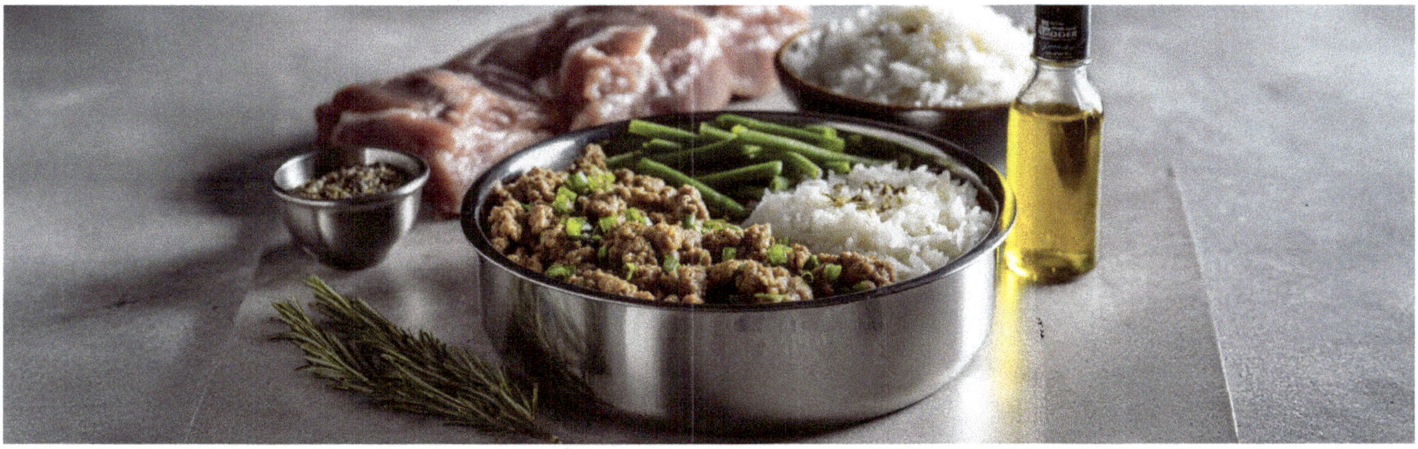

Ingredients:

- 1 lb. ground lamb (85% lean)
- 1 cup steamed green beans (chopped)
- ½ cup cooked white rice
- 1 tsp flaxseed oil
- 1 tsp olive oil

Instructions:

1. Cook lamb thoroughly.
2. Stir in green beans and rice.
3. Mix in oils.
4. Let cool before serving.

Ingredient Substitutions:

- Replace rice with millet.
- Swap green beans with peas.

Nutrition per 500g serving:

Final Weight	~500g
Calories	~600 kcal
Protein	~36g
Fat	~26g
Carbohydrates	~34g

5. Chicken & Carrot Kidney-Friendly Meal

(Lower fat, lower phosphorus, supports kidney function)

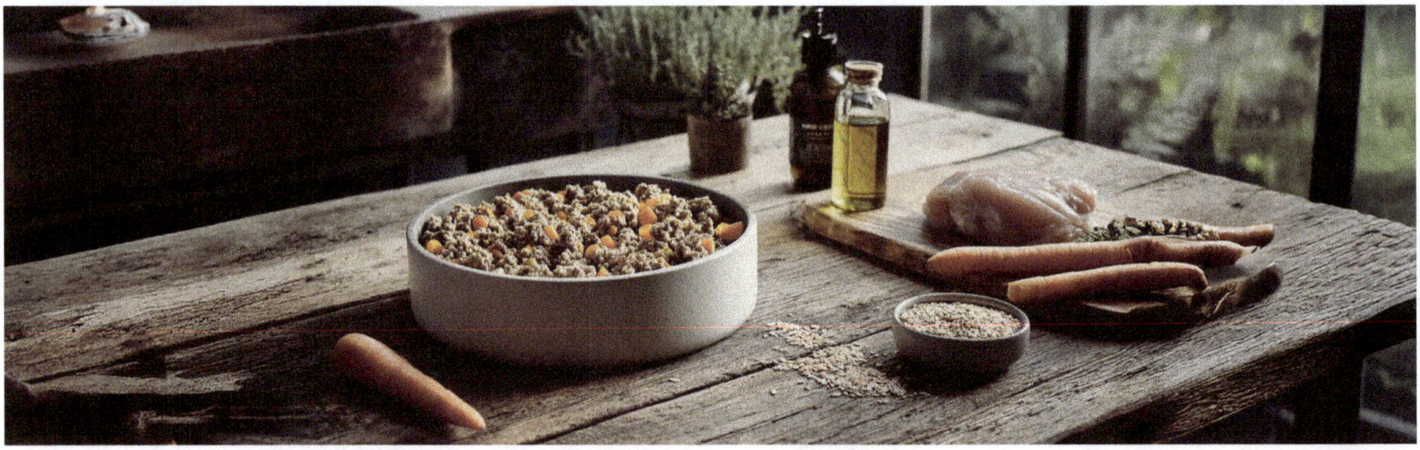

Ingredients:

- 1 lb. ground chicken (93% lean)
- 1 cup steamed carrots (chopped)
- ½ cup cooked millet
- 1 tsp flaxseed oil
- 1 tsp olive oil

Instructions:

1. Cook chicken thoroughly.
2. Stir in carrots and millet.
3. Mix in oils.
4. Let cool before serving.

Ingredient Substitutions:

- Replace millet with white rice.
- Swap carrots with zucchini.

Nutrition per 500g serving:

Final Weight	~500g
Calories	~540 kcal
Protein	~36g
Fat	~20g
Carbohydrates	~34g

6. Venison & Spinach Kidney Comfort Meal

(Low-phosphorus, novel protein, gentle on kidneys and digestion)

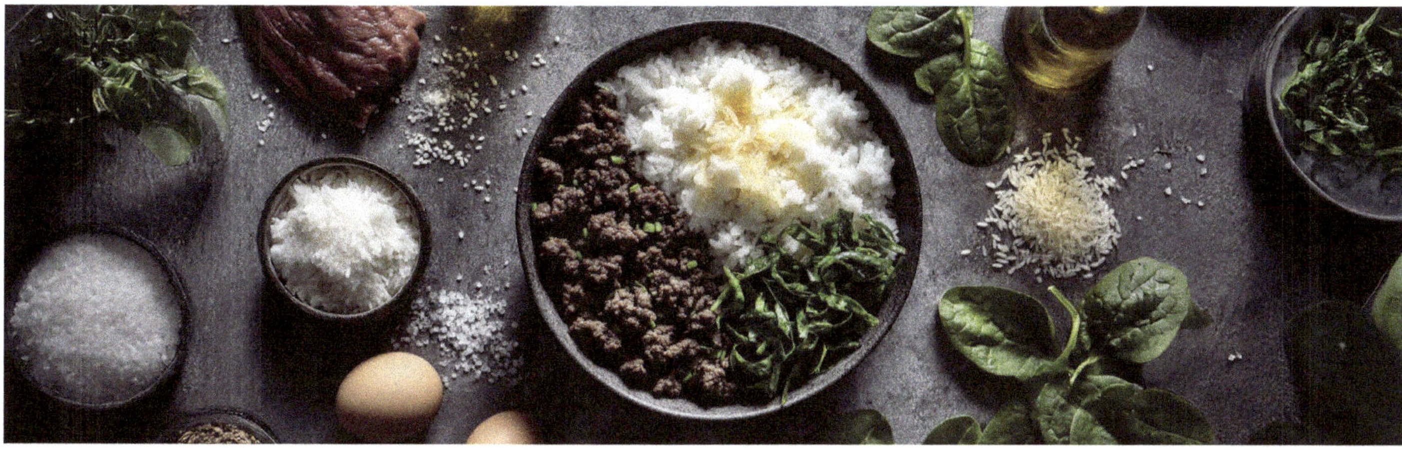

Ingredients:

- 1 lb. ground venison (90% lean)
- 1 cup cooked white rice
- ½ cup steamed spinach (chopped)
- 2 tsp olive oil
- 1 tsp ground eggshells OR 2 crushed calcium tablets
- ½ tsp iodized salt

Instructions:

1. In a pan, cook the ground venison until browned (no added oil).
2. Add the cooked white rice and chopped spinach. Mix thoroughly.
3. Stir in olive oil, ground eggshells (or calcium tablets), and iodized salt.
4. Cool before serving.

Ingredient Substitutions:

- Replace white rice with millet.
- Use ground rabbit instead of venison.

Nutrition per 500g serving:

Final Weight	~500g
Calories	~650 kcal
Protein	~50g
Fat	~25g
Carbohydrates	~35g

7. Pork & Rice Kidney Support Meal

(Low-phosphorus, lean protein, gentle on kidneys)

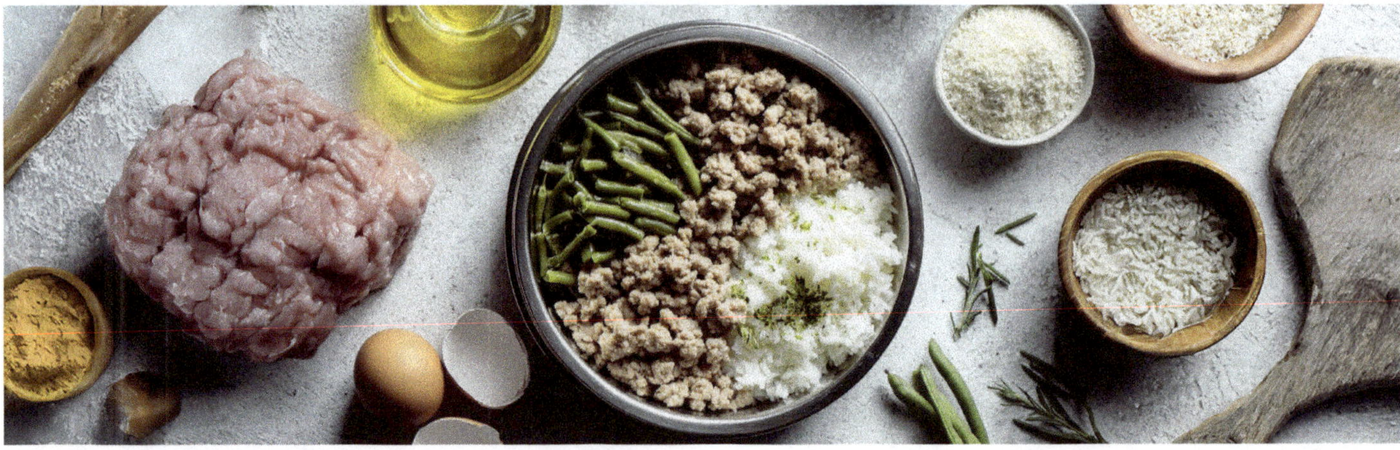

Ingredients:

- 1 lb. ground pork (90% lean)
- 1 cup cooked white rice
- ½ cup steamed green beans (chopped)
- 2 tsp olive oil
- 1 tsp ground eggshells OR 2 crushed calcium tablets
- ½ tsp iodized salt

Instructions:

1. In a pan, cook the ground pork until fully browned (no added oil).
2. Add the cooked white rice and chopped green beans. Mix thoroughly.
3. Stir in olive oil, ground eggshells (or calcium tablets), and iodized salt.
4. Cool before serving.

Ingredient Substitutions:

- Replace white rice with millet.
- Use ground chicken instead of pork.

Nutrition per 500g serving:

Final Weight	~500g
Calories	~700 kcal
Protein	~45g
Fat	~35g
Carbohydrates	~30g

Anti-Inflammatory Foods for Arthritis and Skin Issues

1. Salmon & Spinach Inflammation Support Bowl

(Omega-3 powerhouse, supports joint and skin health)

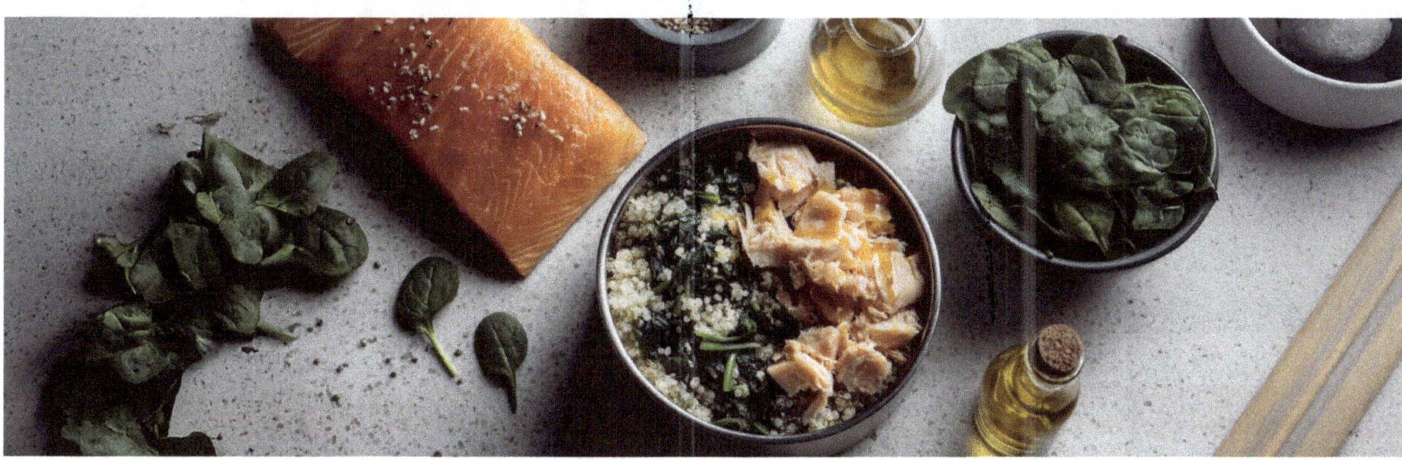

Ingredients:

- 1 lb. boneless salmon (steamed)
- 1 cup cooked quinoa
- ½ cup steamed spinach (chopped)
- 1 tsp fish oil
- 1 tsp olive oil

Instructions:

1. Steam salmon, flake into small pieces.
2. Mix in quinoa and spinach.
3. Stir in oils.
4. Let cool before serving.

Ingredient Substitutions:

- Replace quinoa with brown rice.
- Swap spinach with broccoli.

Nutrition per 500g serving:

Final Weight	~500g
Calories	~610 kcal
Protein	~42g
Fat	~26g
Carbohydrates	~36g

2. Turkey & Broccoli Joint Relief Meal

(Lean, antioxidant-rich, ideal for joint inflammation control)

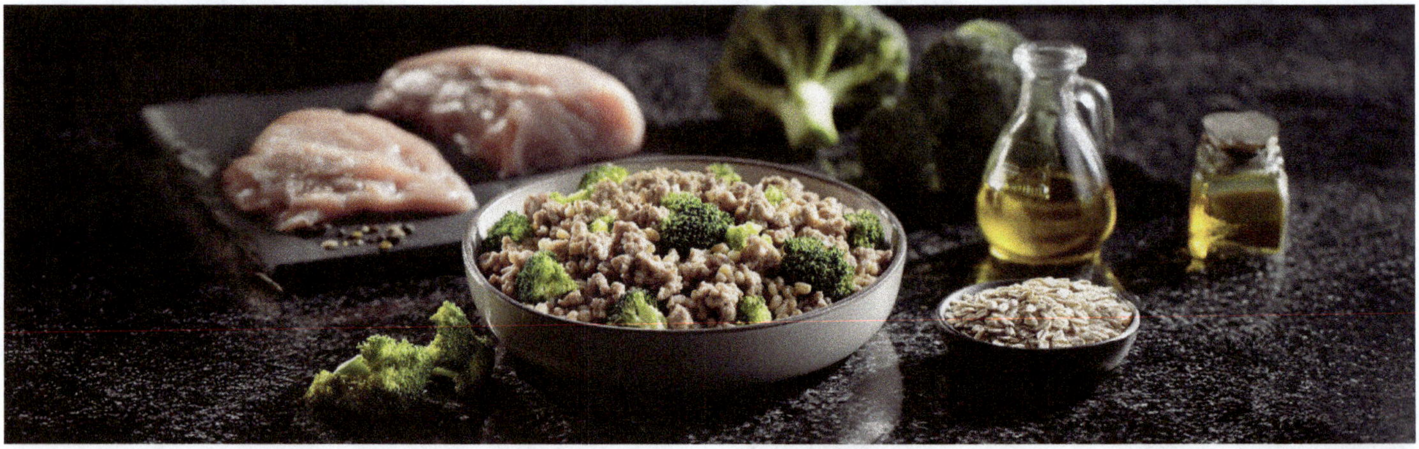

Ingredients:

- 1 lb. ground turkey (93% lean)
- 1 cup cooked barley
- ½ cup steamed broccoli (chopped)
- 1 tsp flaxseed oil
- 1 tsp olive oil

Instructions:

1. Cook turkey thoroughly.
2. Stir in barley and broccoli.
3. Mix in oils.
4. Let cool before serving.

Ingredient Substitutions:

- Replace barley with oats.
- Swap broccoli with spinach.

Nutrition per 500g serving:

Final Weight	~500g
Calories	~580 kcal
Protein	~38g
Fat	~22g
Carbohydrates	~34g

3. Shrimp & Couscous Anti-Inflammatory Meal

(Low-fat, rich in omega-3s, gentle on joints and digestion)

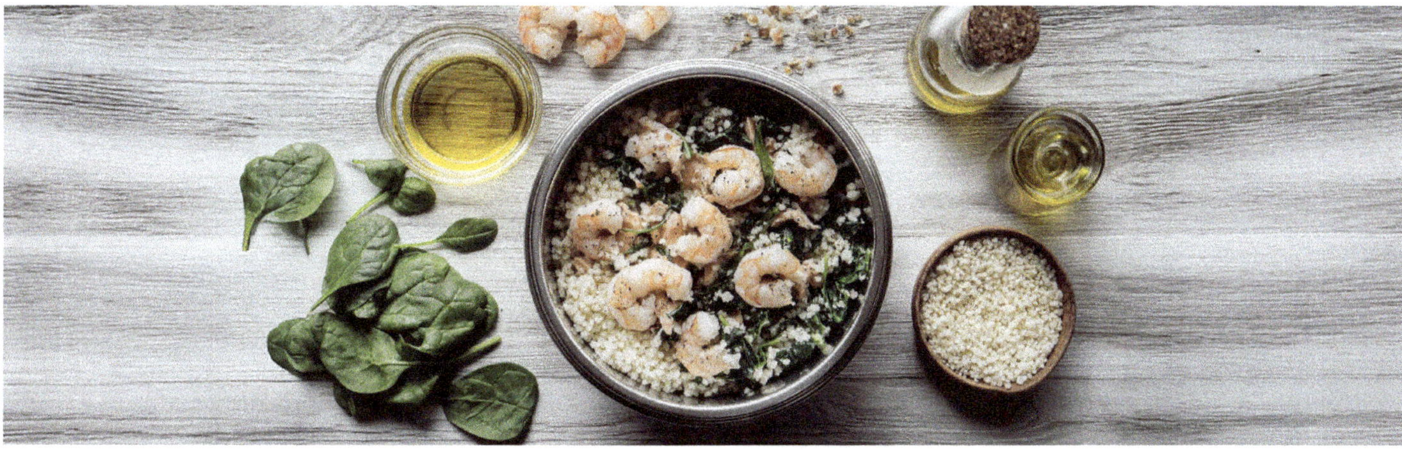

Ingredients:

- 1 lb. (450g) shrimp (steamed, peeled)
- 1 cup (175g) cooked couscous
- ½ cup (75g) steamed spinach (chopped)
- 1 tsp fish oil
- 1 tsp olive oil

Instructions:

1. Steam shrimp, then flake into small pieces.
2. Mix in couscous and spinach
3. Stir in oils.
4. Let cool before serving.

Ingredient Substitutions:

- Replace spinach with steamed zucchini.
- Swap couscous with millet

Nutrition per 500g serving:

Final Weight	~500g
Calories	~650 kcal
Protein	~85g
Fat	~20g
Carbohydrates	~40g

4. Egg & Pumpkin Inflammation Relief Bowl

(Soft-textured, high in antioxidants and healthy fats)

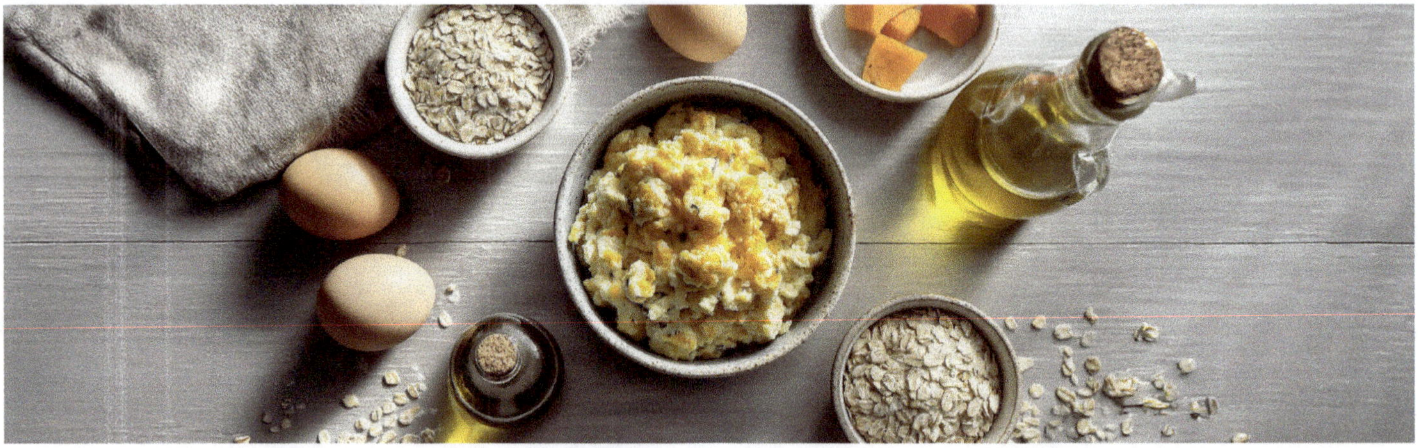

Ingredients:

- 3 large scrambled eggs
- 1 cup mashed pumpkin
- ½ cup cooked oats
- 1 tsp flaxseed oil
- 1 tsp olive oil

Instructions:

1. Scramble eggs gently.
2. Stir in pumpkin and oats.
3. Mix in oils.
4. Let cool before serving.

Ingredient Substitutions:

- Replace oats with quinoa.
- Swap pumpkin with sweet potato.

Nutrition per 500g serving:

Final Weight	~500g
Calories	~540 kcal
Protein	~34g
Fat	~20g
Carbohydrates	~32g

5. Lamb & Carrot Anti-Inflammatory Stew

(Rich in minerals, antioxidant-loaded veggies for inflammation support)

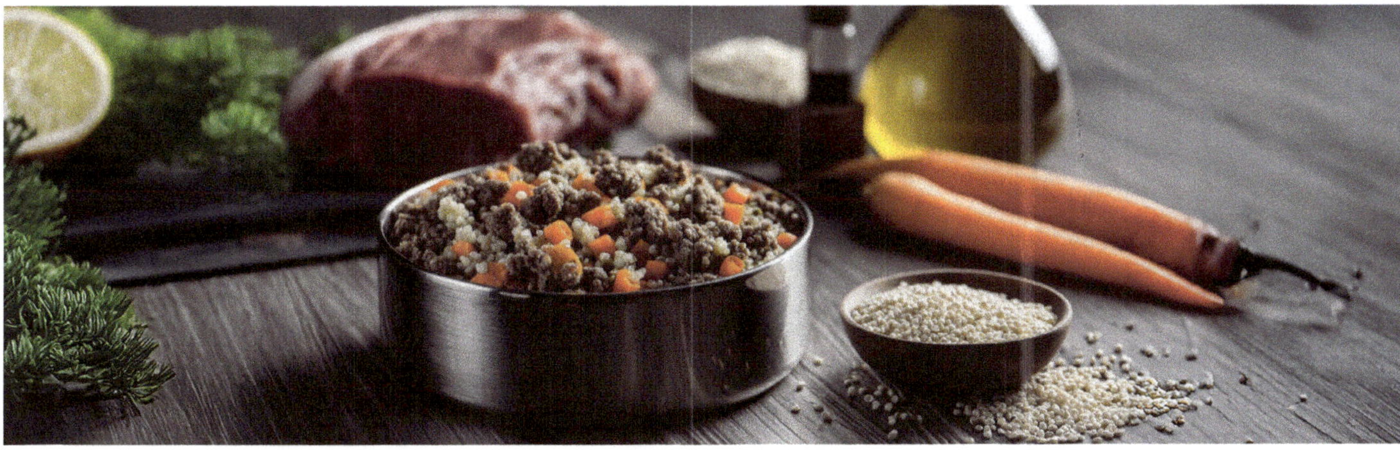

Ingredients:

- 1 lb. ground lamb (85% lean)
- 1 cup steamed carrots (chopped)
- ½ cup cooked millet
- 1 tsp flaxseed oil
- 1 tsp olive oil

Instructions:

1. Brown lamb thoroughly.
2. Stir in carrots and millet.
3. Mix in oils.
4. Let cool before serving.

Ingredient Substitutions:

- Replace millet with oats.
- Swap carrots with green beans.

Nutrition per 500g serving:

Final Weight	~500g
Calories	~620 kcal
Protein	~40g
Fat	~26g
Carbohydrates	~38g

6. Duck & Blueberry Anti-Inflammatory Bowl

(Novel protein, antioxidant-rich, supports joint and skin health)

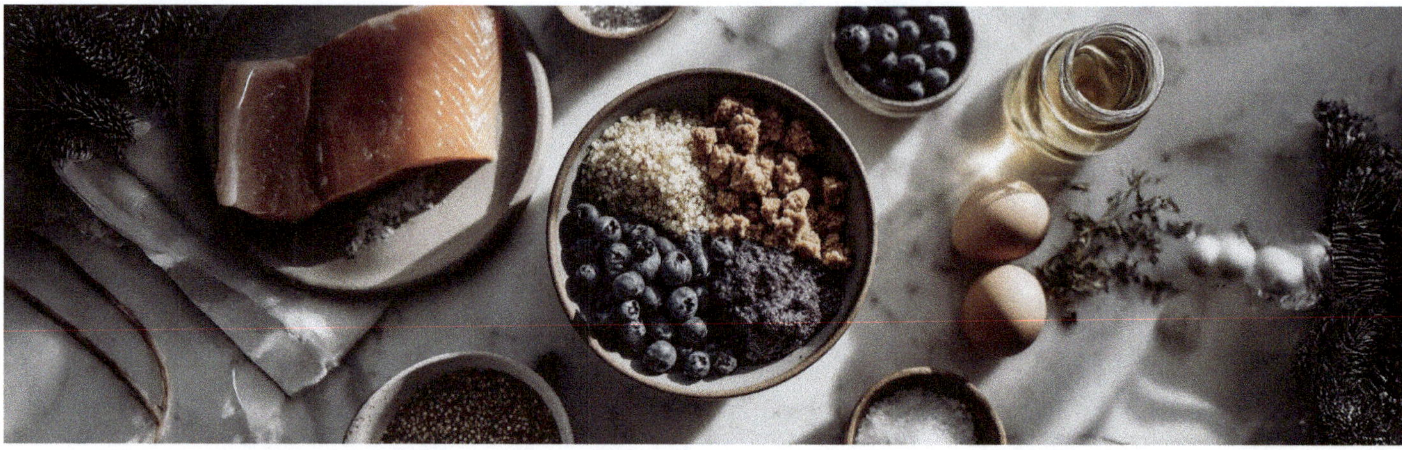

Ingredients:

- 1 lb. ground duck (skin removed, 90% lean)
- 1 cup cooked quinoa
- ½ cup fresh blueberries (mashed)
- 2 tsp fish oil
- 1 tsp ground eggshells OR 2 crushed calcium tablets
- ½ tsp iodized salt

Instructions:

1. In a pan, cook the ground duck until fully browned (no added oil).
2. Add the cooked quinoa and mashed blueberries. Mix well.
3. Stir in fish oil, ground eggshells (or calcium tablets), and iodized salt.
4. Cool before serving.

Ingredient Substitutions:

- Replace quinoa with millet.
- Use ground turkey instead of duck.

Nutrition per 500g serving:

Final Weight	~500g
Calories	~700 kcal
Protein	~45g
Fat	~30g
Carbohydrates	~35g

7. Mackerel & Quinoa Joint Care Meal

(Omega-3 powerhouse, supports joints and inflammation control)

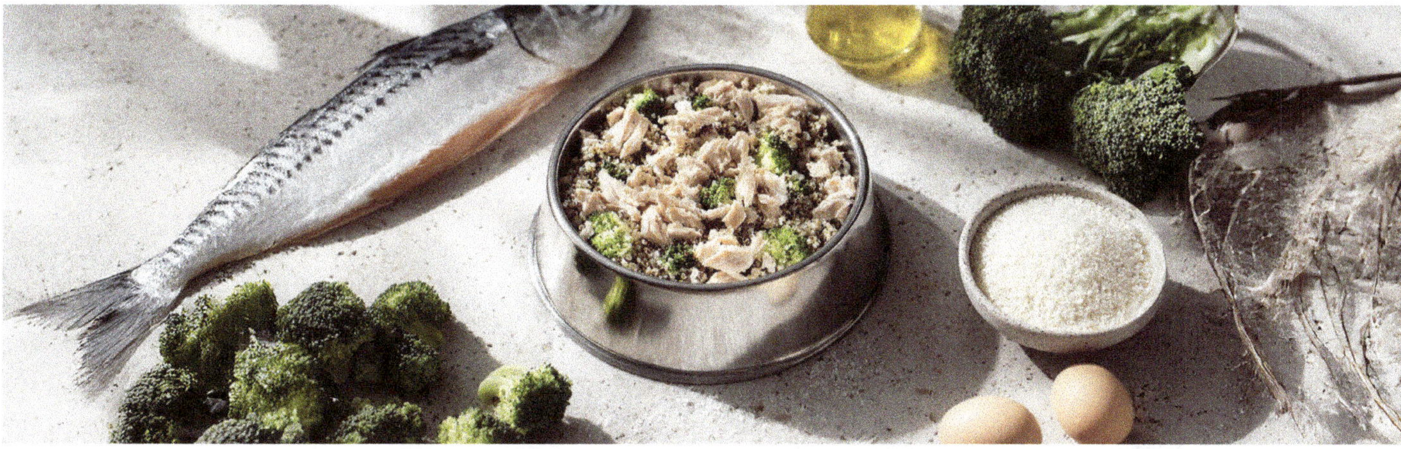

Ingredients:

- 1 lb. boneless mackerel (steamed and flaked)
- 1 cup cooked quinoa
- ½ cup steamed broccoli (chopped)
- 2 tsp fish oil
- 1 tsp ground eggshells OR 2 crushed calcium tablets
- ½ tsp iodized salt

Instructions:

1. Steam the mackerel until fully cooked, then flake into small pieces.
2. Mix in the cooked quinoa and chopped broccoli.
3. Stir in fish oil, ground eggshells (or calcium tablets), and iodized salt.
4. Cool before serving.

Ingredient Substitutions:

- Replace quinoa with millet.
- Use sardines instead of mackerel.

Nutrition per 500g serving:

Final Weight	~500g
Calories	~750 kcal
Protein	~45g
Fat	~35g
Carbohydrates	~30g

Meals for Diabetic Dogs

1. Turkey & Lentil Blood Sugar Support Meal

(Lean, high in fiber, low-glycemic and energy-sustaining)

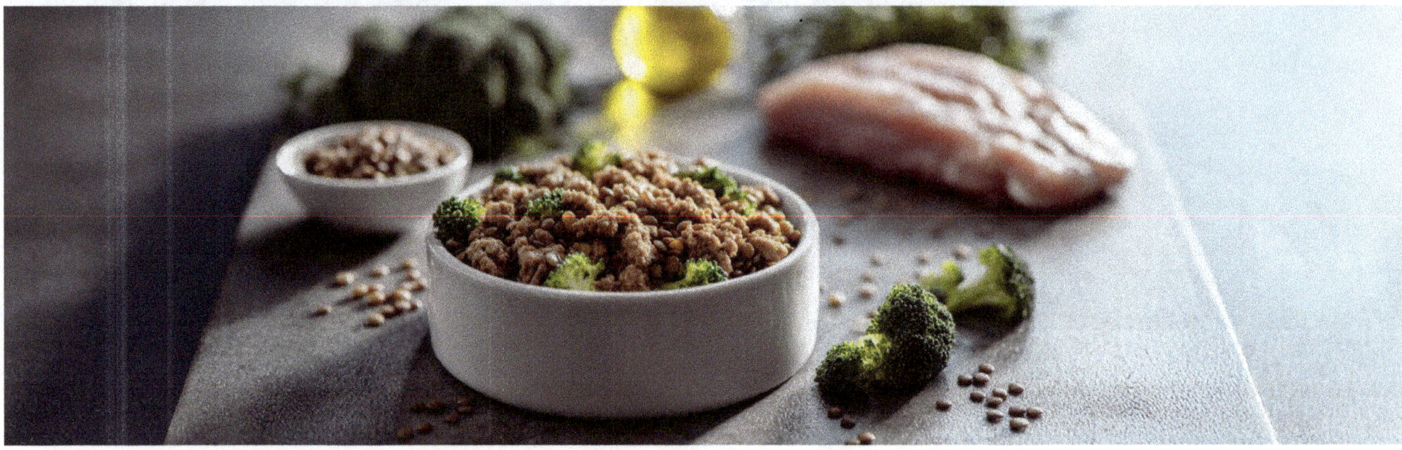

Ingredients:

- 1 lb. ground turkey (93% lean)
- 1 cup cooked lentils
- ½ cup steamed broccoli (chopped)
- 1 tsp flaxseed oil
- 1 tsp olive oil

Instructions:

1. Cook turkey thoroughly.
2. Stir in cooked lentils and steamed broccoli.
3. Mix in oils.
4. Let cool before serving.

Ingredient Substitutions:

- Replace lentils with chickpeas.
- Swap broccoli with green beans.

Nutrition per 500g serving:

Final Weight	~500g
Calories	~560 kcal
Protein	~40g
Fat	~22g
Carbohydrates	~32g

2. Whitefish & Quinoa Glycemic Control Bowl

(Low-fat, fiber-rich, loaded with omega-3s and antioxidants)

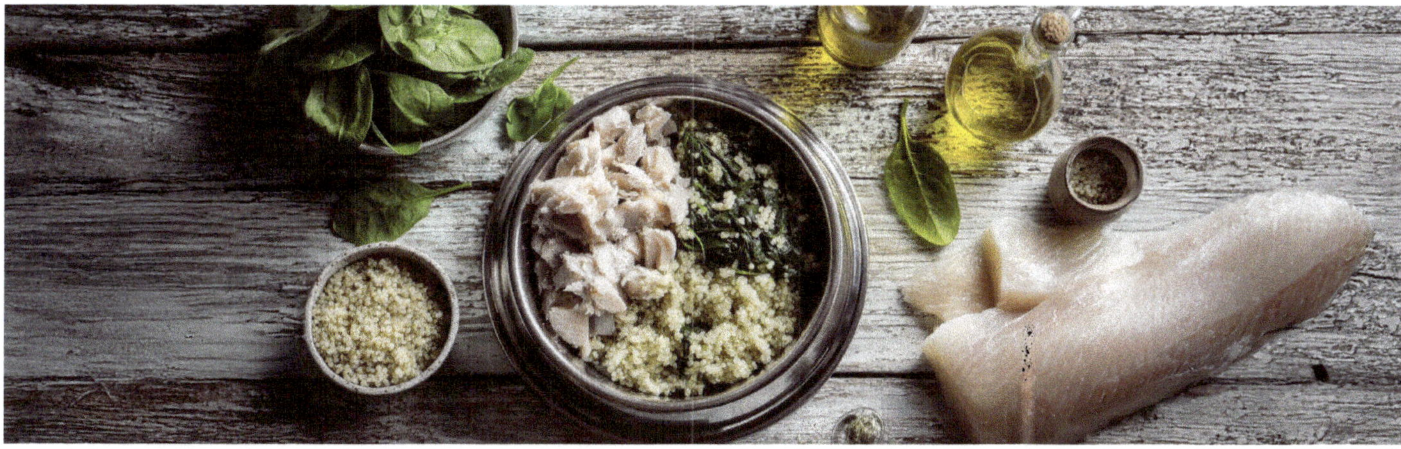

Ingredients:

- 1 lb. boneless whitefish (cod or tilapia, steamed)
- 1 cup cooked quinoa
- ½ cup steamed spinach (chopped)
- 1 tsp fish oil
- 1 tsp olive oil

Instructions:

1. Steam fish until fully cooked, flake.
2. Mix in quinoa and spinach.
3. Stir in oils.
4. Let cool before serving.

Ingredient Substitutions:

- Replace quinoa with millet.
- Swap spinach with broccoli.

Nutrition per 500g serving:

Final Weight	~500g
Calories	~550 kcal
Protein	~38g
Fat	~20g
Carbohydrates	~32g

3. Beef & Chickpea Diabetic-Friendly Meal

(Rich in fiber and iron, helps with blood sugar stability)

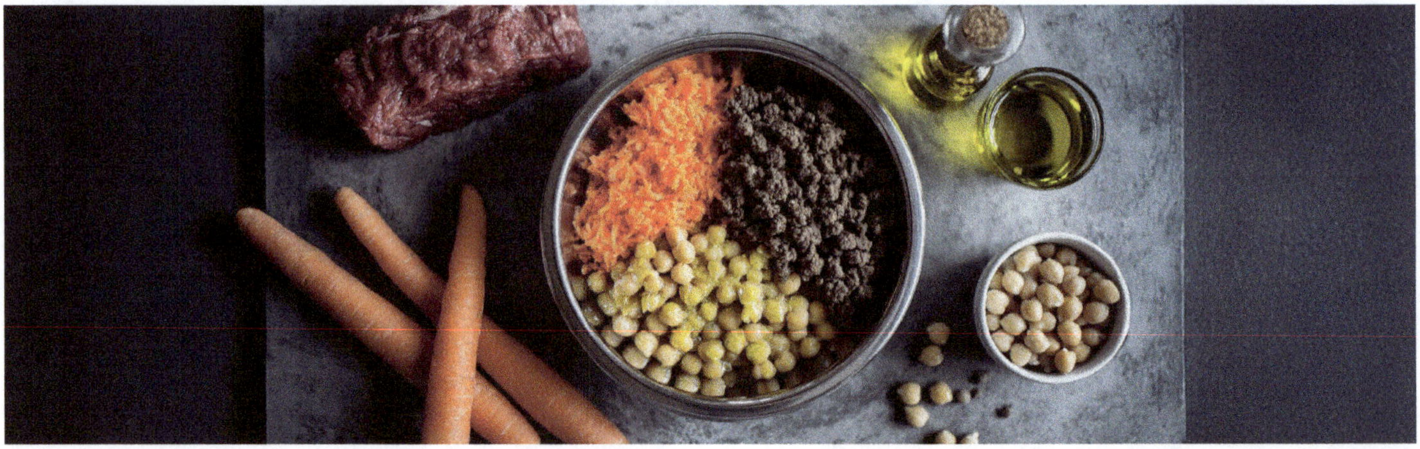

Ingredients:

- 1 lb. lean ground beef (90% lean)
- 1 cup cooked chickpeas (mashed slightly)
- ½ cup steamed carrots (chopped)
- 1 tsp flaxseed oil
- 1 tsp olive oil

Instructions:

1. Brown beef thoroughly.
2. Stir in chickpeas and carrots.
3. Mix in oils.
4. Let cool before serving.

Ingredient Substitutions:

- Replace chickpeas with lentils.
- Swap carrots with spinach.

Nutrition per 500g serving:

Final Weight	~500g
Calories	~600 kcal
Protein	~40g
Fat	~26g
Carbohydrates	~36g

4. Chicken & Barley Glycemic Balance Bowl

(High-fiber, low-glycemic barley to slow sugar absorption)

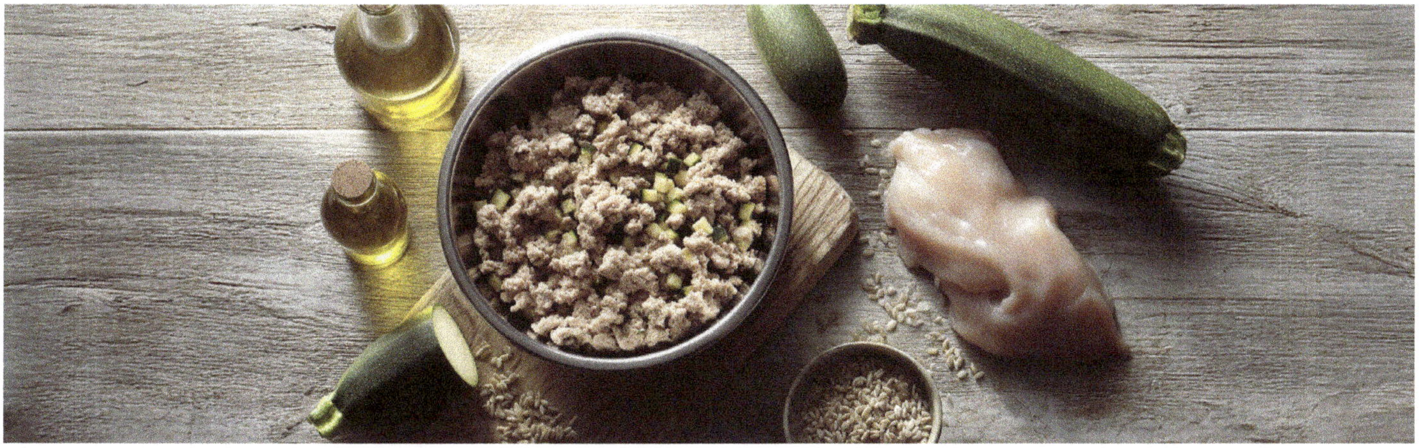

Ingredients:

- 1 lb. ground chicken (93% lean)
- 1 cup cooked barley
- ½ cup steamed zucchini (chopped)
- 1 tsp flaxseed oil
- 1 tsp olive oil

Instructions:

1. Cook chicken thoroughly.
2. Stir in barley and zucchini.
3. Mix in oils.
4. Let cool before serving.

Ingredient Substitutions:

- Replace barley with quinoa.
- Swap zucchini with broccoli.

Nutrition per 500g serving:

Final Weight	~500g
Calories	~540 kcal
Protein	~38g
Fat	~22g
Carbohydrates	~32g

5. Egg & Green Bean Low Glycemic Bowl

(Soft, nutrient-dense, low-carb and high-fiber option)

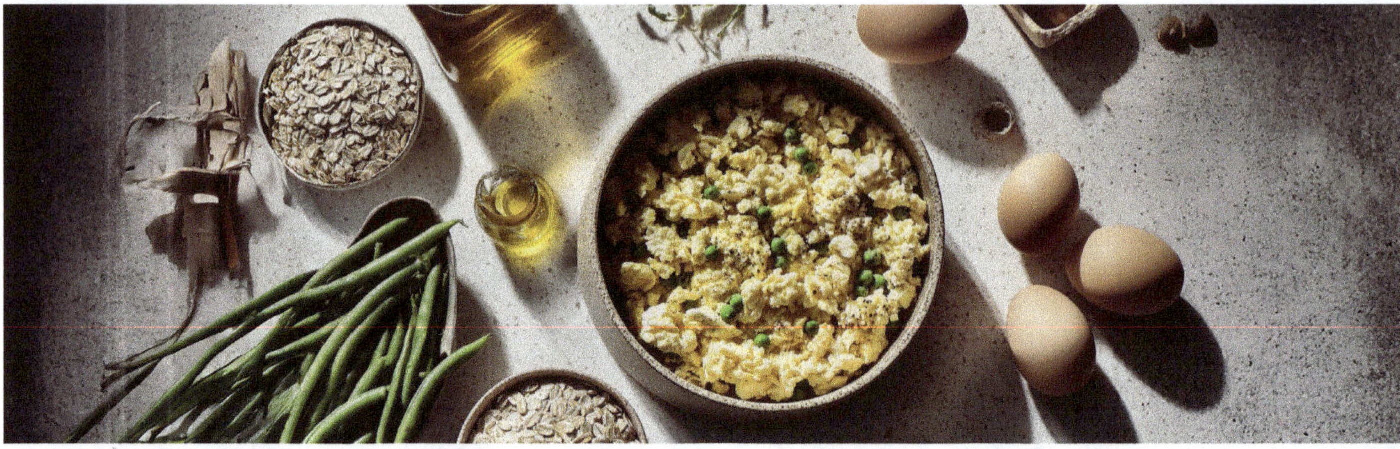

Ingredients:

- 3 large scrambled eggs
- 1 cup steamed green beans (chopped)
- ½ cup cooked oats
- 1 tsp flaxseed oil
- 1 tsp olive oil

Instructions:

1. Scramble eggs gently.
2. Stir in green beans and oats.
3. Mix in oils.
4. Let cool before serving.

Ingredient Substitutions:

- Replace oats with millet.
- Swap green beans with spinach.

Nutrition per 500g serving:

Final Weight	~500g
Calories	~530 kcal
Protein	~34g
Fat	~20g
Carbohydrates	~30g

6. Beef & Lentil Glycemic Stability Meal

(High-fiber, low-glycemic, supports blood sugar control)

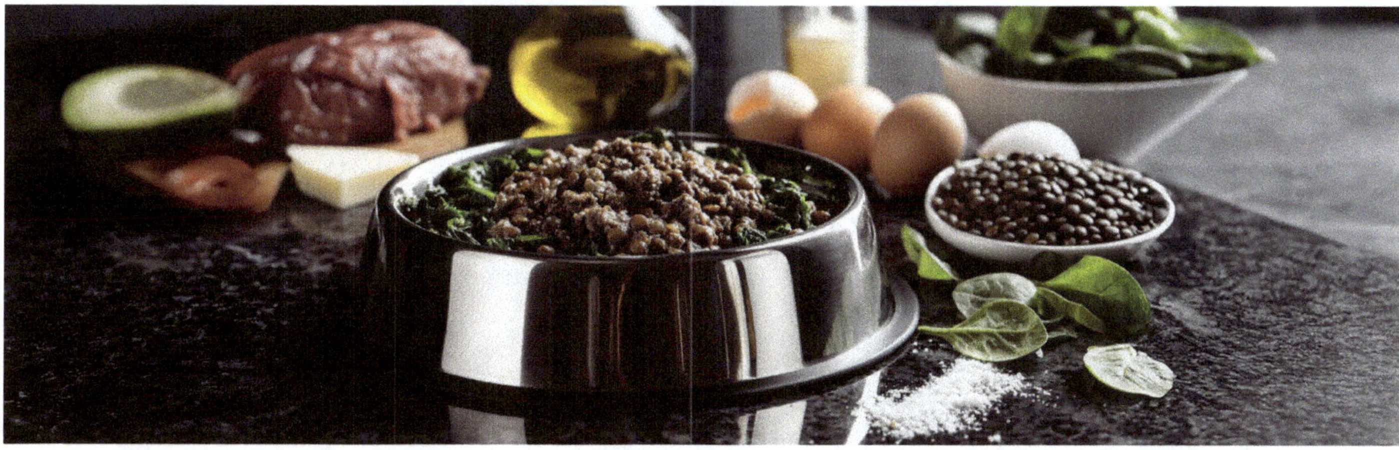

Ingredients:

- 1 lb. lean ground beef (90% lean)
- 1 cup cooked lentils
- ½ cup steamed spinach (chopped)
- 2 tsp flaxseed oil
- 1 tsp ground eggshells OR 2 crushed calcium tablets
- ½ tsp iodized salt

Instructions:

1. In a pan, cook the ground beef until fully browned (no added oil).
2. Add the cooked lentils and chopped spinach. Mix well.
3. Stir in flaxseed oil, ground eggshells (or calcium tablets), and iodized salt.
4. Cool before serving.

Ingredient Substitutions:

- Replace lentils with chickpeas.
- Use ground turkey instead of beef.

Nutrition per 500g serving:

Final Weight	~500g
Calories	~7o0 kcal
Protein	~50g
Fat	~30g
Carbohydrates	~35g

Key Takeaways:

- Beef, chicken, and grains are the most common food allergens in dogs.
- Symptoms of food allergies include itchy skin, ear infections, digestive upset, and chronic itching.
- Food allergies and food intolerances are different, requiring different management strategies.
- Allergies involve an immune system response, while intolerances stem from digestive issues.
- Food allergies require complete avoidance, while intolerances may be managed with portion control or cooking adjustments.
- The elimination diet method helps identify whether a dog has an allergy or intolerance.
- Dogs with a safe previous diet should be introduced to new ingredients one at a time to identify allergens.
- Dogs with known allergies should start fresh with a single protein and carb diet before reintroducing old ingredients.
- A food trial should last 7–14 days per new ingredient to monitor reactions.
- Any ingredient causing symptoms should be removed immediately, with a waiting period before testing another.
- Keeping an elimination diet tracking chart helps monitor symptoms, severity, and safe foods.
- Testing should start with proteins, then move to carbohydrates, dairy, eggs, legumes, fats, and vegetables.

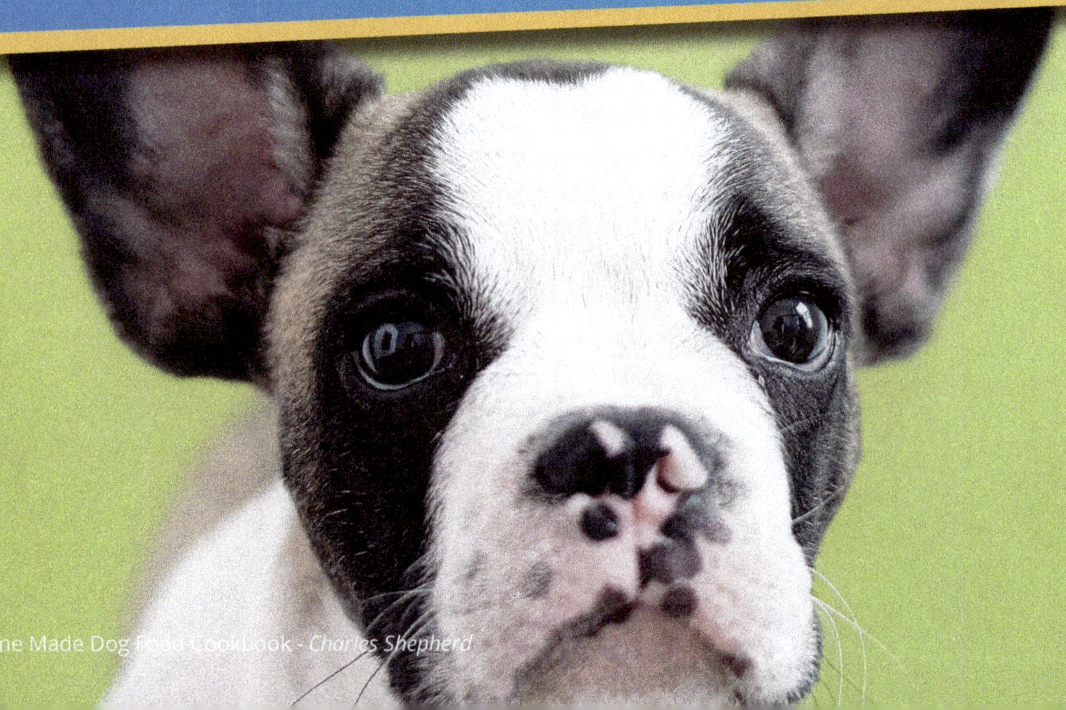

Get the most of what you have just learned:

- Start an elimination diet by feeding your dog a simple meal with one protein and one carbohydrate for 2–4 weeks.
- Keep a tracking chart to record each new ingredient introduced, and any symptoms or reactions.
- Introduce one new ingredient every 7–14 days, monitoring for itching, vomiting, diarrhea, or other signs of allergies.
- If a reaction occurs, remove the ingredient immediately and allow symptoms to heal before trying another ingredient after recovery.
- Gradually build a safe, balanced homemade diet by testing proteins, grains, dairy, eggs, and vegetables gradually.

Now that you can manage food allergies and intolerances, let's focus on making meal prep easier and budget-friendly. Preparing homemade meals for your pup doesn't have to be time-consuming or expensive. In the next chapter, we'll explore smart strategies to save time in the kitchen, affordable ingredient swaps, and meal-planning tips that keep your dog's diet nutritious without breaking the bank. With these practical hacks, you'll create healthy, homemade meals while saving time and money.

Let's go!

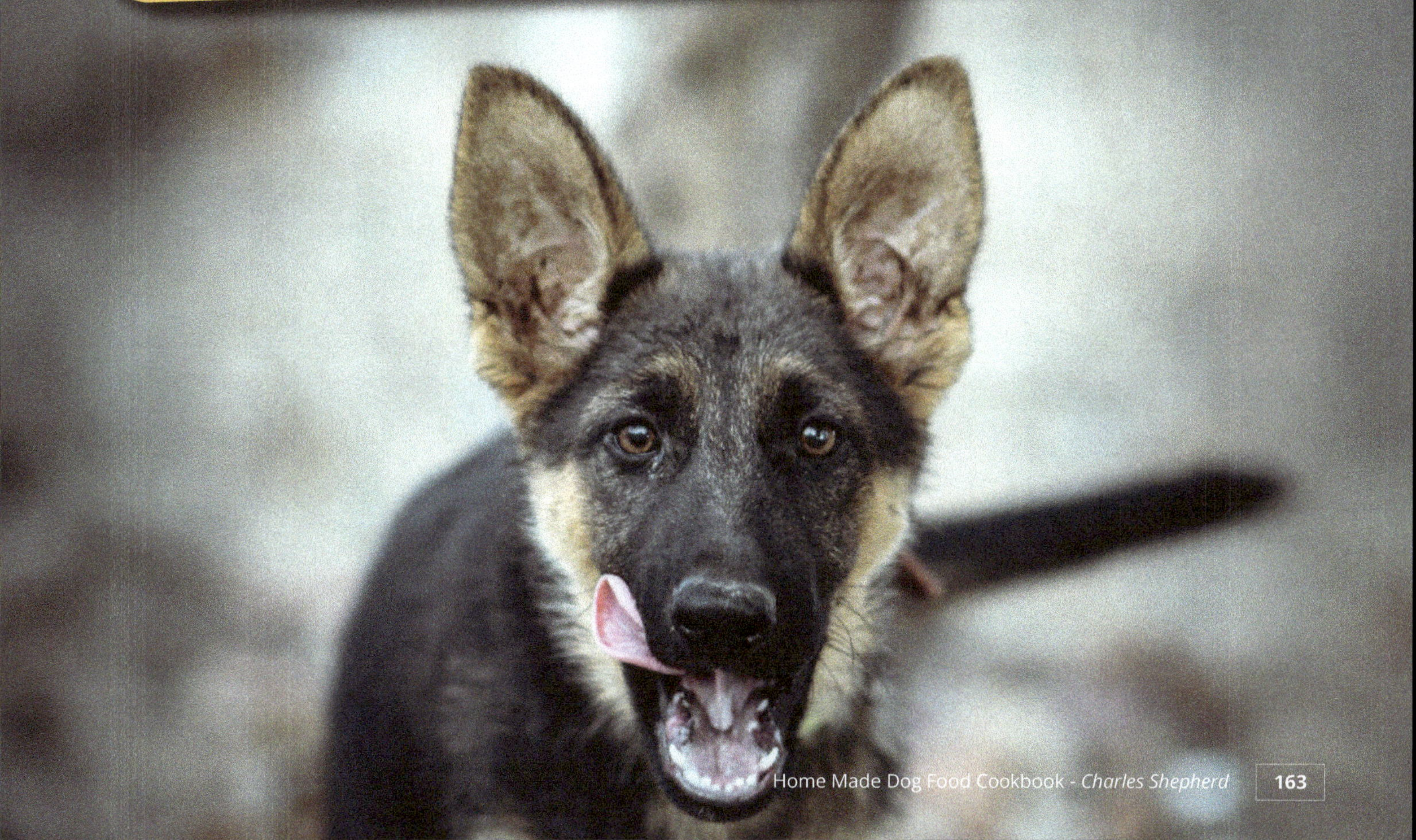

CHAPTER 5:

Time-Saving Meal Prep & Budget-Friendly Tips

"You don't need a gourmet kitchen or hours of free time to feed your dog well."

Keeping your pup's food fresh is the key to providing nutritionally balanced meals. While I always recommend preparing a fresh meal, there is nothing wrong with cooking beforehand–just ensure proper storage.

Always remember... your pup's food should never be exposed to factors like air, moisture, and heat. Which means, if you leave the meal outside the freezer, these external factors can break down nutrients over time. As a result, the food will lose nutrition and may even get spoiled if you let it stay on the counter for too long.

The best way to preserve nutrients is to store meals in airtight containers and keep them in the fridge or freezer. Refrigerated meals should be used within 3-5 days, while frozen meals can last up to 3 months. Avoid frequent thawing and refreezing, as this can cause nutrient loss and spoilage. If you need to thaw frozen food, let it defrost in the fridge overnight or use the cold water method instead of microwaving, which can destroy some nutrients.

Likewise, the storage container also matters. Here are some great options that you can use instead of plastic for long-term storage:

- Airtight containers – Prevent moisture and bacteria from getting in.
- Glass containers – Preserve food quality without absorbing odors or chemicals.
- BPA-free plastic containers – A lightweight, safe option for freezing and refrigerating meals.
- Silicone freezer trays – Great for portioning and easy thawing.
- Vacuum-sealed bags – Prevent freezer burn and keep food fresh longer.
- Mason jars – A good option for storing small portions in the fridge.

No matter which container you choose, always label it with the date to track freshness and avoid using expired meals.

Budget-Friendly and Meal Prep Recipes

Feeding your pup homemade meals shouldn't break your bank. In this section, we are going to cover some really great budget-friendly and time-saving recipes that you can cook for your furry friend.

1. Chicken & Rice Bulk Meal

(Affordable, simple, easily scalable for batch cooking)

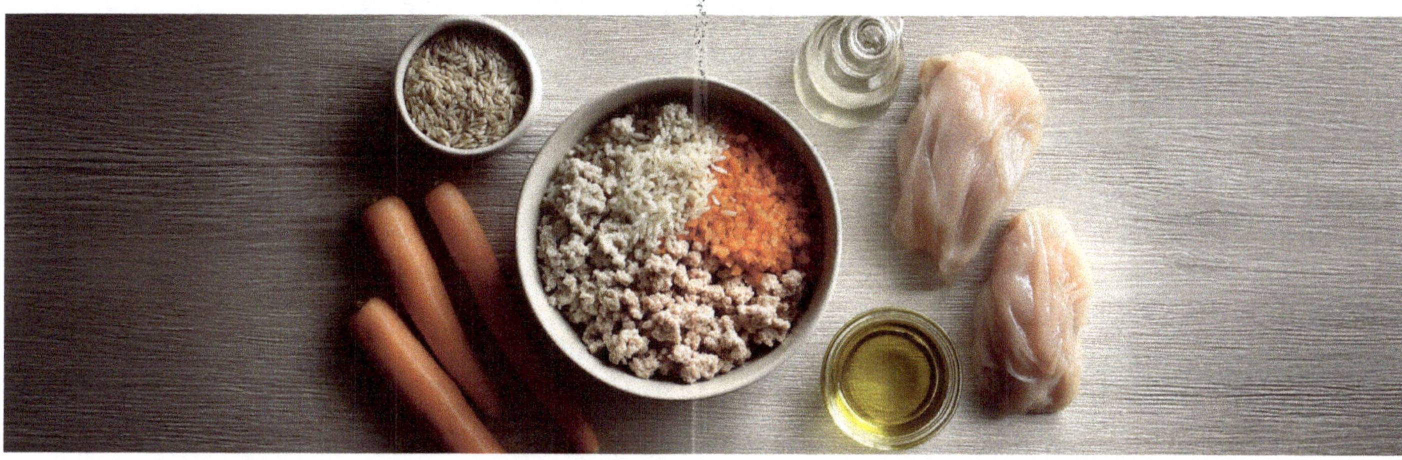

Ingredients:

- 2 lbs. ground chicken (93% lean)
- 3 cups cooked brown rice
- 1½ cups steamed carrots (chopped)
- 2 tsp flaxseed oil
- 2 tsp olive oil

Instructions:

1. Cook chicken thoroughly in a large pan without using any oil.
2. Stir in brown rice and carrots.
3. Mix in oils.
4. Portion into containers and freeze for up to 3 months.

Ingredient Substitutions:

- Replace rice with oats.
- Swap carrots with peas.

Nutrition per 500g serving:

Final Weight	~500g
Calories	~580 kcal
Protein	~38g
Fat	~22g
Carbohydrates	~36g

2. Beef & Lentil Freezer-Friendly Meal

(Cost-effective protein with fiber-rich lentils, batch-cook ready)

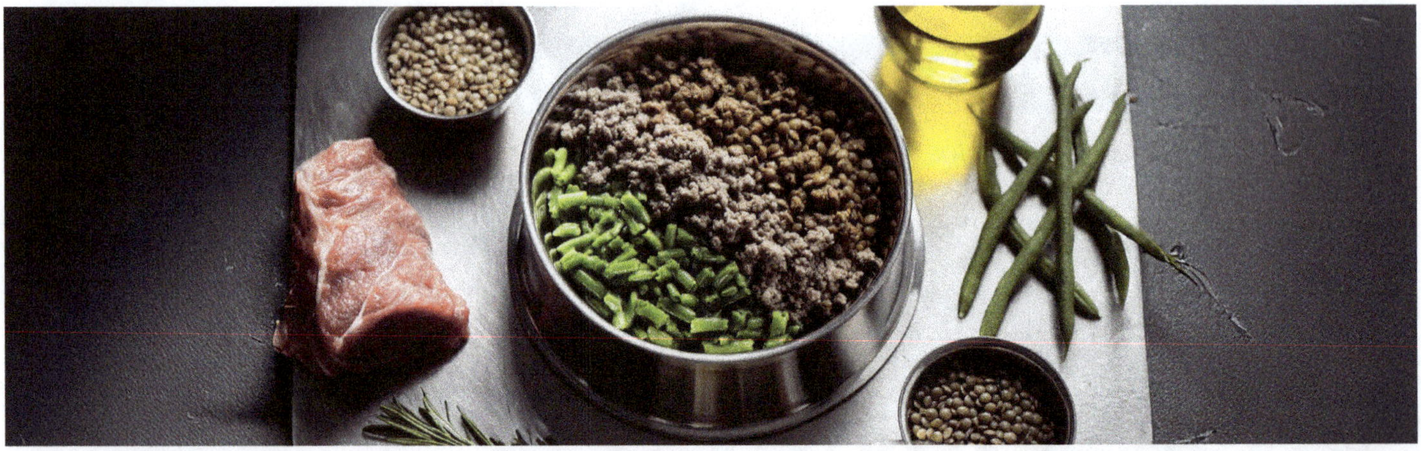

Ingredients:

- 2 lbs. lean ground beef (90% lean)
- 3 cups cooked lentils
- 1½ cups steamed green beans (chopped)
- 2 tsp olive oil
- 2 tsp flaxseed oil

Instructions:

1. In a non-stick pan, brown beef in bulk without any oil.
2. Stir in cooked lentils and green beans.
3. Mix in oils properly.
4. Cool completely, divide into freezer containers, and store for up to 3 months.

Ingredient Substitutions:

- Replace lentils with chickpeas.
- Swap green beans with carrots.

Nutrition per 500g serving:

Final Weight	~500g
Calories	~620 kcal
Protein	~40g
Fat	~24g
Carbohydrates	~40g

3. Egg & Oats Quick Batch Meal

(Inexpensive, quick-prep, great for freezer storage)

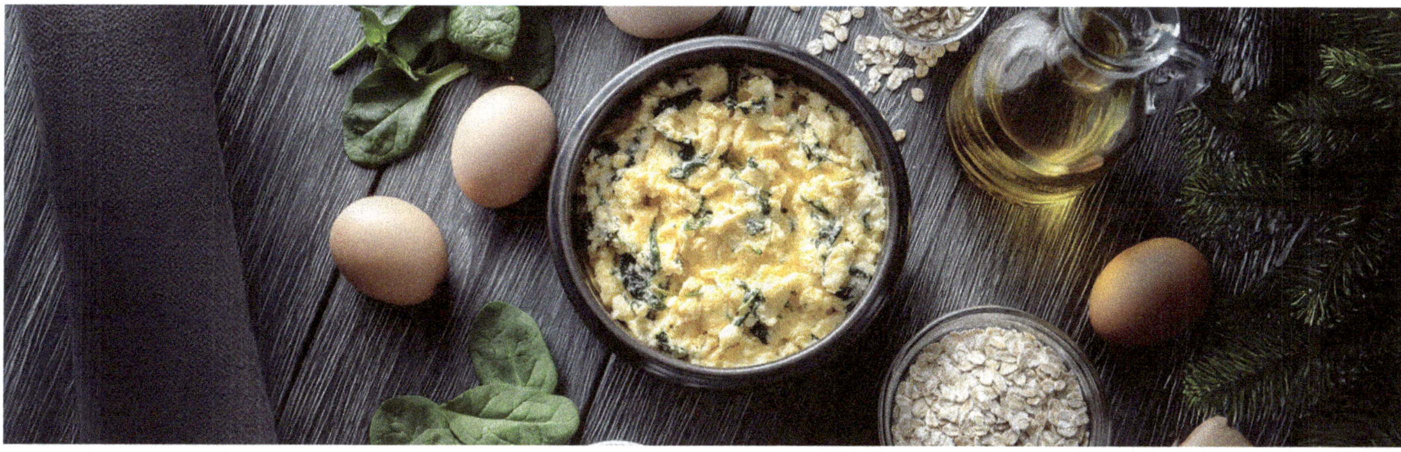

Ingredients:

- 6 large scrambled eggs
- 3 cups cooked oats
- 1½ cups steamed spinach (chopped)
- 2 tsp flaxseed oil
- 2 tsp olive oil

Instructions:

1. Scramble eggs in bulk in the pan with no oil.
2. Mix in oats and spinach and stir well.
3. Add oils.
4. Portion into containers, freeze portions for up to 2 months.

Ingredient Substitutions:

- Replace oats with brown rice.
- Swap spinach with broccoli.

Nutrition per 500g serving:

Final Weight	~500g
Calories	~560 kcal
Protein	~34g
Fat	~22g
Carbohydrates	~36g

4. Turkey & Sweet Potato Budget Bowl

(Lean, budget-friendly, filling and freezer-safe)

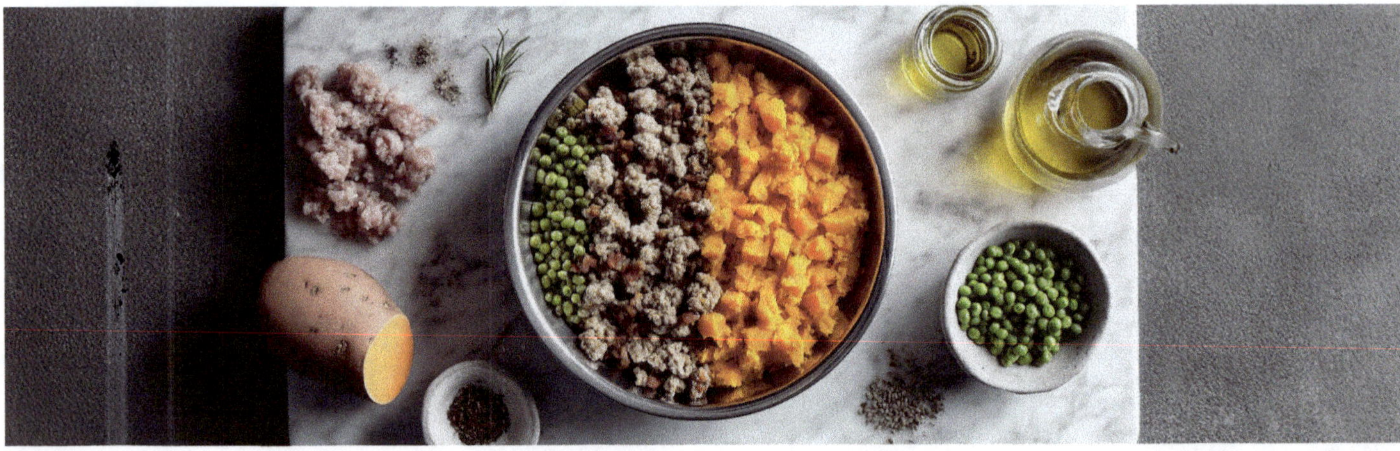

Ingredients:

- 2 lbs. ground turkey (93% lean)
- 3 cups mashed sweet potato
- 1½ cups steamed peas
- 2 tsp flaxseed oil
- 2 tsp olive oil

Instructions:

1. Cook turkey in bulk. Again, no oil needed.
2. Stir in mashed sweet potato and peas.
3. Mix in oils.
4. Cool, divide into portions, and freeze for up to 3 months.

Ingredient Substitutions:

- Replace sweet potato with pumpkin.
- Swap peas with carrots.

Nutrition per 500g serving:

Final Weight	~500g
Calories	~590 kcal
Protein	~40g
Fat	~22g
Carbohydrates	~38g

5. Whitefish & Barley Large Batch Meal

(Low-cost whitefish with hearty barley, ideal for big prep days)

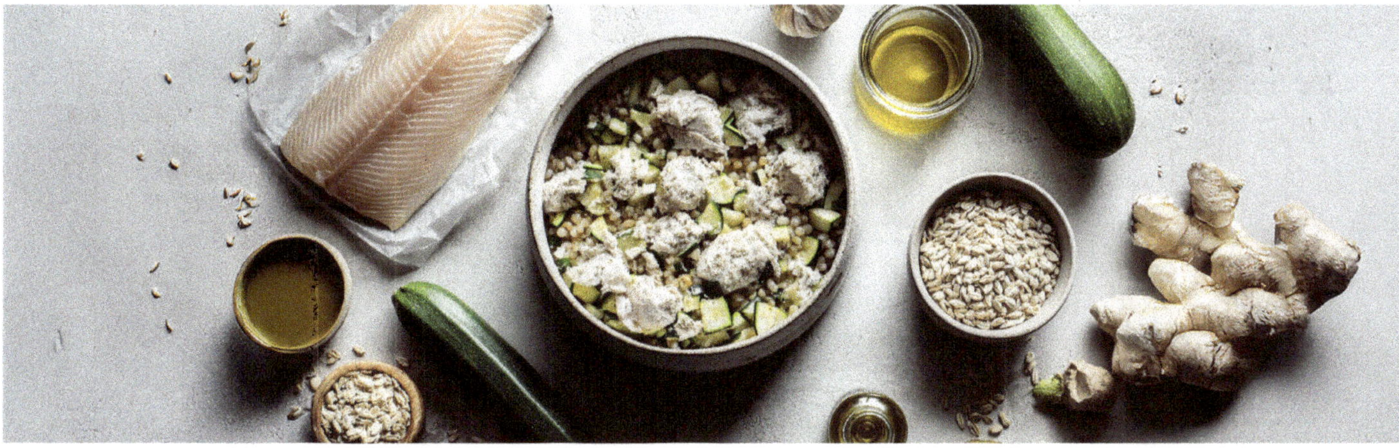

Ingredients:

- 2 lbs. boneless whitefish (steamed and flaked)
- 3 cups cooked barley
- 1½ cups steamed zucchini (chopped)
- 2 tsp fish oil
- 2 tsp olive oil

Instructions:

1. Steam fish in bulk, then flake into a large mixing bowl.
2. Stir in barley and zucchini.
3. Add oils and mix well.
4. Portion into containers, and freeze for up to 3 months.

Ingredient Substitutions:

- Replace barley with oats.
- Swap zucchini with green beans.

Nutrition per 500g serving:

Final Weight	~500g
Calories	~540 kcal
Protein	~38g
Fat	~20g
Carbohydrates	~34g

6. Chicken & Green Bean Bulk Meal

(Simple, lean protein with fiber-rich veggies for large batch prep)

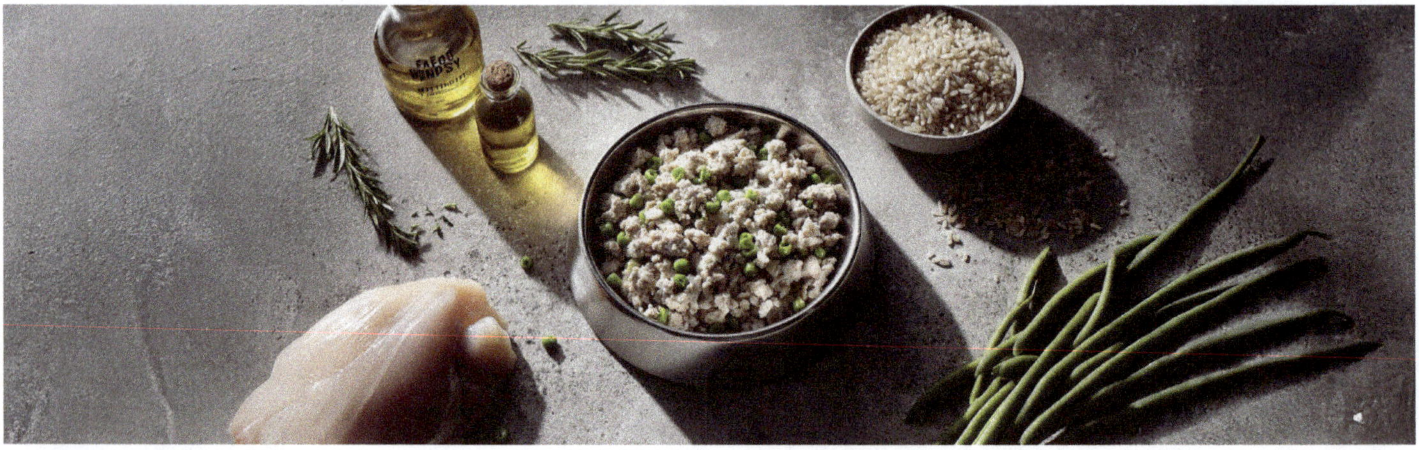

Ingredients:

- 2 lbs. ground chicken (93% lean)
- 3 cups cooked brown rice
- 1½ cups steamed green beans (chopped)
- 2 tsp olive oil
- 2 tsp flaxseed oil

Instructions:

1. Cook chicken in a large pan without using any oil.
2. Stir in brown rice and green beans. Mix well.
3. Add oils.
4. Cool, portion, and freeze for up to 3 months.

Ingredient Substitutions:

- Replace brown rice with oats.
- Swap green beans with peas.

Nutrition per 500g serving:

Final Weight	~500g
Calories	~580 kcal
Protein	~38g
Fat	~22g
Carbohydrates	~36g

7. Beef & Barley Freezer-Friendly Bowl

(Cost-effective, filling, and easy to batch-cook)

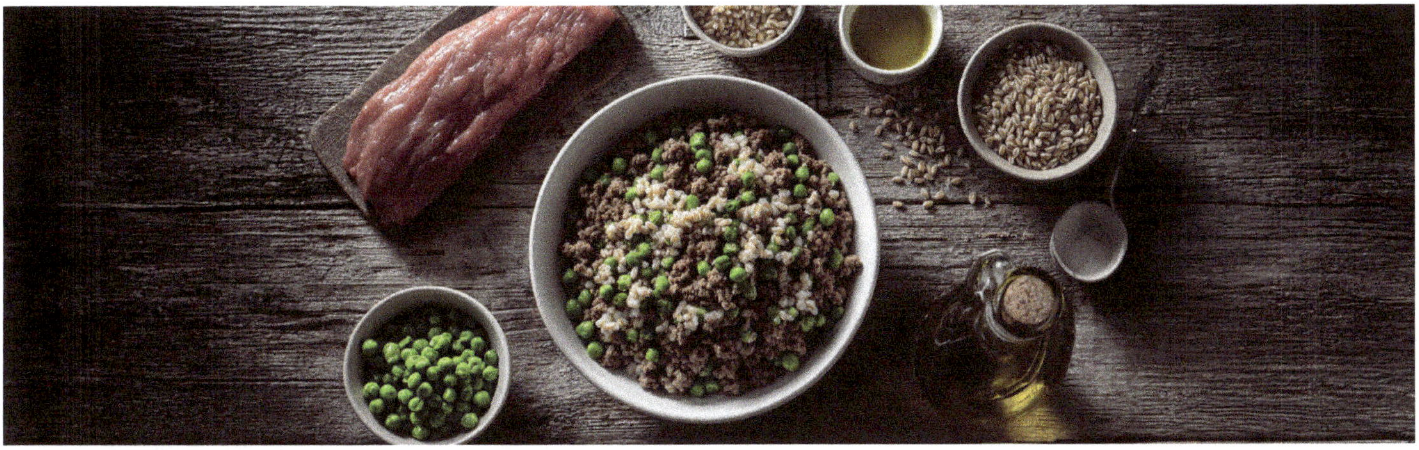

Ingredients:

- 2 lbs. lean ground beef (90%)
- 3 cups cooked barley
- 1½ cups steamed peas
- 2 tsp flaxseed oil
- 2 tsp olive oil

Instructions:

1. Brown beef in bulk in a non-stick pan without any oil.
2. Stir in barley and peas.
3. Mix in oils.
4. Cool, divide into freezer containers, and store for up to 3 months.

Ingredient Substitutions:

- Replace barley with oats.
- Swap peas with carrots.

Nutrition per 500g serving:

Final Weight	~500g
Calories	~620 kcal
Protein	~40g
Fat	~26g
Carbohydrates	~38g

8. Egg & Brown Rice Batch Meal

(Affordable, quick-prep, nutrient-dense, great for freezing)

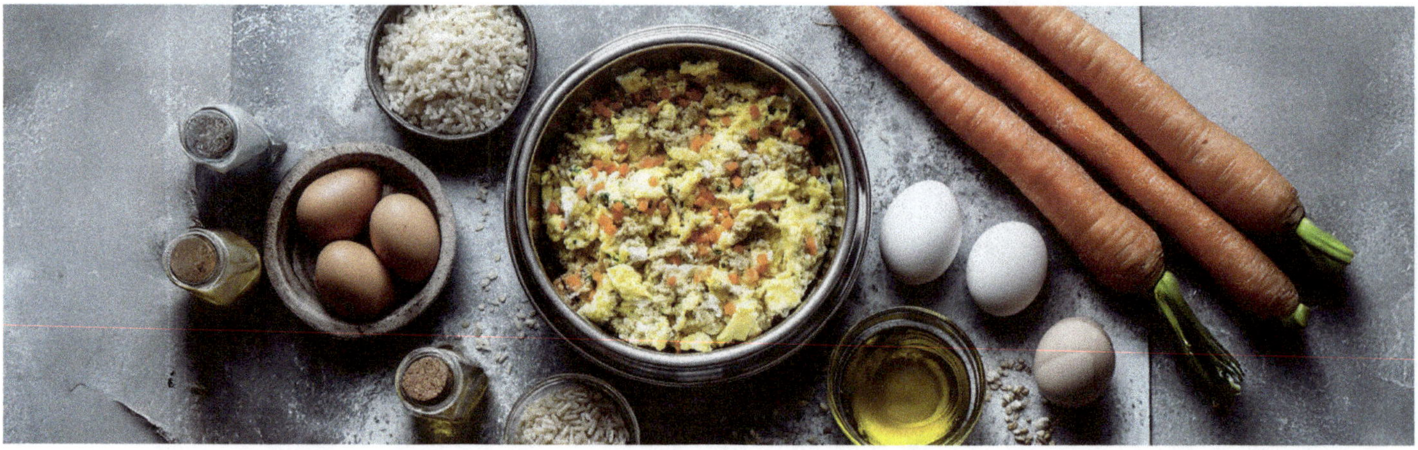

Ingredients:

- 6 large scrambled eggs
- 3 cups cooked brown rice
- 1½ cups steamed carrots (chopped)
- 2 tsp olive oil
- 2 tsp flaxseed oil

Instructions:

1. Scramble eggs in a large pan. No oil required.
2. Mix in brown rice and carrots.
3. Stir in oils.
4. Cool, portion, and freeze for up to 2 months.

Ingredient Substitutions:

- Replace brown rice with quinoa.
- Swap carrots with green beans.

Nutrition per 500g serving:

Final Weight	~500g
Calories	~570 kcal
Protein	~34g
Fat	~22g
Carbohydrates	~38g

9. Turkey & Oats Budget-Friendly Bowl

(Lean, affordable, filling and batch-friendly)

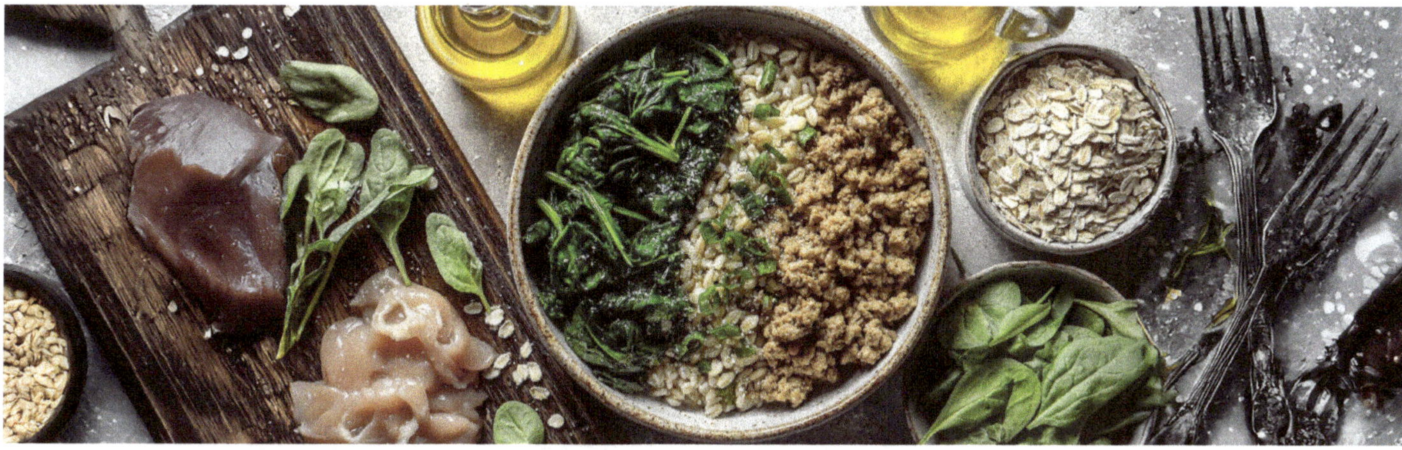

Ingredients:

- 2 lbs. ground turkey (93% lean)
- 3 cups oats
- 1½ cups steamed spinach (chopped)
- 2 tsp olive oil
- 2 tsp flaxseed oil

Instructions:

1. Cook turkey thoroughly in bulk in a non-stick pan (no oil).
2. Stir in oats and spinach. Give everything a good mix.
3. Add oils.
4. Cool, portion, and freeze for up to 3 months.

Ingredient Substitutions:

- Replace oats with brown rice.
- Swap spinach with broccoli.

Nutrition per 500g serving:

Final Weight	~500g
Calories	~580 kcal
Protein	~40g
Fat	~22g
Carbohydrates	~36g

10. Whitefish & Millet Meal Prep Bowl

(Affordable fish option, rich in omega-3, perfect for batch cooking)

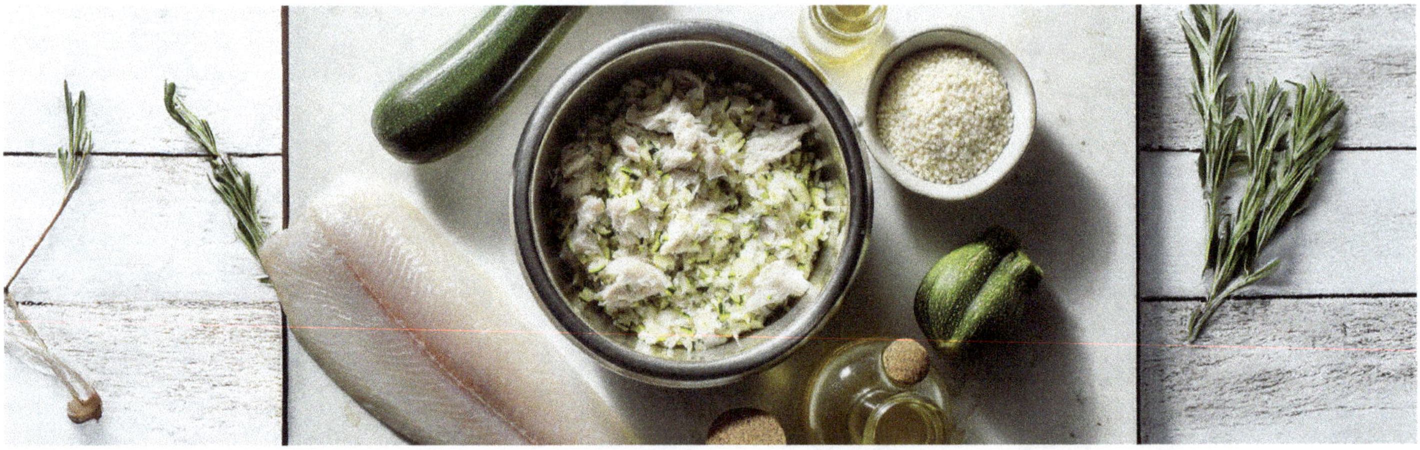

Ingredients:

- 2 lbs. boneless whitefish (steamed and flaked)
- 3 cups cooked millet
- 1½ cups steamed zucchini (chopped)
- 2 tsp fish oil
- 2 tsp olive oil

Instructions:

1. Steam fish in bulk, then flake in a large bowl.
2. Add the millet and zucchini to the bowl and stir well.
3. Mix in oils.
4. Cool, portion, and freeze for up to 3 months.

Ingredient Substitutions:

- Replace millet with oats.
- Swap zucchini with green beans.

Nutrition per 500g serving:

Final Weight	~500g
Calories	~540 kcal
Protein	~38g
Fat	~20g
Carbohydrates	~34g

11. Chicken & Sweet Potato Bulk Meal

(Affordable, digestible, easy to prepare and freeze)

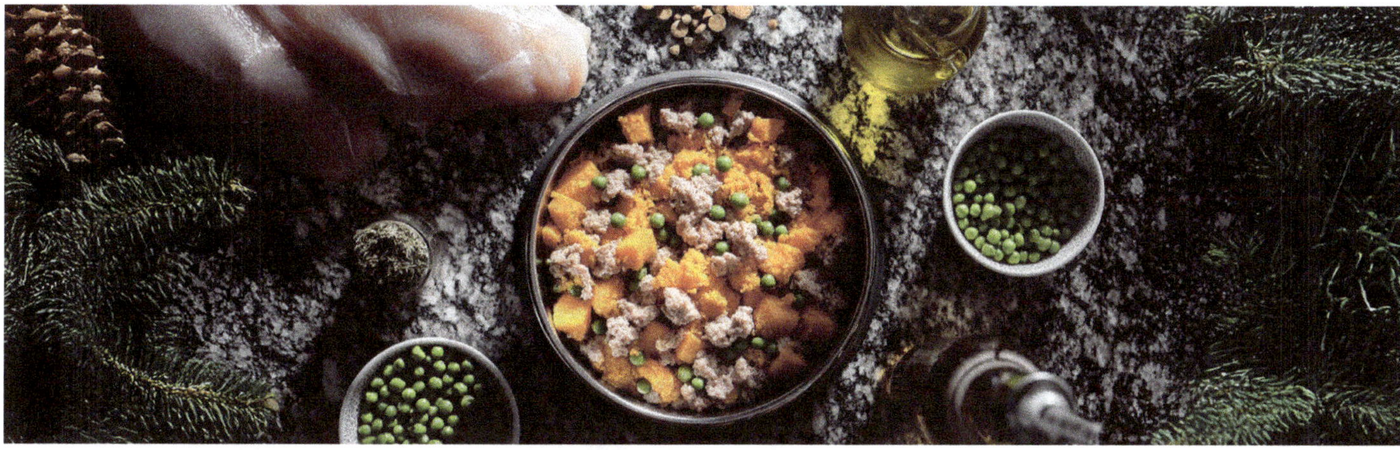

Ingredients:

- 2 lbs. ground chicken (93% lean)
- 3 cups mashed sweet potato
- 1½ cups steamed peas
- 2 tsp olive oil
- 2 tsp flaxseed oil

Instructions:

1. Cook chicken thoroughly without adding oil.
2. Stir in mashed sweet potato and peas.
3. Mix in oils.
4. Cool, divide into freezer portions, store for up to 3 months.

Ingredient Substitutions:

- Replace sweet potato with pumpkin.
- Swap peas with carrots.

Nutrition per 500g serving:

Final Weight	~500g
Calories	~580 kcal
Protein	~38g
Fat	~22g
Carbohydrates	~38g

12. Beef & Oats Bulk Energy Bowl

(Simple, hearty, freezer-friendly for cost-saving meal prep)

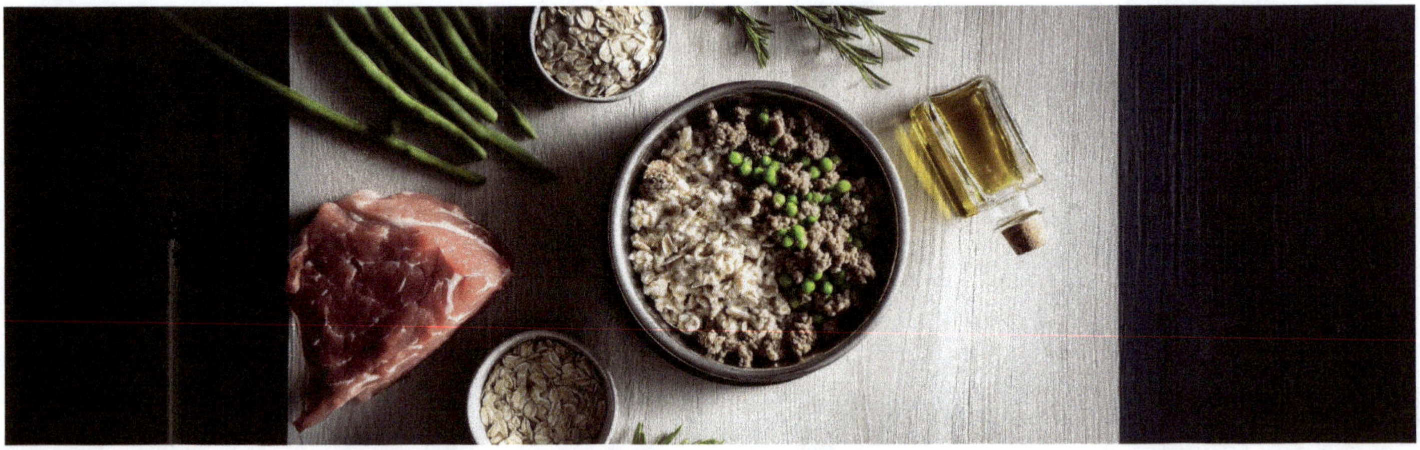

Ingredients:

- 2 lbs. lean ground beef (90% lean)
- 3 cups cooked oats
- 1½ cups steamed green beans (chopped)
- 2 tsp flaxseed oil
- 2 tsp olive oil

Instructions:

1. Brown beef thoroughly in a non-stick pan. No oil required.
2. Stir in oats and green beans.
3. Mix in oils.
4. Cool and freeze in containers for up to 3 months.

Ingredient Substitutions:

- Replace oats with barley.
- Swap green beans with spinach.

Nutrition per 500g serving:

Final Weight	~500g
Calories	~620 kcal
Protein	~40g
Fat	~26g
Carbohydrates	~38g

13. Egg & Rice Freezer Batch Meal

(Affordable protein option, easy-to-prepare in bulk)

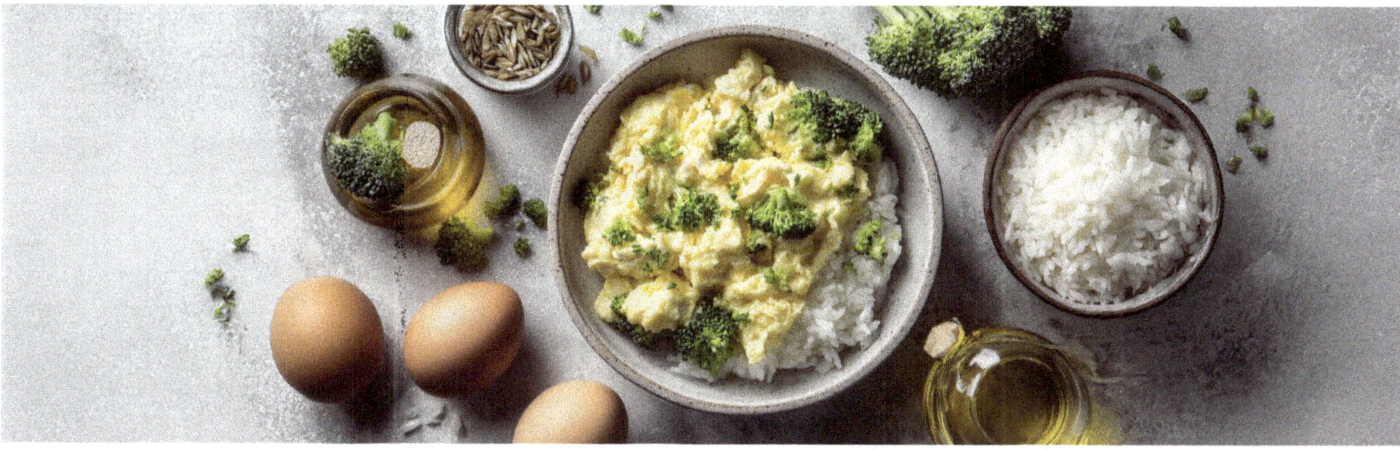

Ingredients:

- 6 large scrambled eggs
- 3 cups cooked white rice
- 1½ cups steamed broccoli (chopped)
- 2 tsp olive oil
- 2 tsp flaxseed oil

Instructions:

1. Scramble eggs in bulk (no oil).
2. Stir in rice and broccoli.
3. Mix in oils.
4. Cool and freeze in portions for up to 2 months.

Ingredient Substitutions:

- Replace rice with oats.
- Swap broccoli with carrots.

Nutrition per 500g serving:

Final Weight	~500g
Calories	~570 kcal
Protein	~34g
Fat	~23g
Carbohydrates	~36g

14. Turkey & Barley Large Batch Bowl

(Lean, affordable protein with hearty carbs, freezer-friendly)

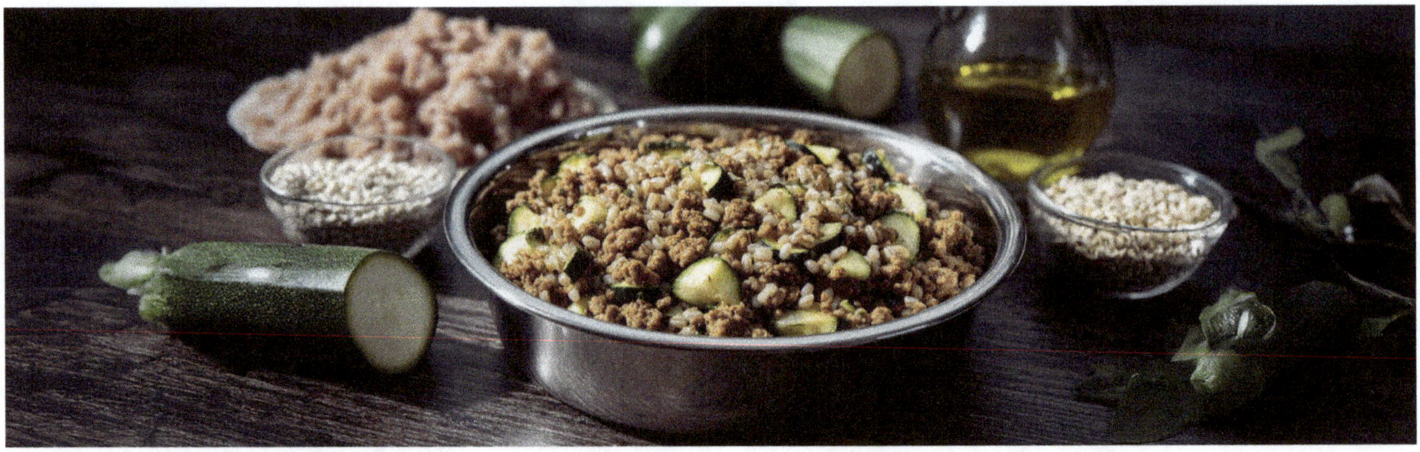

Ingredients:

- 2 lbs. ground turkey (93% lean)
- 3 cups cooked barley
- 1½ cups steamed zucchini (chopped)
- 2 tsp flaxseed oil
- 2 tsp olive oil

Instructions:

1. Cook turkey in bulk in a non-stick pan; no oil.
2. Stir in barley and zucchini.
3. Mix in oils.
4. Cool, portion, freeze for up to 3 months.

Ingredient Substitutions:

- Replace barley with oats.
- Swap zucchini with green beans.

Nutrition per 500g serving:

Final Weight	~500g
Calories	~580 kcal
Protein	~40g
Fat	~22g
Carbohydrates	~38g

15. Whitefish & Brown Rice Freezer Bowl

(Low-cost, omega-3 rich, perfect for batch prep days)

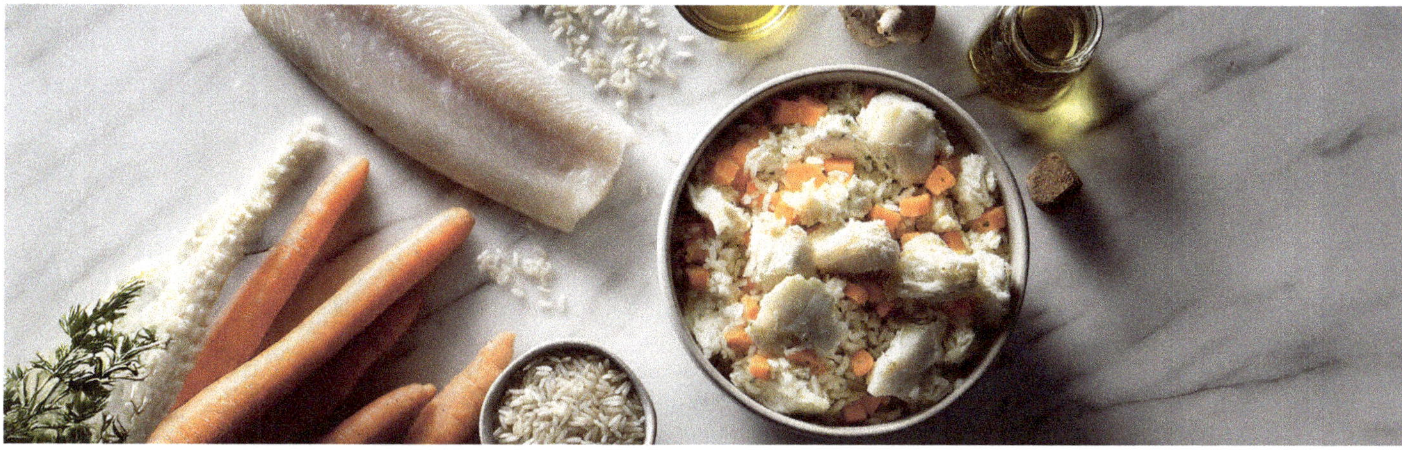

Ingredients:

- 2 lbs. boneless whitefish (steamed and flaked)
- 3 cups cooked brown rice
- 1½ cups steamed carrots (chopped)
- 2 tsp fish oil
- 2 tsp olive oil

Instructions:

1. Steam fish, flake.
2. Stir in brown rice and carrots.
3. Mix in oils.
4. Cool and portion; freeze up to 3 months.

Ingredient Substitutions:

- Replace rice with millet.
- Swap carrots with green beans.

Nutrition per 500g serving:

Final Weight	~500g
Calories	~550 kcal
Protein	~38g
Fat	~22g
Carbohydrates	~34g

16. Chicken & Millet Freezer-Friendly Meal

(Simple, cost-effective, ideal for big batch cooking)

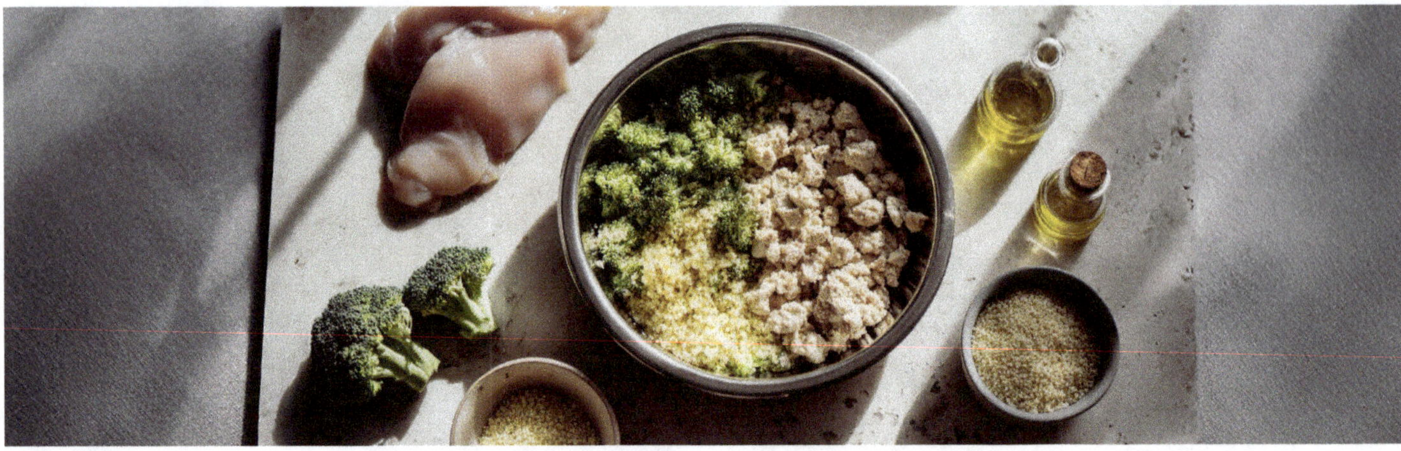

Ingredients:

- 2 lbs. ground chicken (93% lean)
- 3 cups cooked millet
- 1½ cups steamed broccoli (chopped)
- 2 tsp olive oil
- 2 tsp flaxseed oil

Instructions:

1. In a non-stick pan, cook chicken thoroughly in bulk. Don't use any oil.
2. Stir in millet and broccoli.
3. Add oils, mix well.
4. Portion and freeze for up to 3 months.

Ingredient Substitutions:

- Replace millet with oats.
- Swap broccoli with peas.

Nutrition per 500g serving:

Final Weight	~500g
Calories	~580 kcal
Protein	~38g
Fat	~22g
Carbohydrates	~36g

17. Beef & Sweet Potato Bulk Prep Bowl

(Hearty, affordable, easy for meal prepping)

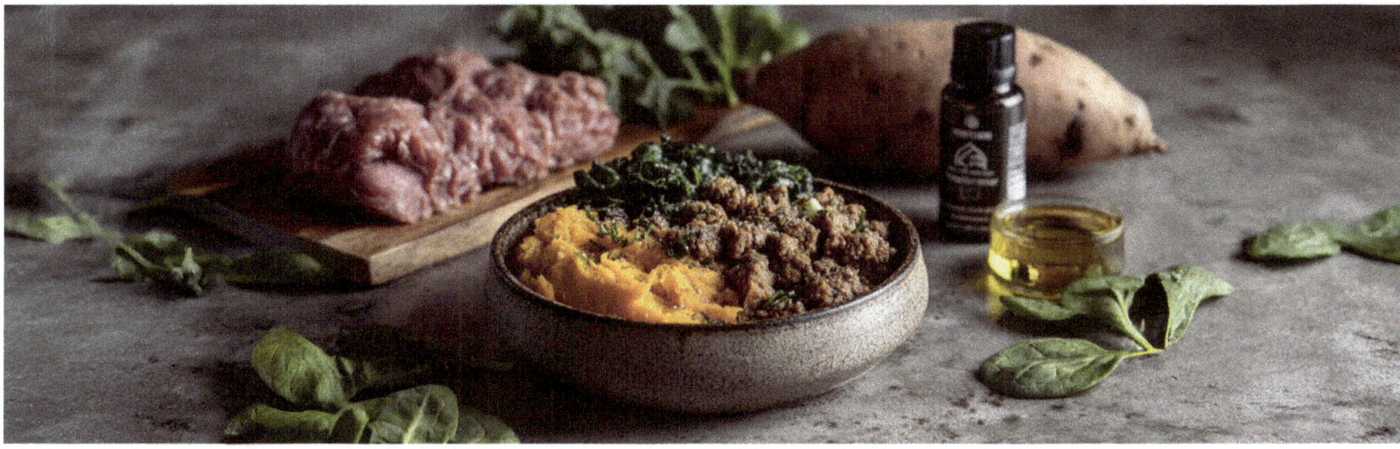

Ingredients:

- 2 lbs. lean ground beef (90% lean)
- 3 cups mashed sweet potato
- 1½ cups steamed spinach (chopped)
- 2 tsp flaxseed oil
- 2 tsp olive oil

Instructions:

1. Brown beef thoroughly in a non-stick pan without using any oil.
2. Stir in sweet potato and spinach.
3. Add oils, mix well.
4. Cool and portion, freeze for up to 3 months.

Ingredient Substitutions:

- Replace sweet potato with pumpkin.
- Swap spinach with carrots.

Nutrition per 500g serving:

Final Weight	~500g
Calories	~620 kcal
Protein	~40g
Fat	~26g
Carbohydrates	~40g

18. Egg & Quinoa Batch Prep Bowl

(Low-cost, nutrient-dense, easy to freeze and serve)

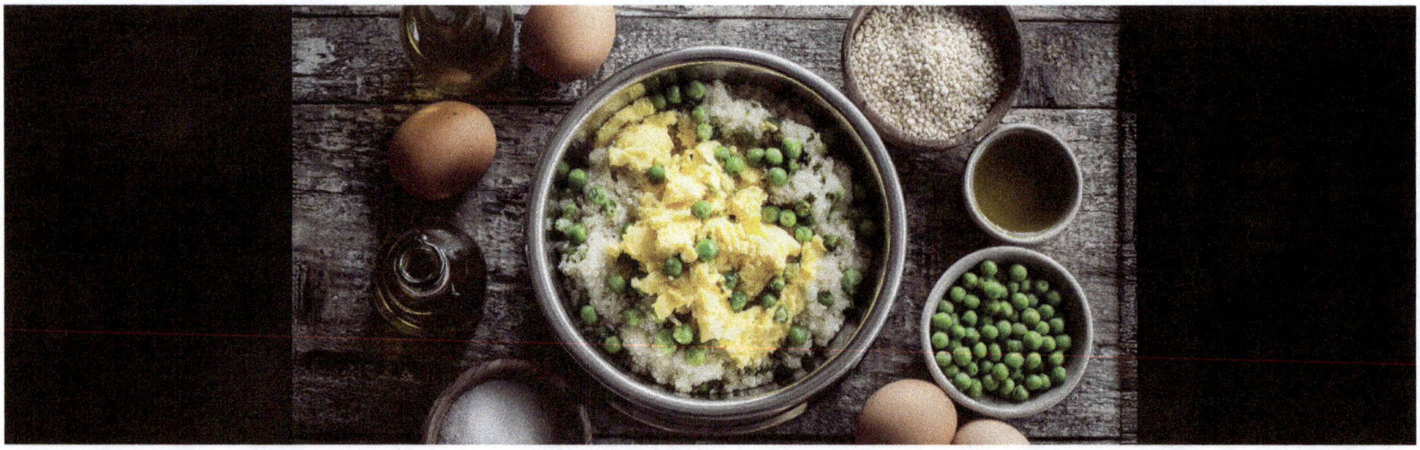

Ingredients:

- 6 large scrambled eggs
- 3 cups cooked quinoa
- 1½ cups steamed peas
- 2 tsp olive oil
- 2 tsp flaxseed oil

Instructions:

1. Scramble eggs in bulk. No oil needed.
2. Stir in quinoa and peas.
3. Mix in oils.
4. Cool and freeze in containers for up to 2 months.

Ingredient Substitutions:

- Replace quinoa with oats.
- Swap peas with carrots.

Nutrition per 500g serving:

Final Weight	~500g
Calories	~580 kcal
Protein	~34g
Fat	~22g
Carbohydrates	~36g

19. Turkey & Oats Freezer-Friendly Bowl

(Lean, affordable, simple meal-prep recipe)

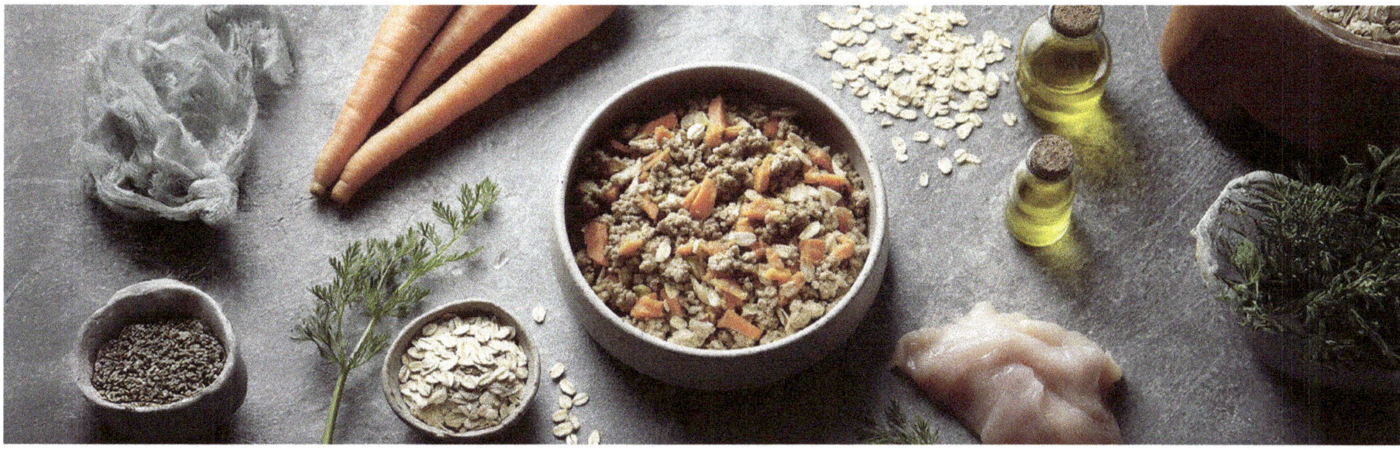

Ingredients:

- 2 lbs. ground turkey (93% lean)
- 3 cups cooked oats
- 1½ cups steamed carrots (chopped)
- 2 tsp olive oil
- 2 tsp flaxseed oil

Instructions:

1. Cook turkey thoroughly in bulk (without using any oil).
2. Stir in oats and carrots.
3. Add oils, mix.
4. Portion and freeze for up to 3 months.

Ingredient Substitutions:

- Replace oats with brown rice.
- Swap carrots with green beans.

Nutrition per 500g serving:

Final Weight	~500g
Calories	~580 kcal
Protein	~40g
Fat	~22g
Carbohydrates	~36g

20. Whitefish & Spinach Meal Prep Bowl

(Low-cost whitefish with nutritious greens, perfect for freezing)

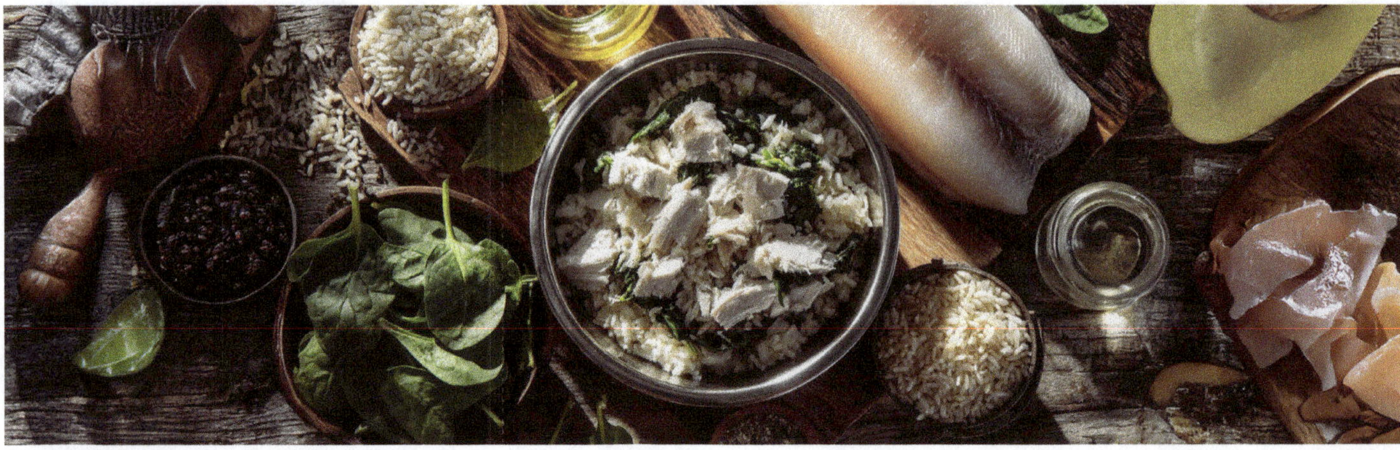

Ingredients:

- 2 lbs. boneless whitefish (steamed and flaked)
- 3 cups cooked brown rice
- 1½ cups steamed spinach (chopped)
- 2 tsp fish oil
- 2 tsp olive oil

Instructions:

1. Steam fish, then flake in a bowl.
2. Stir in brown rice and spinach.
3. Add oils, mix well.
4. Portion, freeze up to 3 months.

Ingredient Substitutions:

- Replace rice with millet.
- Swap spinach with peas.

Nutrition per 500g serving:

Final Weight	~500g
Calories	~550 kcal
Protein	~38g
Fat	~22g
Carbohydrates	~34g

Saving Money on Ingredients

High-quality protein doesn't have to be expensive if you know where to look. Local butchers often sell meat at lower prices than big grocery stores, and you can even ask for scraps or organ meats, which are both nutritious and budget-friendly.

Farmer's markets are also a great option, especially for fresh eggs and lean meats. Buying in bulk from wholesale stores or online retailers can also save you money in the long run. If you're open to variety, canned fish like sardines or salmon (in water, no added salt) can be an affordable and healthy protein source for your pup.

In short, there are plenty of options to find ingredients that cost half the price of expensive stores. Yes, it takes some time to find out where you can find the best value for money, but it will save you in the long run!

DIY supplements vs. store-bought.

Just like ingredients, you can save a lot of money by making your own supplements. Ingredients like eggshell powder for calcium, bone broth for joint support, and pureed veggies for added vitamins are easy and cost-effective options. These are great sources of your dog's nutritional needs and cost almost nothing. However, store-bought supplements are carefully formulated and tested for proper dosage, which can be important for certain nutrients like omega-3s or probiotics. If you choose to go the DIY route, consult your vet to avoid over- or under-supplementing.

Key Takeaways:

- Storing homemade dog food properly keeps it fresh and nutrient-rich for longer.
- Airtight containers, glass jars, and vacuum-sealed bags keep food safe from moisture, bacteria, and nutrient loss.
- Refrigerated meals should be eaten within 3-5 days, while frozen meals can last up to 3 months.
- Buying ingredients from local butchers, farmer's markets, or in bulk can help save money on high-quality protein.
- DIY supplements like eggshell powder and bone broth are budget-friendly, but some nutrients may require store-bought options.
- Always label stored food with dates to track freshness and avoid feeding expired meals to your pup.

Get the most of what you have just learned:

- Store homemade dog food in airtight containers and label them with the date to keep track of freshness.
- Buy high-quality protein from local butchers, farmer's markets, or bulk stores to save money.
- If making DIY supplements, consult your vet to ensure your dog is getting the right nutrients in safe amounts.

With a little planning and smart shopping, you can make delicious, healthy meals without overspending. In the next chapter, we'll cover simple meal-prep tips to keep you organized, save time, and ensure your pup gets nutritious, homemade meals without any waste!

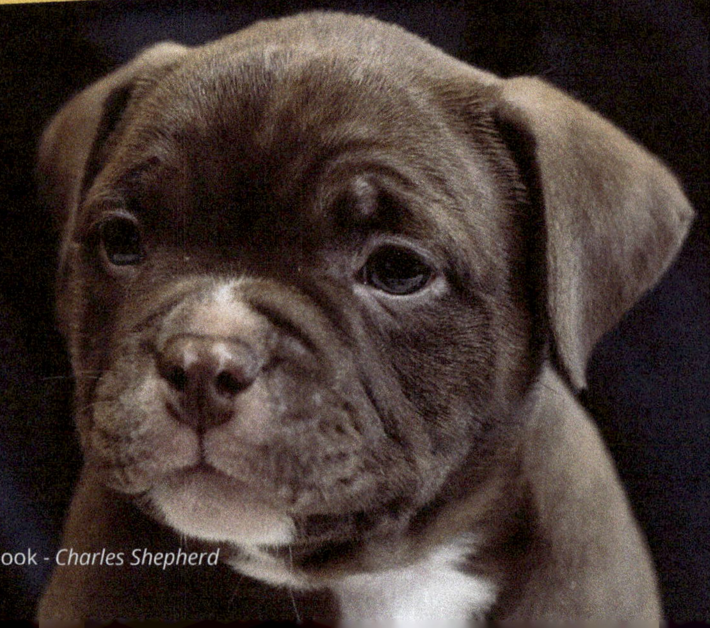

Day	Recipe	Morning Portion	Evening Portion	Notes
1	Beef & Sweet Potato Power Bowl	250g	250g	
2	Chicken & Rice Energy Boost	250g	250g	
3	Turkey & Pumpkin Power Mix	250g	250g	
4	Lamb & Brown Rice Strength Meal	250g	250g	
5	Salmon & Quinoa Vitality Meal	250g	250g	
6	Chicken & Rice Bulk Meal	250g	250g	
7	Turkey & Green Bean Trim Mix	250g	250g	
8	Beef & Lentil Energy Meal	250g	250g	
9	Whitefish & Millet Energy Boost Bowl	250g	250g	
10	Egg & Brown Rice Protein Bowl	250g	250g	
11	Turkey & Sweet Potato Budget Bowl	250g	250g	
12	Salmon & Oats Shine Meal	250g	250g	
13	Chicken & Barley Stamina Bowl	250g	250g	
14	Beef & Oats Bulk Energy Bowl	250g	250g	
15	Turkey & Quinoa Skin Health Bowl	250g	250g	
16	Lamb & Pumpkin Daily Energy Meal	250g	250g	
17	Whitefish & Brown Rice Freezer Bowl	250g	250g	
18	Chicken & Sweet Potato Energy Meal	250g	250g	
19	Egg & Cottage Cheese Shine Boost Meal	250g	250g	
20	Turkey & Barley Energy Booster	250g	250g	
21	Beef & Sweet Potato Grain-Free Bowl	250g	250g	
22	Chicken & Green Bean Bulk Meal	250g	250g	
23	Lamb & Sweet Potato Endurance Meal	250g	250g	
24	Whitefish & Sweet Potato Glow Meal	250g	250g	
25	Turkey & Oats Budget-Friendly Bowl	250g	250g	
26	Beef & Brown Rice Power Bowl	250g	250g	
27	Salmon & Quinoa Allergy-Free Meal	250g	250g	
28	Chicken & Barley Strength Mix	250g	250g	
29	Turkey & Green Bean Lean Meal	250g	250g	
30	Egg & Quinoa Batch Prep Bowl	250g	250g	

CHAPTER 6:

Structured Meal Plans for Dogs

"A balanced meal plan means a healthier, happier pup—one bowl at a time."

Planning your dog's meals every single day can be overwhelming, as you're not always going to be sure of what to make. To make things easier, here are two 30-day meal plans to give you a head start. These are simple, stress-free guides with daily recipes and portion suggestions so you can confidently feed your dog without second-guessing.

Select a meal plan that suits your pup and keep it in your kitchen, and now you'll always know what your furry friend is eating each day for the next 30 days!

30-Day Meal Plan 1 for a Healthy Dog:

30-Day Meal Plan 2 for a Healthy Dog:

Day	Recipe	Morning Portion	Evening Portion	Notes
1	Chicken & Sweet Potato Energy Meal	250g	250g	
2	Beef & Lentil Freezer-Friendly Meal	250g	250g	
3	Turkey & Barley Energy Booster	250g	250g	
4	Whitefish & Millet Energy Boost Bowl	250g	250g	
5	Lamb & Brown Rice Skin Nourish Bowl	250g	250g	
6	Egg & Oats Quick Batch Meal	250g	250g	
7	Salmon & Quinoa Vitality Meal	250g	250g	

8	Chicken & Broccoli Light Meal	250g	250g
9	Turkey & Sweet Potato Power Meal	250g	250g
10	Beef & Oatmeal Muscle Fuel	250g	250g
11	Whitefish & Barley Large Batch Meal	250g	250g
12	Turkey & Green Bean Lean Meal	250g	250g
13	Lamb & Oatmeal Hydration Mix	250g	250g
14	Chicken & Millet Freezer-Friendly Meal	250g	250g
15	Beef & Brown Rice Power Bowl	250g	250g
16	Salmon & Spinach Inflammation Support Bowl	250g	250g
17	Turkey & Oats Freezer-Friendly Bowl	250g	250g
18	Whitefish & Zucchini Slim Bowl	250g	250g
19	Chicken & Rice Energy Boost	250g	250g
20	Egg & Brown Rice Batch Meal	250g	250g
21	Lamb & Pumpkin Daily Energy Meal	250g	250g
22	Turkey & Quinoa Skin Health Bowl	250g	250g
23	Beef & Sweet Potato Bulk Prep Bowl	250g	250g
24	Whitefish & Sweet Potato Anti-Inflammatory Meal	250g	250g
25	Chicken & Barley Stamina Bowl	250g	250g
26	Turkey & Pumpkin Grain-Free Meal	250g	250g
27	Beef & Spinach Weight Control Bowl	250g	250g
28	Salmon & Oats Shine Meal	250g	250g
29	Chicken & Sweet Potato Bulk Meal	250g	250g
30	Turkey & Barley Large Batch Bowl	250g	250g

Customized Meal Plans Based on Activity Level

Active pups need more nutrients than less energetic dogs. If your dog likes to play a lot, feed them meals that are rich in proteins and healthy fats. But if they are less active, you'll find plenty of healthy meals with balanced portions.

Again, pick a meal plan that best fits your pup and keep it in your kitchen for easy access.

30-Day Meal Plan for a Low-Activity Dog

Day	Recipe	Morning Portion	Evening Portion	Notes
1	Turkey & Green Bean Lean Meal	200g	200g	Lean protein, low calorie
2	Whitefish & Zucchini Slim Bowl	200g	200g	Light fish, low fat
3	Chicken & Broccoli Light Meal	200g	200g	High fiber, low calorie
4	Beef & Spinach Weight Control Bowl	200g	200g	Nutrient-dense, moderate fat
5	Egg & Pumpkin Slim Meal	200g	200g	Soft, low calorie
6	Turkey & Zucchini Light Meal	200g	200g	Low-fat, easy digest
7	Whitefish & Green Bean Lean Meal	200g	200g	Omega-3s, low calorie
8	Chicken & Carrot Grain-Free Energy Bowl	200g	200g	Lean, moderate energy
9	Turkey & Pumpkin Grain-Free Meal	200g	200g	Gentle, low calorie
10	Egg & Spinach Lean Meal	200g	200g	Soft, nutrient-rich
11	Beef & Cauliflower Fat-Burn Mix	200g	200g	Low carb, weight control
12	Whitefish & Pumpkin Hypoallergenic Meal	200g	200g	Light, low fat
13	Turkey & Oats Budget-Friendly Bowl	200g	200g	Affordable, moderate energy
14	Chicken & Green Bean Bulk Meal	200g	200g	Lean, simple prep
15	Lamb & Cabbage Weight Control Meal	200g	200g	Fiber-rich, low calorie
16	Egg & Rice Freezer Batch Meal	200g	200g	Affordable, light
17	Turkey & Green Bean Trim Mix	200g	200g	Skin health, low calorie
18	Whitefish & Sweet Potato Glow Meal	200g	200g	Light, coat support

19	Chicken & Barley Glycemic Balance Bowl	200g	200g	Steady energy, moderate
20	Egg & Green Bean Low Glycemic Bowl	200g	200g	Low carb, nutrient-dense
21	Turkey & Sweet Potato Kidney Care Meal	200g	200g	Gentle, moderate protein
22	Whitefish & Quinoa Glycemic Control Bowl	200g	200g	Light, omega-3 rich
23	Chicken & Rice Bulk Meal	200g	200g	Simple, low energy
24	Beef & Lentil Freezer-Friendly Meal	200g	200g	Fiber-rich, moderate
25	Turkey & Broccoli Joint Relief Meal	200g	200g	Anti-inflammatory, light
26	Whitefish & Brown Rice Freezer Bowl	200g	200g	Affordable, low calorie
27	Egg & Oats Quick Batch Meal	200g	200g	Easy prep, light
28	Chicken & Millet Freezer-Friendly Meal	200g	200g	Lean, moderate energy
29	Turkey & Lentil Blood Sugar Support Meal	200g	200g	High fiber, steady energy
30	Whitefish & Spinach Meal Prep Bowl	200g	200g	Light, nutrient-rich

30-Day Meal Plan for a Moderate-Activity Dog

Day	Recipe	Morning Portion	Evening Portion
1	Beef & Sweet Potato Power Bowl	250g	250g
2	Chicken & Rice Energy Boost	250g	250g
3	Turkey & Pumpkin Power Mix	250g	250g
4	Lamb & Brown Rice Strength Meal	250g	250g
5	Salmon & Quinoa Vitality Meal	250g	250g
6	Chicken & Green Bean Bulk Meal	250g	250g
7	Turkey & Green Bean Trim Mix	250g	250g
8	Beef & Lentil Energy Meal	250g	250g
9	Whitefish & Millet Energy Boost Bowl	250g	250g
10	Egg & Brown Rice Protein Bowl	250g	250g
11	Turkey & Sweet Potato Budget Bowl	250g	250g
12	Salmon & Oats Shine Meal	250g	250g
13	Chicken & Barley Stamina Bowl	250g	250g
14	Beef & Oats Bulk Energy Bowl	250g	250g
15	Turkey & Quinoa Skin Health Bowl	250g	250g
16	Lamb & Pumpkin Daily Energy Meal	250g	250g
17	Whitefish & Brown Rice Freezer Bowl	250g	250g
18	Chicken & Sweet Potato Energy Meal	250g	250g
19	Egg & Cottage Cheese Shine Boost Meal	250g	250g
20	Turkey & Barley Energy Booster	250g	250g
21	Beef & Sweet Potato Grain-Free Bowl	250g	250g
22	Chicken & Millet Freezer-Friendly Meal	250g	250g

23	Lamb & Sweet Potato Endurance Meal	250g	250g
24	Whitefish & Sweet Potato Glow Meal	250g	250g
25	Turkey & Oats Budget-Friendly Bowl	250g	250g
26	Beef & Brown Rice Power Bowl	250g	250g
27	Salmon & Quinoa Allergy-Free Meal	250g	250g
28	Chicken & Barley Strength Mix	250g	250g
29	Turkey & Green Bean Lean Meal	250g	250g
30	Egg & Quinoa Batch Prep Bowl	250g	250g

30-Day Meal Plan for a High-Activity Dog

Day	Recipe	Morning Portion	Evening Portion
1	Beef & Sweet Potato Power Bowl	300g	300g
2	Chicken & Rice Energy Boost	300g	300g
3	Turkey & Pumpkin Power Mix	300g	300g
4	Lamb & Brown Rice Strength Meal	300g	300g
5	Salmon & Quinoa Vitality Meal	300g	300g
6	Beef & Oatmeal Muscle Fuel	300g	300g
7	Chicken & Barley Stamina Bowl	300g	300g
8	Turkey & Sweet Potato Power Meal	300g	300g
9	Lamb & Pumpkin Daily Energy Meal	300g	300g
10	Whitefish & Millet Energy Boost Bowl	300g	300g
11	Beef & Lentil Energy Meal	300g	300g
12	Chicken & Sweet Potato Energy Meal	300g	300g
13	Turkey & Barley Energy Booster	300g	300g

14	Lamb & Sweet Potato Endurance Meal	300g	300g
15	Beef & Brown Rice Power Bowl	300g	300g
16	Chicken & Barley Strength Mix	300g	300g
17	Salmon & Quinoa Allergy-Free Meal	300g	300g
18	Beef & Oats Bulk Energy Bowl	300g	300g
19	Turkey & Sweet Potato Budget Bowl	300g	300g
20	Whitefish & Barley Large Batch Meal	300g	300g
21	Chicken & Rice Bulk Meal	300g	300g
22	Beef & Sweet Potato Grain-Free Bowl	300g	300g
23	Lamb & Brown Rice Allergy Support Meal	300g	300g
24	Turkey & Oats Budget-Friendly Bowl	300g	300g
25	Chicken & Millet Freezer-Friendly Meal	300g	300g
26	Beef & Lentil Freezer-Friendly Meal	300g	300g
27	Whitefish & Brown Rice Freezer Bowl	300g	300g
28	Turkey & Barley Large Batch Bowl	300g	300g
29	Chicken & Sweet Potato Bulk Meal	300g	300g
30	Beef & Sweet Potato Bulk Prep Bowl	300g	300g

Adjusting Meal Plans Over Time

As dogs get older, their nutrition requirements change due to slower metabolism. Senior pups need less calories than young or adult dogs to prevent weight issues. Likewise, they need more joint supporting nutrients like omega-3s and glucosamine, so they can easily walk without pain.

Therefore, you should feed your old furry friend soft, easy-to-digest meals with lean protein and fiber to keep them healthy and comfortable. Always keep an eye on their appetite and weight, and adjust meals as needed. If you suspect your senior dog is gaining weight, try giving smaller portions and more fiber to keep them full. On the other hand, underweight dogs need extra calories from healthy fats and protein to maintain a healthy weight.

Also, remember to make seasonal adjustments to your senior pup's diet. In colder months, give them extra calories to stay warm, while in summer, lighter meals with more hydration keep them cool.

Monitoring Weight Changes

The easiest way to monitor your dog's weight is by checking their Body Condition Score (BCS). Run your hands over their ribs—if you can't feel them, they may be overweight; if they're too visible, they might be underweight. Yes, it's that simple!

Once you know your dog's weight and BCS, you can tweak their meal portions. If they need to lose weight, slightly reduce portions while keeping meals balanced. If they need to gain, add extra calories from healthy sources like lean meats or healthy fats. Likewise, watch for signs like low energy or sudden weight changes to make sure your pup is getting the right amount.

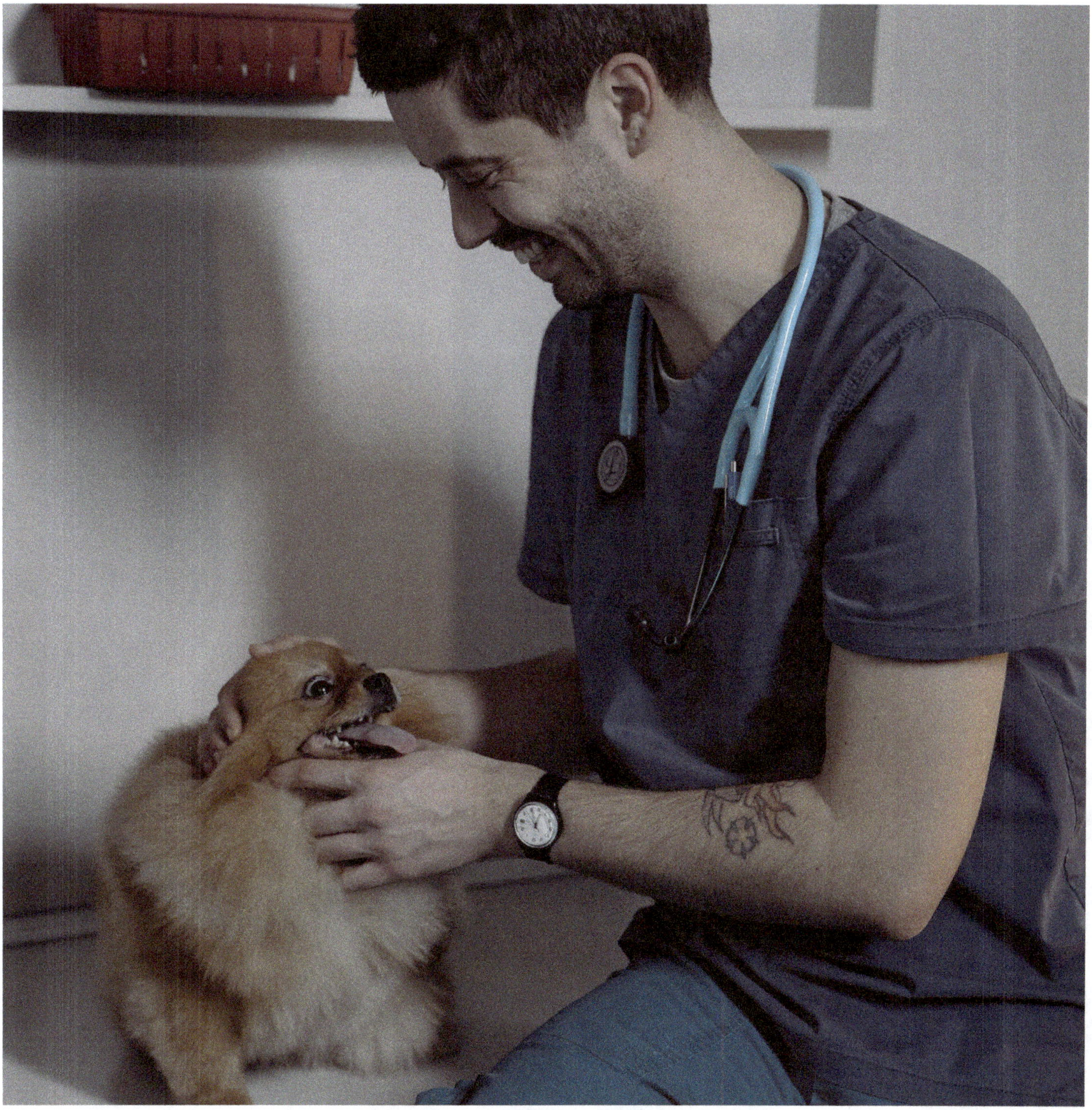

Key Takeaways:

- A 30-day meal plan takes the guesswork out of feeding your dog and makes mealtime stress-free.
- Choose a meal plan that matches your dog's activity level to keep them healthy and full of energy.
- Senior dogs need fewer calories but more joint-supporting nutrients to stay comfortable and active.
- Adjust your dog's portions based on their weight and body condition to prevent overfeeding or underfeeding.
- Seasonal changes impact your pup's diet, so increase calories in winter and hydration in summer.
- Regularly check your dog's weight and body condition to keep their meals balanced and health in check.

Get the most of what you have just learned:

- Pick a 30-day meal plan that fits your dog's needs and keep it in your kitchen for easy reference.
- Check your dog's weight and body condition regularly and adjust meal portions as needed.
- Make seasonal changes to their diet by adding more calories in winter and keeping meals light in the summer.

Figuring out the right meals for your pup is one thing, but making sure you have the right tools and resources is just as important. The next chapter is packed with helpful charts, guides, and conversion tables to make meal prep super handy. Let's make feeding time stress-free!

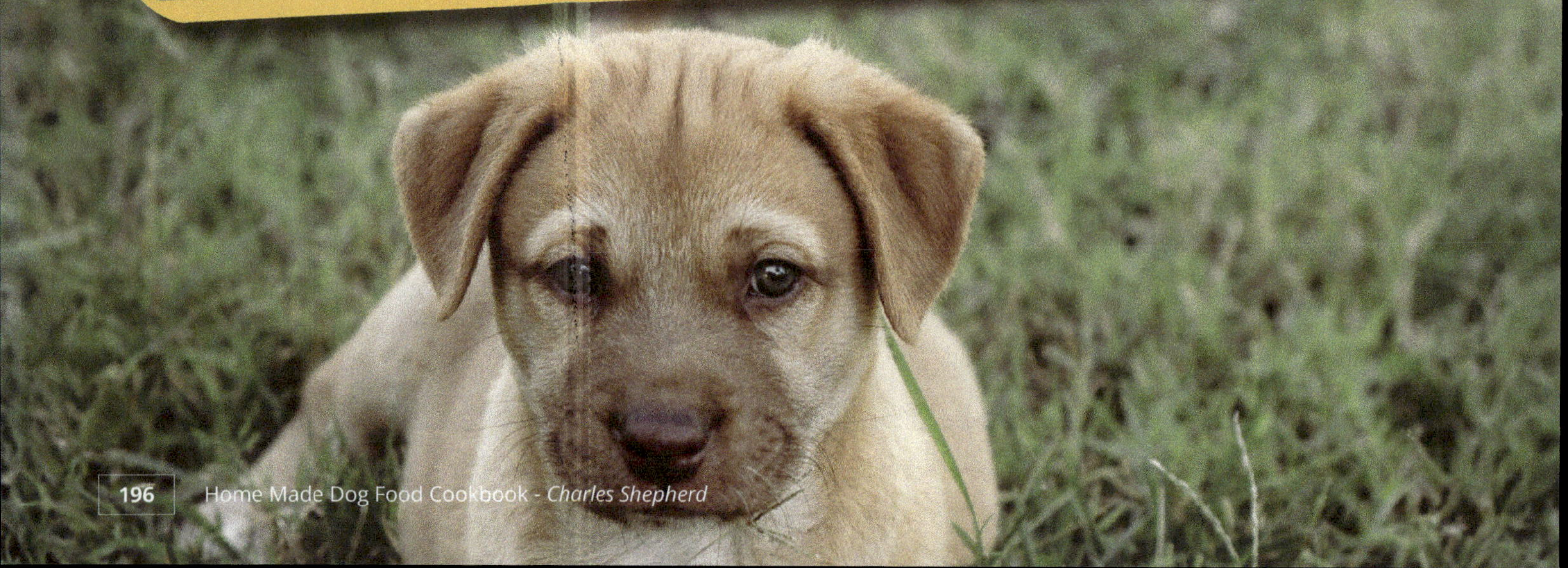

CHAPTER 7:

Tools and Resources for Success

"Creating nutritious dog food at home isn't just about effort it's about having the right tools and resources to make every meal safe, balanced, and delicious."

Conversion tables make cooking homemade meals easier. When you know how much of an ingredient is required in a recipe, you can easily measure it, avoid mistakes, and ensure your dog gets the right balance of nutrients in every meal. As even slight miscalculation can impact portion sizes, nutrient balance, and digestion, conversion tables make it easier to follow recipes and adjust portion sizes as needed. Likewise, they:

- Prevent overfeeding or underfeeding.
- Make following recipes easier. No guessing or estimating when switching between measurement systems.
- Help with portion control with weight differences between raw and cooked food.
- Prevent nutrient imbalances, so your dog gets the right amount of protein, fat, and carbs.

In this section, we will dive deeper into conversion tables for common ingredient measurements, including weight, volume, and temperature. I have explained it in as much detail and easy way as possible, so your pup can enjoy nutritionally balanced meals.

1. Weight Conversions: Ounces, Pounds, and Grams

The first thing you need to understand are weight conversions, which are ounces, pounds, and grams. Some dog food recipes list ingredients in ounces, while others use grams or pounds. You can use this table to convert between these units easily.

Weight (US Customary & Metric)	Equals to
1 ounce (oz)	28.35 grams (g)
4 ounces (oz)	113.4 grams (g) or ¼ pound (lb.)
8 ounces (oz)	226.8 grams (g) or ½ pound (lb.)
16 ounces (oz)	453.6 grams (g) or 1 pound (lb.)
1 kilogram (kg)	2.2 pounds (lbs.)

Example Use:

If a recipe calls for 500 grams of chicken, you can use approximately **1.1 pounds** of chicken instead.

2. Liquid Volume Conversions: Cups, Milliliters, and Fluid Ounces

Liquid ingredients like bone broth, oil, or milk are often measured in different units. Use this table to convert liquid volumes.

Liquid Volume (US & Metric)	Equivalent
1 teaspoon (tsp)	5 milliliters (ml)
1 tablespoon (tbsp)	15 milliliters (ml)
¼ cup	60 milliliters (ml)
½ cup	120 milliliters (ml)
1 cup	240 milliliters (ml) or 8 fluid ounces (Fl oz)

Example Use:

If a recipe requires **500 ml of bone broth**, you can measure 2 cups instead.

3. Dry Ingredient Conversions: Cups to Grams & Ounces

Dry ingredients like flour, rice, or kibble have different weights per cup. You can use the following table to get approximate conversions for commonly used ingredients.

Ingredient	1 Cup (US)	Weight in Grams (g)
Cooked Rice	175 g	6.2 oz
Oats	90 g	3.2 oz
Whole Wheat Flour	120 g	4.2 oz
All-Purpose Flour	125 g	4.4 oz
Peanut Butter	258 g	9.1 oz
Canned Pumpkin	225 g	8 oz
Grated Cheese	113 g	4 oz
Raw Meat (Chicken, Beef, Fish)	227 g	8 oz

Example Use:

If a recipe needs 2 **ounces of peanut butter**, you can measure about **¼ cup.**

4. Temperature Conversions: Fahrenheit to Celsius

If you're baking treats or cooking homemade meals for your dog, you will need to convert oven temperatures between Fahrenheit (°F) and Celsius (°C).

Liquid Volume (US & Metric)	Equivalent
200°F	93°C
250°F	121°C
300°F	149°C
350°F	177°C
375°F	190°C
400°F	204°C

425°F	218°C
450°F	232°C

Example Use:

If a dog treat recipe says to bake at **350°F**, you should set your oven to **177°C** for your Celsius-based oven.

5. Meat & Protein Conversions: Raw to Cooked Weight

Since raw meat loses moisture when cooked, it's important to know how much to start with to get the right portion.

Raw Meat Weight (g)	Cooked Meat Weight (g)	Raw Meat Weight (oz)	Cooked Meat Weight (oz)
100 g	75 g	3.5 oz	2.6 oz
200 g	150 g	7 oz	5.3 oz
300 g	225 g	10.6 oz	8 oz
400 g	300 g	14 oz	10.6 oz

Example Use:

If a recipe requires 100 grams of cooked chicken, you should start with about 130-140 grams of raw chicken before cooking.

Tips for Measuring Accuracy

When making homemade meals for your dog, measuring ingredients can make or break the entire recipe. Too much or too little of certain ingredients, and the meal can upset your pup's health. However, the good news is that with a few simple tricks, you can make sure every meal is just right. Keep in mind the following tips to save your recipes!

1. Use the Right Measuring Tools

Not all measuring cups and spoons are the same. If you're eyeballing ingredients or using random kitchen spoons, your meals will always be different. The result? Your pup will be getting a different meal every time, which can impact their health.

To avoid giving your dog too much or too little of an ingredient, you should:

- Use dry measuring cups for ingredients like flour, rice, or kibble.
- Use liquid measuring cups for things like broth, oils, or yogurt.
- Stick to measuring spoons for small amounts of powders, spices, or supplements.

2. Level Off Dry Ingredients

This is one of the most common mistakes dog owners make: they don't level off dry ingredients, which means the measurement is never the same! If you scoop up a cup of flour or kibble and don't level it off, you could be adding more than the recipe calls for. To be on the safer side, you should always:

- Use the back of a knife to smooth out the top of the measuring cup.
- Avoid shaking or tapping the cup, as this can pack down the ingredient and add extra weight.

3. Weigh Ingredients for Best Accuracy

If you want to be extra precise, a kitchen scale is your best friend! Measuring by weight instead of volume is more accurate, especially for ingredients that don't scoop evenly (like chopped meat, vegetables, or soft foods). Likewise, if a recipe gives measurements in grams or ounces, using a scale is the easiest way to get it right.

4. Be Careful with Sticky or Liquid Ingredients

Some ingredients, like peanut butter, honey, or oils, can be tricky to measure because they stick to the spoon or cup. This can alter a recipe's portion and nutrition; to get an accurate amount, try these simple tricks:

- **Use a non-stick spray:** Lightly spray your measuring spoon or cup with cooking spray before scooping sticky ingredients. This will slide out the sticky ingredients easily, so you get the right amount without wasting any.
- **Try the dip-and-level method:** For thick liquids like peanut butter, scoop it into the measuring cup, then use a flat edge (like a knife) to level off the top. This removes extra product, but be careful about creating a mess.
- **Use a digital scale:** If a recipe gives weight instead of volume, weigh the ingredient directly. This is the most precise way to measure sticky foods.

5. Avoid Guessing or Estimating

It's easy to think, "that looks about right," but believe me, it can be disastrous! If you're not sure how much to use, you should:

- Refer to conversion tables if you need to switch between cups, tablespoons, or grams.
- Stick to the exact measurements given in a recipe to maintain proper nutrient balance.
- When in doubt, measure again. It's always better to take an extra second to be sure!

6. Keep a Consistent Routine

Homemade meals are different from dry/wet food because the chances of altering portions accidentally are always high. Measuring accuracy is not about one meal because you have to feed your pup equal portions every day. Here are some tips to help you achieve the same consistency every time you cook meals:

- Use the **same measuring tools** each time to avoid variations.

If you prepare meals in bulk, pre-portion servings before storing them.

- Write down ingredient amounts or create a simple meal plan to keep track of what works best for your pup.

Serving Size Charts for Different Breeds and Weights

Every dog is different, which means their nutritional needs are also unique. Too little food can leave your pup undernourished, while too much can lead to obesity and health issues. That's where serving size charts come in handy! They help you figure out exactly how much food your furry friend needs based on their breed, weight, and activity level.

How to Use a Serving Size Chart?

Serving size charts are usually based on weight, so step one is to know your dog's weight. Once you know how much your pup weighs, you can check the following feeding chart to see how much food your dog should be eating daily.

- **Small Breeds (Under 20 lbs.)** → ½ to 1½ cups of food per day
- **Medium Breeds (20–50 lbs.)** → 1½ to 2½ cups of food per day
- **Large Breeds (50–100 lbs.)** → 2½ to 4 cups of food per day
- **Giant Breeds (Over 100 lbs.)** → 4+ cups of food per day

However, these amounts also depend on your dog's energy level. A couch potato pup will need less calories than an active dog who runs around all day. One way to ensure you are not giving your dog too little or too much is to adjust their portions based on their needs.

Adjusting Portions for Your Dog's Needs

While serving sizes help, they are not one-size-fits-all. If you need to adjust portions based on your dog's lifestyle and metabolism, here are some tips:

- **If your dog is gaining weight**, slightly reduce portion sizes and monitor their activity level.
- **If your dog seems hungry all the time but maintains a healthy weight**, try adding fiber-rich veggies like pumpkin or carrots to meals.
- **If your dog is highly active**, like a working or sporting breed, they will need extra food to fuel their energy levels.

In short, it's always best to monitor your dog's body condition rather than just following the numbers on a chart. If you can feel their ribs without them being too bony, they're likely at a good weight.

Key Takeaways:

- Conversion tables make it super easy to measure ingredients accurately, so your dog gets the right nutrients in every meal.
- Even small measurement mistakes can mess with portion sizes, digestion, and nutrient balance.
- Conversion tables help prevent overfeeding or underfeeding, so your pup stays at a healthy weight.
- No need to guess or estimate when switching between measurement systems—just check the table!
- Raw and cooked food weigh differently, so knowing the right conversions keeps up with portion control.
- Accurate measuring tools (cups, spoons, and scales) make a huge difference in getting portions just right.
- Sticky ingredients like peanut butter or honey can be tricky to measure, but a little non-stick spray or a digital scale helps.
- Serving size charts are a good way to figure out how much food your dog needs based on breed, weight, and activity level.
- Active dogs need extra food, while couch-potato pups might need a little less to stay healthy.

Get the most of what you have just learned:

- Keep a handy conversion chart in your kitchen or save one on your phone to quickly switch between grams, ounces, cups, and tablespoons.
- Get a digital kitchen scale, measuring cups, and spoons to ensure precise portions for your dog's meals.
- Use a feeding guide in this chapter to avoid overfeeding or underfeeding.
- Stick to the same measurement method (weight vs. volume) to keep your pup's diet balanced and avoid nutrient imbalances.
- Remember that raw and cooked foods weigh differently, so use the right conversion to portion meals correctly.

Keeping your dog's meals nutritious is important, but so is making sure they're prepared safely. After all, a healthy diet isn't just about the right ingredients—it's also about proper hygiene and food handling. In the next chapter, we'll cover simple steps to keep your kitchen clean, prevent contamination, and store homemade dog food the right way. With these easy habits, you can ensure every meal is as safe as it is healthy.

CHAPTER 8:

Hygiene and Safety in Homemade Dog Food

"Healthy food isn't just about ingredients it's also about safety. As they say... clean prep, safe storage, happy pup!"

You could be making the yummiest, nutritious meals for your dog, but without proper hygiene, they could carry harmful bacteria. Every time you are in kitchen to prepare a meal for your pup, follow these food handling practices to keep the food safe:

- Always wash your hands before and after handling food. Use warm, soapy water for at least 20 seconds to kill any bacteria or germs that could contaminate the meal. If you are dealing with raw meat, always wash your hands before touching anything.
- A messy kitchen means home to bacteria. Always wipe down counters and cutting boards (and knives, cutlery, and bowls) with hot, soapy water before and after preparing food.
- Don't mix cutting boards for meats and veggies. Using separate boards prevents cross-contamination.
- Wash all utensils, bowls, and food containers thoroughly after each use.
- Store raw meat in a sealed container and keep it separate from other foods. Properly clean the counter after thawing it.
- If you are reusing a cooked meal, heat it properly. If meat is involved, heat it to at least **165°F (74°C)** to kill bacteria.
- Never use old or expired food, as it can make your dog sick. Always check expiration dates before using ingredients.
- Inspect fresh foods like meat and vegetables for signs of spoilage (bad smell, discoloration, or mold).
- Store perishable ingredients properly to keep them fresh longer.

Preventing Cross-Contamination

You'd be surprised how common cross-contamination is in home-cooked meals. Not only can it put your pup's health at risk, but it can also affect you physically. Generally, cross-contamination happens when bacteria from raw food spread to other ingredients, surfaces, or even your hands. To prevent this from happening, keep these things in mind when cooking in the kitchen:

- As mentioned earlier, keep the raw and cooked foods separate. Reserve one cutting board for raw meat and another for vegetables or cooked food.
- Likewise, keep separate knives and utensils when handling different types of food.
- To make things even easier, you can color-code cutting boards, like one for meats, one for veggies, and one for treats.
- After using any cutting board, wash it with hot, soapy water. Better yet, sanitize it with a mix of one tablespoon of bleach in a gallon of water for extra safety.
- Similarly, when storing food in the fridge or freezer, keep raw ingredients away from ready-to-eat or cooked food.
- Always place raw meat in sealed containers or plastic bags to prevent juices from leaking. If possible, store raw food on the bottom shelf of the fridge so it doesn't drip onto other items.
- Keep homemade dog food in a separate section of the fridge to avoid mixing with human food. This is really important as many dog owners mix the two, which results in adverse health reactions for the dog and their owner.
- It may be tempting to taste your dog's food while preparing it, but using the same spoon for stirring and tasting can introduce bacteria. You should use separate spoons for tasting and mixing; better if you use a separate dish rather than dipping the spoon into the main batch.
- Remember this: If you're making raw meals, never ever taste the food before cooking—it could contain harmful bacteria.

Proper Storage Techniques for Homemade Dog Food

Just like human food, dog food needs to be stored correctly to stay safe and tasty. Improper storage can lead to food spoilage, bacterial growth, and nutrient loss. Luckily, there are ways to properly store your dog's meals; just follow these guidelines:

- Use the right container, like airtight containers for keeping out moisture, bacteria, and odors, glass/ BPA-free plastic containers, and portion-sized containers for easy thawing and unfreezing.
- Never use flimsy plastic bags or open bowls, as they don't provide enough protection from harmful bacteria.
- Homemade dog food doesn't have preservatives like store-bought kibble, so it needs to be refrigerated or frozen. If you are using the fridge, store the meal in airtight containers and use it within **3-5 days.** For the freezer, always store meals in portion-sized containers and use them within **3 months.**
- Pro Tip: **Label containers with the date** so you always know when to use them!
- Keep dry ingredients in a cool, dark place (like a pantry). It's even better to use airtight containers to prevent moisture from getting in.

- Always check for expiration dates and use older ingredients first.
- Frequent thawing and refreezing is never a good idea because repeated temperature changes spoil food. Avoid that.
- If you have to thaw frozen food, switch it to the refrigerator overnight. But if you are in a hurry, the best way is to place the food in a sealed bag and submerge it in cold water.
- Never microwave dog food in plastic containers—use glass or ceramic instead.

Detecting Spoiled Food

Even with the best storage methods, always check food before serving it. If you notice:

- A sour or off smell
- Mold or discoloration
- A slimy texture
- Your dog refusing to eat it

...it's time to toss it! Better safe than sorry.

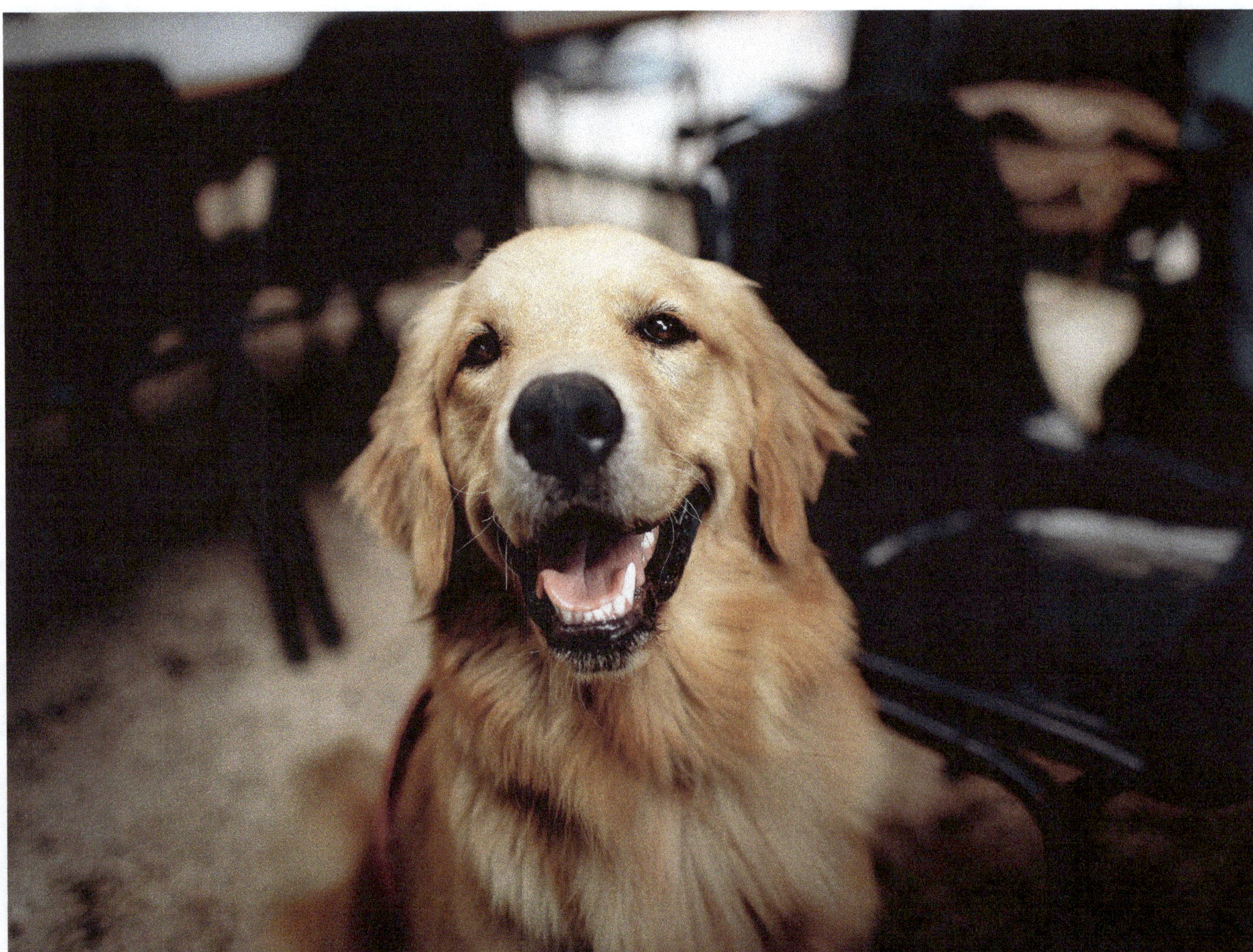

Key Takeaways:

- Good hygiene is just as important as good ingredients when preparing homemade dog food.
- Always wash your hands, utensils, and surfaces before and after handling food to keep bacteria away.
- Use separate cutting boards and knives for raw meat and vegetables to prevent cross-contamination.
- Store raw meat in sealed containers and keep it separate from other foods in the fridge.
- Refrigerate homemade dog food within 3-5 days or freeze it for up to 3 months in airtight containers.
- Always check for signs of spoilage like bad smells, discoloration, or mold before serving food.
- Avoid frequent thawing and refreezing, as it can lead to bacterial growth.
- When in doubt, throw it out. Your pup's health is worth more than a risky meal.

Get the most of what you have just learned:

- Always wash your hands, utensils, and food prep areas before and after handling ingredients to prevent bacteria from spreading.
- Store homemade dog food in airtight containers, refrigerate within 3-5 days, or freeze it in portion-sized servings for up to 3 months.
- Check food for signs of spoilage before serving—if it smells off, looks discolored, or has mold, throw it away.

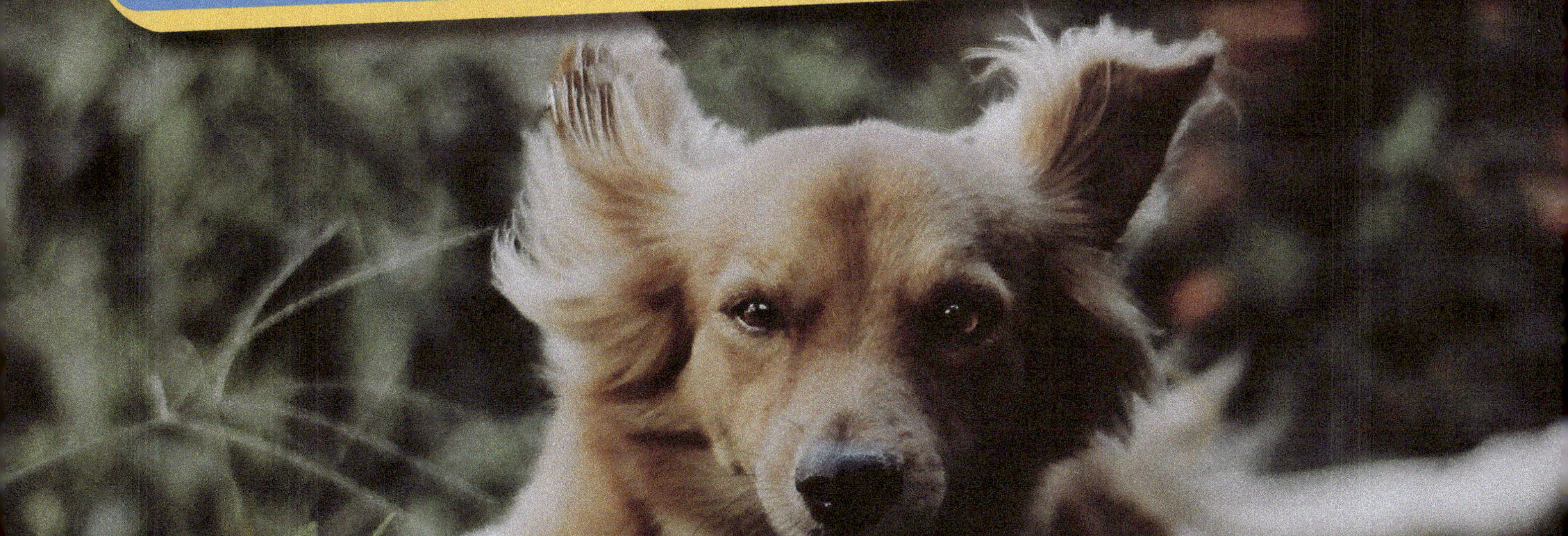

CONCLUSION

"Dogs do speak, but only to those who know how to listen."
Orhan Pamuk

Congrats, you've made it this far! Now you are packed with all the things you need to make the best decisions for your pup's diet. Throughout our journey, we have covered everything about canine nutrition, from the basics of essential nutrients to the proper methods of transitioning your dog to homemade meals. And the best thing? You have a full set of vet-approved recipes, structured meal plans, and even time-saving and budget-friendly strategies to make feeding your pup both practical and sustainable.

One of the biggest takeaways from this book is that feeding your dog is not about following a single rigid plan—it's about understanding their needs and making informed choices. Every dog is different, and their nutritional needs shift over time with age, activity levels, health conditions, sensitivities, and even seasonal changes. For example, puppies require energy-dense meals to support their growth, while senior dogs need softer, nutrient-rich foods to support joint health and digestion. Some dogs thrive on high-protein diets, while others do better with a balanced mix of carbs and fats. Likewise, pups need more water intake in the summer than in winter. In short, no single approach works for all dogs, and now you understand how to assess and adjust accordingly.

Also, remember that homemade dog food, when done right, can be as convenient as store-bought options. Bulk cooking, freezing meals, and using simple storage solutions can save time while still giving your dog access to fresh, healthy meals every day. You can batch cook on a free Sunday and freeze for the entire week. Just make sure to serve at room temperature after thawing and warming frozen food. Avoid cross-contamination by keeping separate cutting boards and utensils, and do the dishes right away. You don't need to break the bank either—affordable ingredient swaps and smart shopping can make homemade dog food more cost-effective than many commercial options.

Beyond meal prep, regularly monitor your dog's weight and health. A simple body condition score check can help you keep their weight in check, and minor adjustments to portion sizes can prevent issues like obesity or malnourishment. Make a habit of running your hands over your dog's ribs—if you can't feel them, limit their portions to prevent obesity; if they're too visible, offer balanced nutrition to help them gain healthy weight.

Pay attention to seasonal needs—keep your dog hydrated and offer cooling foods in the summer and add extra calories in winter. This greatly elevates their comfort and well-being. If your pup is dehydrated, offer homemade meals with more moisture content. Keep fresh, clean water available all the time, so your pup can stay active and healthy throughout the hot seasons.

Feeding your dog, after all, is an act of love. It's not just about what goes into their bowl but also about the care and attention that comes with it. Watching them thrive, seeing their coat shine, and knowing they have the energy to play, explore, and live their best life—that's what makes it all worthwhile.

Now that you have the knowledge, the next step is simple: put it into action. Start small if you need to. Try a recipe, adjust portion sizes based on your dog's needs, or begin incorporating homemade meals alongside their current diet. The goal isn't perfection—it's progress.

Your dog depends on you for their health and happiness, and now you have the tools to make the best choices for them. Every meal you prepare, every adjustment you make, and every effort you put into their diet will pay off in the form of a healthier, happier companion. Even if something goes wrong, it's alright. Keep in touch with your vet and take notes to prevent future reactions. It takes time, but you will get it right.

Thank you so much for taking this journey with me. If you've enjoyed this book, I'd be grateful if you could take a moment to leave a review on Amazon. Your feedback helps others find the book and ensures that more pet owners can benefit from healthy, homemade meals for their dogs.

SCAN THE QR CODE

Here's to many years of tail wags, happy barks, and a well-fed, thriving pup!

Charles Shepherd

REFERENCES

American Veterinary Medical Association. (2015). *Pet supplements trend report*. AVMA.

Ardente, A. (2020). *The impact of nutrition on companion animal health. Journal of Veterinary Nutrition Studies,* 12(3), 44–52.

Coates, J. (2022). *Safe diet transitions for dogs: Gradual vs. immediate switching. Veterinary Health Digest*, 9(1), 21–27.

Kazimierska, M., & Biel, W. (2020). *Micronutrient needs in active dogs: A veterinary perspective. Journal of Animal Nutrition,* 8(4), 78–85.

Koehler, R. (2024). *Understanding canine fasting and hydration. The Modern Veterinarian,* 14(2), 33–39.

McCarthy, G., O'Donovan, J., Jones, B., McAllister, H., & Seed, M. (2007). *Influence of glucosamine and chondroitin sulfate supplementation on canine osteoarthritis. The Veterinary Journal,* 174(1), 54–61.

Mueller, R. S., Olivry, T., & Prélaud, P. (2016). *Critically appraised topic on adverse food reactions of companion animals (2): Common food allergen sources in dogs and cats. BMC Veterinary Research,* 12(1), 9.

National Research Council. (2006). *Nutrient requirements of dogs and cats.* The National Academies Press. https://doi.org/10.17226/10668

Russel, K. (2023). *Comprehensive guide to canine joint supplements. Journal of Veterinary Therapeutics,* 17(2), 89–96.

Tupler, T. (2024). *Canine nutritional requirements across life stages. Veterinary Nutrition Quarterly,* 15(1), 12–18.

Wiese, H. F., Durr, U. M., & Nelson, M. M. (1962). *Effect of dietary fat levels on the development of beagle puppies. Journal of Animal Science,* 21(1), 140–144.

www.ingramcontent.com/pod-product-compliance
Lightning Source LLC
Chambersburg PA
CBHW061355240926
51846CB00007B/1411